Mediating Alzheimer's

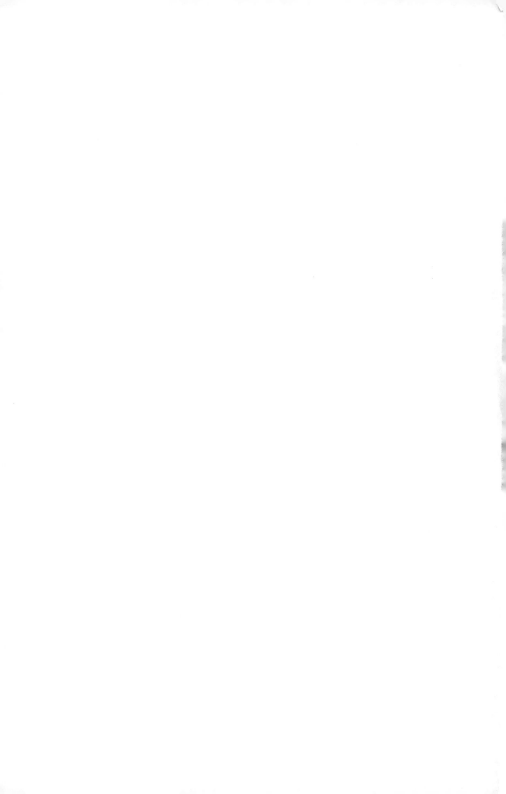

Mediating Alzheimer's

Cognition and Personhood

S<small>COTT</small> S<small>ELBERG</small>

UNIVERSITY OF MINNESOTA PRESS
MINNEAPOLIS • LONDON

A different version of chapter 5 was previously published as "Modern Art as Public Care: Alzheimer's and the Aesthetics of Universal Personhood," *Medical Anthropology Quarterly* 29, no. 4 (2015): 473–91; copyright 2015 by the American Anthropological Association. A different version of chapter 6 was previously published as "Dementia on the Canvas: Art and the Biopolitics of Creativity," in *Popularizing Dementia: Public Expressions and Representations of Forgetfulness,* edited by Mark Schweda and Aagje Swinnen (Bielefeld: transcript, 2015); reprinted by permission of transcript Verlag, Germany (2021).

Published by the University of Minnesota Press
111 Third Avenue South, Suite 290
Minneapolis, MN 55401-2520
http://www.upress.umn.edu

ISBN 978-1-5179-0228-5 (hc)
ISBN 978-1-5179-0229-2 (pb)

Library of Congress record available at https://lccn.loc.gov/2021062863.

Printed in the United States of America on acid-free paper

The University of Minnesota is an equal-opportunity educator and employer.

UMP BmB 2022

Contents

Alzheimer's and Media

As a potential epidemic and the source of significant public fear, Alzheimer's disease has moved to the forefront of U.S. consciousness over the past four decades. This is in part because of the instability and profundity of its symptoms, the increasing number of diagnoses in older adults, and the lack of effective therapy or cure. The popular story of Alzheimer's is sad and heartbreaking: it is the memory disease, the failure to recognize family and loved ones, and the very antithesis of the progress narratives that authorize successful aging. As such, it poses a significant threat to familial and generational survival. It seems as if each of us knows someone living with Alzheimer's, and thus our personal relationships with the disease help cement its pain within larger social narratives of aging, care, loss, and love.

The increased awareness of Alzheimer's has accompanied a substantial spike in the diversity and breadth of its mediation: in medical research, movies and television shows, news coverage, drug advertisements, and advocacy campaigns. A paradox of this heightened mediation, however, rises from the fact that Alzheimer's proves to be a very difficult thing to successfully represent. After more than a century of effort, medical professionals still encounter significant barriers to reliable neuroimaging and biomarkers for diagnostic and research purposes. There is also ongoing disagreement about what actually causes Alzheimer's, the best research strategies that might one day cure the disease, or even its relationship to everyday aging. Common symptoms of the disease, such as memory loss or disorientation, are easily interpreted as more banal "senior moments." As such, in its popular representation, Alzheimer's is often swept up in a more universal narrative of aging and decline.

A common assumption is that as someone with Alzheimer's loses her memory and other cognitive abilities, her very identity or self is lost. What is left if you can't remember your own job, habits, or home? If Alzheimer's robs your ability to recognize your friends and loved ones, on what exactly are those relationships now based? As Pia Kontos frames it, "the presumed loss of selfhood is itself a product of the Western assumption that status as a full human being is completely dependent on cognition and memory. . . . This representation of personhood is itself the legacy of Western philosophy's tendency to split mind from body and to position the former as superior to the latter."[1]

If Alzheimer's is understood to threaten selfhood, then much of the work of treatment and care tries either to rescue that self or to redefine the values of self. Given the way modern selfhood is so wrapped up with media practices and technologies, it should come as no surprise that much of that treatment is oriented around media. The successful industry of digital brain training is only a subset of a broader interest in games, puzzles, and other exercises designed to prevent the disease. Symptoms of Alzheimer's are also treated with a range of media, including photograph-based reminiscence therapy, art therapy, music therapy, and even care facilities that simulate eras of the past. While these technologies ostensibly target specific symptoms of dementia, they are often tethered to a more abstract ideal of self-preservation or rescue. Something like music therapy, for example, which is shown to lessen anxiety and support certain cognitive functions, is often celebrated for its ability to tap into lost or buried identity, or who the person with Alzheimer's "used to be" before disease onset.[2]

Medical descriptions of brain atrophy only reinforce the narrative of diminished selfhood. Indeed, because it is a disease commonly understood to originate in the brain, Alzheimer's is profoundly wed to a more abstract pathology of interiority. Memories, feelings, self, brain: all of that is hidden inside and under threat. It is precisely this abstract ideology of pathologized self and brain that makes the disease so available to stigmas of loss but also open to positive thinking and narratives of a better future. A great deal of that positivity is wrapped up in national optimism in neuroscience and the truths it affords.

The rise of Alzheimer's as a public health crisis in the last decades of the twentieth century accompanied a dramatic rise in public and professional interest in the brain. We now grant the brain all kinds of agency, and a massive industry investigates the ways the brain shapes everything from mood to morality. Neuroimaging technologies like positron emission tomography (PET) and magnetic resonance imaging (MRI) allow us seemingly to peer inside the brain, to map its structures and understand its operations. And yet, the brain is a vastly complicated organ, and many believe we are only just beginning to comprehend its mysteries. Those mysteries are as much an invitation to creative representational practice as they are an obstacle. Hope and progress toward a solution for Alzheimer's are now firmly rooted in the modern industries of neuroscience.

The popular focus on the brain as a site of concern narrates a productive biopolitical tension: the brain is pathologized in large part because it is deemed so agential. That media technologies are popularly used to understand the brain is a correlate to the principle that we increasingly understand the self through its capacity for mediation. In fact, it is through various forms of neuroculture that the Alzheimer's self is both medicalized and rescued. Of course, the rise of the neurosciences did not "create" or socially construct Alzheimer's, but they do offer an authoritative and progressive language for modeling both the pathologies of the disease and its solutions. They also reveal scientific interest in the brain as the most valuable object of inquiry, an interest predicated in part on broader social interest in the brain. As Fernando Vidal points out, the relationship between neuroculture and neuroscience is integral to cerebral subjectivity: "the idea that 'we are our brains' is not a corollary of neuroscientific advances, but a prerequisite of neuroscientific investigation."[3]

Alzheimer's now belongs to a culture of neurofetishism, where cognitive ability is framed as a gateway to economic, spiritual, and emotional success. This is what Nikolas Rose and Joelle Abi-Rached call a "neuro-ontology." They clarify: "it is not that human beings are brains, but that we have brains. And it is in this form—that our selves are shaped by our brains but can also shape those brains—that neuroscientific arguments are affecting conceptions of personhood and practices of self-fashioning."[4] This means not simply that brains determine our lives but that we have some agency over that determinism. Self-improvement is predicated on brain improvement, and the plasticity of the brain allows for the plasticity of one's self.[5] Awareness of this kind neuroagency is only growing, and something like digital brain training is only the tip of the iceberg. Cognitive abilities and their attendant representational frames are claimed as the determinant characteristics of personhood, and those very abilities—agency over one's capacities—are marketed to consumers as an attainable object of desire.

Put more simply, cognitive ability is tightly woven into what it means to belong in the United States. The primary symptoms of Alzheimer's, most popularly articulated as the loss of cognitive abilities like memory, are at odds with a society that requires those abilities for productive membership. However, concordant with the rhetoric of improvement and aspiration, the brain's challenges are increasingly normalized within American life-course narratives. New knowledge of the brain and its functions allows for a better understanding of symptom and risk but also for an opportunity for socialization around or against diagnosis. Autism, for example, is normalized through the discourse of rising diagnoses and neurodiversity movements, and it is pathologized by the search for a cure. Just as autism helps narrate a spectrum of social belonging at an early age, Alzheimer's dominates its ends. Each condition normalizes the brain and its challenges as a central logic of belonging.

Increasingly, that is a logic reinforced through the collective embrace of media technology. It is not just that media provide meaningful narratives or offer the invitation to social participation, but also that we have modeled our media technologies on our own neurocapacities. Memory, for example, is a cognitive ability performed by both humans and technologies. Certain media technologies (computers, for example, or photo albums) are able to remember, but they also help negotiate memory's importance in a social context. Memory loss, then, is a cognitive symptom of Alzheimer's, but it is also a product of the demands that are put on cognitive abilities.

This book's claims about Alzheimer's, then, are founded on the historical integration of cognitive abilities within media environments.[6] Just as media technologies rehearse cognitive abilities, they also promise to save or augment those abilities. For Alzheimer's, these investments in media technologies are still largely an ideological claim, but they are increasingly reinforced through medical and popular practice. The rise of digital brain-training tools like Lumosity is clear evidence of the popular appeal of cognitive enhancement media. In other words, not only do technologies like photographs and computers help authorize and describe cognitive abilities—memory, say, or recognition— but they also participate in a more pervasive cognitive culture, extending cognitive value into a network of media practice and infrastructure. For example, an Alzheimer's researcher recently proposed a digital app that would track poor financial decisions to help diagnose Alzheimer's before the onset of any symptoms, because the "first clinical markers of cognitive decline are found not in the brain but in the bank account."[7] Media technology can be both the environment and the tool with which to understand Alzheimer's.

While cognitive values may seem to be the product of new digital environments or popular narratives of smart technology, cognitive culture is not new. Cognitive abilities and media technology have a long, interdependent history—eventually coinciding with modernity itself. Memory is a dominant logic of that media history, as we have long sought to externalize our ability to remember through writing, painting, sculpture, and other representational tools. And yet, the last century of modern life has seen an incredible rise in the sophistication of machine learning and artificial intelligence. Media technologies now perform a diverse set of cognitive tasks, such as decision-making, problem solving, reasoning, and recognition. The rise of personal computing and algorithmic culture integrates these operations into everyday life. Furthermore, the emergence of "cognition" within popular and scientific discourse over the past half century has naturalized and mythologized cognitive value. Whether they are engaged as a part of neuroculture or through popular practices of self, media technologies help enact and remediate that value.

This book, then, provides a genealogy of the mediation of Alzheimer's in the United States, analyzing how the subject of Alzheimer's is constructed, contested, produced, and reproduced through different media technologies and epistemologies. This includes a range of media, such as neuroimaging, art therapy, social media, and popular film and television. But it also addresses the media context of the cognitive symptom: brain training, the labor of caregiving and scientific research, and a national economy increasingly dependent on cognitive ability and cognitively oriented media infrastructures. It describes some different ways cognitively oriented media shapes self and person—indeed, how it helps make the self a condition of personhood. This cognitive quotient has less to do with what might be described as intelligence and instead with a capacity for media integration.

So while empirically, this book focuses on traditional forms of media, theoretically and politically, it reinvigorates its study through the social optic of cognition. This is in part because the popular culture of cognition—that is, popular understanding of what cognition is—defines Alzheimer's as much as it more broadly underwrites the form and use of media environments. From pathology to progress, investments in representational value define the limits of an otherwise overdetermined disease. That is the dominant narrative of this book: one cannot understand how Alzheimer's has become a national health crisis without understanding the history of its mediation. This is because media provide the very logic and context for understanding, treating, and living with the disease.

What Is Alzheimer's? Aging and the Brain

The question of what exactly Alzheimer's *is* can be quite divisive. Theories of a cause and how exactly Alzheimer's "happens" in the brain drive research as to possible interventions, but they also shape perspectives on best-care practices and how limited money and resources should be used. Given the overlap of Alzheimer's and discourses of aging, they also contribute to both gerontological and popular theories of how to grow old successfully.

According to the dominant medical model, Alzheimer's is a progressive, degenerative brain disorder that always ends in death. There is no known cure, though some drugs and therapies can help alleviate some of its symptoms and perhaps forestall the rate of cognitive decline. There is no known cause of Alzheimer's, though research pointing toward risk factors for the disease seems to grow daily. The biggest risk factor for Alzheimer's is age. People diagnosed with the disease are most often over the age of sixty-five, and it is therefore generally understood as a disease of the elderly. However, given that certain disease biomarkers can in fact predate the appearance of symptoms, many believe that Alzheimer's in fact begins much earlier in life. Aside from age, other risk factors are often environmental or lifestyle related, including aspects of diet, exercise, social activity, and emotional health. A smaller proportion of people with Alzheimer's have the early- or younger-onset variety of the disease. It generally begins between the ages of thirty and sixty, and it is more strongly associated with genetic predisposition. The difference between early- and late-onset Alzheimer's has been a subject of debate since the disease was named more than a century ago.

Physically, Alzheimer's is usually associated with an accumulation of what are called "plaques and tangles" in the brain—essentially accretions of amyloid and tau proteins around dying cells. According to the most prominent model of Alzheimer's etiology (or cause), fragments of these amyloid plaques called beta-amyloid build up in the brain, causing the brain to atrophy severely. The rate of degeneration varies greatly, and how these degenerative changes correspond to symptoms is still unclear. Some of these changes can also be found in the brains of asymptomatic people, complicating causal arguments. The instability of these disease models has not, however, led to the diminution of the science that addresses them. Instead, most researchers continue to search for cause and cure on the basis of the plaques and tangles, with beta-amyloid being the most common target.

For most of the last century since its discovery, this atrophy and pathology were only identifiable postmortem, and any diagnosis of living people relied on clinically identifiable but somewhat unreliable symptoms. Recent developments in neuroimaging, however, have demonstrated successful "in vivo" detection of Alzheimer's biomarkers. This accompanies a wave of new diagnostic technology aimed at detecting the disease earlier and earlier in life. In essence, these biomarkers are aimed at establishing the presence of the disease in people without disease symptoms. While there are now tests for biomarkers in cerebrospinal fluid and blood that correspond to various aspects of brain pathology, the majority of the research in diagnostics and therapeutics of the last forty to fifty years has relied on PET, MRI, and other neuroimaging technologies combined with clinical evaluation. The U.S.-based, open-access Alzheimer's Disease Neuroimaging Initiative (ADNI) has been the primary orchestration of these efforts in the twenty-first century.

Symptoms of the disease include a range of changes to cognition, mood, emotion, judgment, and personality. People with Alzheimer's are more prone to apathy, anxiety, and depression, and they can have trouble sleeping and eating.[8] Moderate Alzheimer's can also be characterized by hallucinations, aggression, and paranoia. Adding to that, people with dementia are usually dealing with a host of other health issues—these are often related to aging—creating complicated problems for care and medication. In later-stage Alzheimer's, the body begins to lose its functions, leading to incontinence, seizures, and loss of mobility. Problems with swallowing can lead to weight loss, pneumonia, or other infections. Eventually the heart or lungs can shut down, leading to death.

Despite this broad range of symptoms, the disease is most popularly articulated as a disease of memory and recognition. Memory loss can be quite profound. For example, people with Alzheimer's might forget where their keys are, but they might also forget what their keys do. This kind of memory loss eventually affects one's ability to recognize other people, even family members and friends. The discourse of memory even describes the Alzheimer's care industry, as "memory care" has come to stand in for Alzheimer's care more generally. The association of memory loss with Alzheimer's is now so profound that the disease popularly signifies the general loss of memory associated with aging. Who hasn't heard someone, upon losing or forgetting something, subsequently complain of their early-onset Alzheimer's?

It should be no surprise that part of the difficulty in diagnosing Alzheimer's rests in the banality of its symptoms, especially in its early stages. "Normal" forgetting is easily confused with "Alzheimer's" forgetting. Symptoms do not strike suddenly but instead manifest gradually over many years, like many aspects of aging. In fact, an entirely new diagnostic category, called mild cognitive impairment (MCI), has evolved in response to the tenuity of symptomatic origin and debates over how to schematize the progression of the disease over stages. MCI can also be attributed to increased interest in the earliest symptoms of the disease as a part of the structural prioritization of diagnostics, early medical intervention, and drug development. It is now argued that Alzheimer's can begin to affect a person up to twenty years before the onset of any behavioral symptoms.[9]

The ordinary nature of early symptoms is also responsible for much of the fear of Alzheimer's. Risk is universalized by the association with aging, so it seems like Alzheimer's could be in anyone's future. Along with cancer, Alzheimer's is now the most feared disease in the country, and the lack of a cure only exacerbates this fear.[10] Not surprisingly, the consumer market for Alzheimer's prevention is booming. And because of debates over disease etiology, countless strategies are marketed to older adults to help them negotiate disease threat. This is despite clear warnings from the National Institutes of Health (NIH) and the National Institute on Aging (NIA) that nothing can prevent disease onset. Over the past decade, cognitive risk management has become an important part of successful aging in the United States, whether it is through diet, exercise, or brain training.

Another reason for the widespread fear of Alzheimer's is the seemingly unstoppable trend in rising prevalence. That prevalence is most certainly linked to the rising number of older people. In fact, some studies have shown that incidence numbers are actually going down, but that fact is overshadowed by the rising prevalence due to an aging population.[11] The NIA estimates that more than five million Americans currently live with the disease. The primary U.S. advocacy organization, the Alzheimer's Association, estimates that one-third of all Americans older than eighty-five years have Alzheimer's. The NIH estimates it as the sixth leading cause of death in the United States. Alzheimer's Disease International, another advocacy organization, estimates that worldwide, forty-six million people currently have dementia.[12] These numbers all depend, of course, on how you understand the disease and its pathological processes.

This diagnostic trajectory echoes the substantial rise in disease visibility in the media. These numbers are a standard component of advocacy and education, news reports, and public health outreach. While they are indeed alarming and deserve attention, it is critical to recognize that the narrative of an epidemic should be considered alongside other kinds of narratives, such as narratives of aging, scientific progress, and the promise of a cure. Epidemics normalize certain bodies just as they pathologize others, and I understand the epidemic of Alzheimer's as—at least in part—a meaningful narrative of the kinds of value societies place on cognition and aging more generally.

Alzheimer's is the most common form of dementia, but there are many other diagnostic categories with similar kinds of symptoms, such as vascular dementia, dementia with Lewy bodies, frontotemporal dementia, Parkinson's, and Creutzfeldt–Jakob disease. My exclusive use of the term *Alzheimer's* in the book reflects the way that the eponym has come to stand in for or eclipse other forms of dementia in the popular imagination. It is frequently used as a reference point by scientists and doctors hoping to educate the public about other degenerative brain diseases. Alzheimer's is invoked by athletes to publicize problems with repeated head trauma in their sports, and researchers often use Alzheimer's neuropathology to frame the degeneration associated with chronic traumatic encephalopathy.[13] It is now a primary reference point for any kind of cognitive decline associated with aging and the brain.

As I discuss in chapter 2, several factors helped bring Alzheimer's to the forefront of national consciousness, many of them intentional efforts to articulate advocacy, research, and legislation around a unifying "health politics of anguish."[14] Because of this history and its discursive focus, I specifically address Alzheimer's rather than the various categories of dementia with which it is often confused or collapsed. While attentive to important differences between these conditions, I am more concerned with the ways Alzheimer's dominates the public consciousness of aging. Along with cancer, it harnesses the lion's share of research dollars and media attention. It gets steady coverage in newspapers, magazines, and radio. It has its own nationally oriented task force, massive research initiatives, and powerful advocacy organizations. Movie stars, athletes, and at least one president have famously had the disease. It shows up in the plotlines of novels, television shows, and films. We see pharmaceutical ads for its therapy on television and in social media. Alzheimer's has become so germane to the processes of aging that it increasingly stands in for aging itself. That trend is not only an ideological one; it historically permeates the political economy of research and care. This narrow focus on Alzheimer's is part of a trend that Richard Adelman has famously called the "Alzheimerization of Aging."[15] Adelman argued that exaggerated public attention to the disease tends to encourage disproportionate research funding, legislation, and advocacy. He raised that claim in 1995, and it is still true today.

The uneasy overlap of Alzheimer's and aging is one reason why the biomedical model of Alzheimer's is so divisive. In fact, a strong contingent of medical professionals, historians, and social scientists maintains that the pathologies of Alzheimer's are a normal part of aging. Some seek to dispel the biomedicalization of what was known for a long time simply as senility. Rather than a distinct disease pathology, some argue that Alzheimer's might be a mix of different conditions associated with brain aging. If bodies break down with aging, then why not brains? One of the more outspoken advocates of this position, Peter Whitehouse, argues that "Alzheimer's disease represents our culture's attempt to make sense of a natural process (brain aging) that we cannot control."[16] According to this perspective, the "myth of Alzheimer's" is not that brain pathology does not exist but rather simply that the biomedical approach to that pathology sets up an unreasonable expectation that we will identify a cause and a cure.

The Alzheimer's establishment, of course, is deeply invested in identifying a cause and discovering a cure—or at the very least preventing the disease. The NIH, the Alzheimer's Association, the pharmaceutical industry, and almost every major health organization in the United States are opposed to a normalization model of Alzheimer's. According to their research and advocacy priorities, that makes sense: if Alzheimer's is a normal part of aging, then there can be no cure, leaving a nation without hope, without a future. Thus the majority of government and private funding goes to research on disease description, diagnostics, and medical interventions. The possibility of a successful medical intervention is in many ways dependent on the idea that Alzheimer's is a discrete disease, describable at molecular levels of the brain. While some scientists believe that Alzheimer's might be an amalgam of conditions caused by a range of factors, the majority of disease research is geared toward a more localized model of biological or material etiology.

This optimistic approach to biomedical research can ironically disenfranchise those who suffer disproportionately from the disease in the day to day.[17] Economics aside, a medical model that privileges the molecular operations of the brain is ill suited to accommodate the ways environmental or social considerations in fact structure the lived experiences of Alzheimer's.[18] Even understanding Alzheimer's as a discrete set of symptoms undermines the way the experience of the disease is in many ways dependent on environmental factors.

One of the problems with dominant dementia culture is the way in which it visibly universalizes risk while undermining the very real, often invisible marginalization that occurs along lines of race, ethnicity, gender, and class. Though biomedicine argues that Alzheimer's is in fact an abnormal occurrence, the threat of the disease is deeply normalized, drawing the disease into an anticipatory net for all. But make no mistake: Alzheimer's disproportionately affects people living in the United States. Two-thirds of those diagnosed are women (as are two-thirds of caregivers). Studies show that compared to whites, the risk of Alzheimer's doubles for Black Americans and that Latinos are 50 percent more likely than non-Latino whites to get the disease. With so many potential risk factors, and given the preponderance of attention paid to etiology at the molecular level, we don't know why.[19]

Beyond diagnosis, access to good care is also tied to a range of practical, often economic considerations. Because resources are limited, a medical model dedicated to prevention and a cure is also often at odds with the sustainability of care. Instead, people living with Alzheimer's and their caregivers are asked to hold on the best they can until the cure arrives. They are told by the medical establishment that the solution is just around the corner. They were told this in the 1980s, in the 1990s, in the 2000s, and in the 2010s, and now, in the fifth decade of Alzheimer's-oriented public health, the rhetoric is more powerful than ever before. To the research community's credit, the condition is enormously complicated, and quite a lot of descriptive progress has been made over the last century. The question, of course, is, progress toward what? And at the expense of what other kinds of progress? Clearly the world would be a better place if Alzheimer's were not around, but it is debatable whether that dream should eclipse the demands of people living with the symptoms of the disease right now.

Mediated Personhood

This debate between care and cure is as old as the public life of Alzheimer's in the United States—dating roughly to the end of the 1970s—and it is not likely to go away any time soon. It is bound up with a host of other Alzheimer's debates, including environmental versus molecular approaches to disease pathology, medical versus disability approaches to symptoms, and pharmacological versus psychosocial approaches to care. These divides are reinforced through the scarcity of resources as much as through epistemological difference. One of the most powerful historical splits in the national culture of Alzheimer's is between personhood movements and biomedicine.

Personhood has long been a concern of philosophers, anthropologists, and bioethicists, but it has a special place in the history and politics of Alzheimer's care—primarily because of this dominant stigma of the pathologized self. The 1990s saw the rise of efforts to restore or recognize the person in the Alzheimer's patient, often represented as pathologically absent in popular and medical culture.[20] Annette Leibing describes how the crisis of Alzheimer's personhood originally grew out of first-person accounts from caregivers and scientists in the 1980s struggling with few resources and little information.[21] Those early descriptions of empty shells and vacant selves met with resistance, however, by the founder of the person-centered movement in dementia care, psychiatrist Tom Kitwood.[22] Kitwood helped spawn a movement, still active today, that works to secure personhood for people with dementia. Kitwood and others have argued that we should recognize the many different ways people with dementia maintain personhood despite symptomatology that seems to threaten that status.[23] This often involves practicing caregiving methods that do not force the person with Alzheimer's to adjust to cognitive demands.

Not surprisingly, this movement in care and research often differentiates itself from the labor of biomedicine.[24] Annette Leibing argues that the goal of good critique should not be to repair this epistemological split—as that instability can be productive for Alzheimer's research; rather, the goal should be to show how these different perspectives are able to exist at the same time.[25] She argues for a turn from the "tired and unproductive dichotomies" that inform these debates—specifically personhood versus biomedicine—and advocates for more complexity in those accounts.[26] Certainly reparative efforts would not be unhelpful, especially because good faith attempts to integrate ideas perhaps at odds with one's own approach can lead to collaborative new research paths and break down entrenched research paradigms. It is increasingly evident that just as Alzheimer's can be defined in many different ways, its solutions will come not from a miracle drug or procedure but from various approaches and collaborative alliances over time.

Of course, a range of important work has already helped negotiate these divides, much of it written by historians, anthropologists, sociologists, gerontologists, philosophers, and care professionals. Some have worked to recover the subjective experiences of Alzheimer's from these restrictive versions of lost selfhood; they do this in part by describing how notions of self are structured through particular social values.[27] These efforts often address the consequences of a hypercognitive society for personhood. Others weave these debates into autobiographical narratives of family and care, the ethics of genetic identification, or ethnographies of care and biomedicine.[28] These works are informed by a much longer tradition of concern over the importance of cognition in the construction of self, and in their own way, they answer Leibing's call for a kind of complexity to the debate.

This book adds the centrality of media to these accounts. Until now, this is an area that has been treated only as supplemental rather than as an organizing principle. If culture is the mechanism through which societies organize epistemologies and ideologies of interiority—from notions of self and person to love, obligation, and agency to neuroscience and the promises of the brain—then it is through their mediation that those epistemologies take empirically recognizable form. Because of this, social and cultural analysis must specifically address the importance of media practices, technologies, industries, and ethics to Alzheimer's personhood. In fact, another way to answer Leibing's call is to explore how each of these divisive approaches to Alzheimer's invests in media to address or overcome the disease.

Within humanities and social science disciplines like sociology, anthropology, philosophy, and comparative literature, a lot of related work has been accomplished through descriptions of the "subject." *Subjectivity* has been a particularly significant keyword in media and cultural studies because of its focus on representation and power.[29] Personhood is not subjectivity, however, and the fact that I write about subjectivity in this book should not detract from my more specific critique of personhood. Understanding the broader subject of Alzheimer's certainly requires careful attention to both self and person. But the concept of the person is a lot more concrete than the subject. One reason for this is that subjectivity largely remains the purview of academic critique, and it does not command public interest the way debates over personhood often do.

Americans like talking about what makes a person a person. They even fight over it. Look no further than the third rail of abortion rights or so-called death panels to see how operative personhood can be in U.S. politics. These personhood debates are not limited to the beginning or end of life—they also help structure everyday experience for anyone living in the country, citizen or not. Because the U.S. Constitution actually relies on the concept of the "person" to frame rights and responsibilities, legal descriptions of personhood frame voting, immigration, citizenship, and free speech. Even corporations have made a claim to personhood, giving them many of the rights of humans in the United States. Despite its articulation in legal discourse, however, personhood is still socially contentious and under threat.

One clear problem for any evaluation of Alzheimer's personhood is the historical slippage between self and person. What is the difference between these categories, and how are media involved in confusing them? One simple reason for this collapse is the importance of some kind of identity to social participation—especially within digital environments. Contemporary investments in the mediated self are of course not limited to Alzheimer's, and the idea that Americans use media technologies to construct or maintain a sense of identity should now be obvious. After the rise of participatory digital media in the early 2000s, online platforms now allow for full-time performance and curation of self. Despite widespread awareness of problems like surveillance, bullying, and "fake news," social media use continues to grow.[30] Moreover, media platforms as different as Facebook and Fitbit demonstrate just how diversely modeled our digital selves can be. Concepts like users, avatars, and profiles are just some of the ways we mount our digital identities. Whether those selves are enabled through pictures, words, or another form of data, it is clear that identitarian value is increasingly tied to its mediation.

A popular discourse of "self" even accompanies these practices, from the quantified self to self-help to the selfie. That the self now has a popular resonance within media culture encourages social awareness about the self and its values. Ultimately, these practices help shape popular understanding of what a self is. They put pressure on all of us to think about our self, to develop, perform, protect, or share in that self. And they articulate the self as a subject of public concern, even if they also invite debates over the value of its privacy. It is in its public articulation that selfhood begins to look like personhood.

These digital articulations of self are valuable to a host of outside interests, and user data is now harvested and sold with abandon. Data mining and datafication now pervade the full spectrum of American life, including consumer relationships, education, politics, and health care. Data is not just one of the bigger industries in the United States; it is conceivably a part of all industry. Data plays a central role in structuring digital experience, but it can also shape life away from our media technologies. It even helps shape the parameters of the sacred in the United States—within both emergent secular lifestyles and more traditional religious practice.

In fact, the availability of one's personal information to surveillance and tracking does not result in the demise of the authentic self, as one might imagine; rather, these online spaces increasingly shape the very possibility for authenticity.[31] Media technologies may expand our capacities for self-awareness and self-improvement, but they also reinforce the importance of an identity and its constant maintenance. That is because an individual identity is both an interest and an effect of these other actors.[32]

Despite the dispersal of the self's interests, however, we continue to privilege a model of liberal, autonomous selfhood in both popular and medical culture. Rather than a radically new concept of self, these digital trends are a part of a longer, modern tradition of the mediation of self, some of which I explore in this book. From personal photography to celebrity to the institutions of art and creativity, Americans share a long history of the celebration of individuality through technologies of media.

One side effect of the public mediation of self, however, is that its social recognition can be limited to those spaces and activities. Membership or recognition within society (or personhood) often requires some level of media participation. Of course, personhood has a wide spectrum of social, civic, and ethical meanings, but it is clear that a whole range of social institutions now demand media participation for personhood to be recognized. And it is through these diverse media practices that selfhood is most often confused with personhood.[33]

For it is only in its mediation that selfhood acquires value as personhood, and for Alzheimer's in this conjuncture, it is precisely that mediation that increasingly makes the self a condition of personhood. For this reason, this book looks more carefully at *mediated personhood* and the ways it shapes the experience of Alzheimer's in the United States. What are the consequences of a society that mandates a self as a condition of acceptance or membership? What can Alzheimer's teach us about broader patterns of social belonging, as it is evident that mediated personhood far exceeds the experience of symptom or disease? Conversely, then, how can media scholars familiar with technologies and practices of media bring some clarity to the crisis of Alzheimer's? One way to understand the consequences of mediated personhood is to look more closely at cognitive ability and representation.

Representation and Cognition

Alzheimer's media varies considerably in form, but quite a lot of it is visual, especially that designed for public consumption.[34] Visual media dominates the history of American popular and public culture, so that is not unusual. There are of course other forms of media—forms that don't involve pictures or screens. Audio culture is particularly important to certain kinds of Alzheimer's care. However, public understanding of interiority often presupposes some visual encounter. This is especially true in the popular reception of neuroscience, and there is a significant need for careful analysis of how representations of brains can affect personhood. Given the seemingly endless flow of medical discourse currently contributing to the popular imagination of Alzheimer's, this book could have been substantive simply pursuing that element alone. In fact, it is precisely because of the increasing diversity and ubiquity of neuroimaging tools and the circulation of their products in popular culture that addressing representation in medical and scientific practice continues to be of such critical importance.[35] So, before investigating the way cognition is modeled through the broad diversity of media technologies, we must first acknowledge the simple effects these medical images can have in popular culture.

The first step is to destabilize the objective authority of the neuro-image, especially as it helps shape the pathologized self of the person with Alzheimer's.[36] The rhetorical potential of neuroimagery may seem obvious to humanities scholars or social scientists well practiced in representational critique, but it remains surprisingly opaque in its public reception. Despite pervasive suspicion of science in areas like climate change, evolution, and vaccinations, certain forms of scientific representation maintain remarkable authority—images of brains in particular—and biomedicine borrows on that authority. This is not to say that neuroscience is implicitly suspect. But in their public reception, neuroimages often exceed the scope of the research for which they were produced. They also require an expertise or literacy unavailable to the public. Joseph Dumit describes how this works in his ethnography of PET, *Picturing Personhood*: images of brains communicate certain facts about human nature and behavior, facts that can shape social narratives of normal and abnormal.[37] How or whether one accepts the facts of the neuroimage depends, of course, on the context of reception, but it is precisely the objective authority of the neuroimage that engenders a logic of difference and identification. The public is asked to bear witness to those representations, to validate them as a part of shared research goals, or to identify with their diagnoses. As Janelle Taylor makes clear with her analysis of fetal sonograms, "this task, to the extent that it necessarily involves making visible the invisible, revealing and unmasking what has been hidden and obscured, inevitably draws us into a rhetoric and a politics of vision."[38]

As concerns Alzheimer's, that rhetoric both elevates the descriptive expertise of the neuroscientist and contributes to a stigma of loss with respect to the changing brain. Both expertise and stigma are based on the imaging technology's ability to describe changes to the brain that signify the presence of Alzheimer's. Those changes have historically focused on atrophy, but also a range of other biomarkers for the disease, many of which are described in the opening chapters of this book. From the perspective of the untrained witness, however, the proficiency of

the imaging technology and expertise of the neuroscientist authorize
that stigma of pathological loss. Through diagnosis and description,
the physical interiority of the brain collapses into other models of interiority, such as selfhood.

The rhetoric of the image, however, is not merely an exercise in realism, and the neuroimage is only one small part of a diverse media ecosystem invested in the self and its values. Understanding Alzheimer's
relationship to representation requires a more complex understanding of media practice, industry, and technology. This involves analyzing not simply a broad range of media texts but also patterns of use
and interpretation. It means trying to think critically about the different modes of seeing that are historically framed through the logics of
medicine and health. David Serlin argues that "examining the visual
culture of public health from within multiple systems of meaning making relocates analysis of images beyond simple aesthetic or interpretive
claims to focus on how certain health practices are deeply imbedded
in larger networks of visual practices and interrelated genealogies of
visual media."[39] Serlin's argument for framing medical visual culture
in the context of use and practice is an important one because it reinforces the perspective that medical images always operate within a
broader history of media technology.[40] For example, the diagnostic truth
claim offered by a PET brain scan is in many ways predicated on a cultural history of photography and mimetic realism. Not surprisingly,
that photographic history often mixes with neuroimages in the popular culture of Alzheimer's, a pattern that will become more clear in
chapter 4 of this book.

Another valuable idea that Serlin raises is that health media is
not always overtly medicalized. This is particularly important for Alzheimer's, because the representational culture of Alzheimer's is not
always about the disease or its symptoms. It is not even always "about."
In other words, beyond acknowledging the mixture of media practices
and technologies that contribute to understanding the disease, the critical tools of media studies are also good for thinking about representation beyond meaning or signification. This holds special importance

for understanding Alzheimer's, because representation and cognition are so interrelated.

After the so-called material turn, representational critique has fallen out of favor as media scholars increasingly address technology, software, data, infrastructure, industry, and the broad agency of nonhuman actors involved in media environments.[41] As a consequence of these new materialisms, it has become common in media studies to discard representation as a critical concept—especially as it concerns textual or hermeneutic critique. One could argue that this is merely a fashionable turn because of representation's ties to purportedly limited identity criticism and constructivisms, where studying representation is often a claim about meaning making and power. Rather than disparage the concept of representation as too overdetermined for good critique, however, I would argue that it continues to require careful critical attention. This has *always* been true for minoritarian groups seeking access and agency, and it should continue to be a site of critical leadership for academics, activists, and advocates. It is certainly still true that representation of people with Alzheimer's matters more than ever, as it shapes everything from stigma to best practice to disease paradigms and diagnosis. While understanding the ways media is made to mean will always be critically viable (just as it is in this book), addressing representation's material, affective, and infrastructural relationships to agency is perhaps equally important.

This is evident in the contexts of both digital culture and neuroculture, where representation so often exceeds the recognition of human actors. The incidental invisibility of the operations of both brains and digital technology is reason enough to study their representational effects—especially since society is so invested in those effects. From neurons to data, and from synapses to software, the brain and digital media increasingly serve as touchstones for social perspectives on agency. Representation, then, is material both in the embodied, neurological sense and in the ways it exists within media technologies and environments. Clearly representation still matters. It has both material and symbolic consequences. It is critical that media scholars continue to develop the concept as a material concern as well as an ethical, agential one. Instead of thinking about the demise in representational authority, we ought to think about these clear shifts in representational values along the lines of the brain and its logics.

This is especially true for Alzheimer's, because representation is not simply a supportive concept. Particularly in the United States, Alzheimer's is most popularly understood as a crisis of representation and selfhood. Given the public struggles that dominate the politics of disease research in this country, that claim could also be made about other diseases, such as cancer, HIV-AIDS, or really any disease that acquires the popular visage of pathology and loss. But Alzheimer's is different: as the "memory disease," representation is the central paradigm through which we understand the disease. Many of the cognitively oriented symptoms associated with Alzheimer's disease can be understood as threats to representation. These include the progressive loss of memory, the inability to make new memories, failure to recognize friends and family members, altered perception, hallucinations, aphasia, and other cognitive impairments. What is often assumed to be threatened by the sum of those symptoms is some notion of self. Those deeply modern cultural logics that locate notions of selfhood in and through representation fear precisely those symptoms that threaten its security.

But what about representations beyond the operations of the human brain? Cognition is popularly imagined as something that happens in the body, by virtue of the brain's ability. However, cognition is also a distributed and relational practice, increasingly coproduced by media technologies. The more this distributed or systemic cognition pervades our media environments, the more it changes our own relationship to cognitive ability. The negotiation of cognitive demands through the artifacts and processes of media is not new. It is as old as the media. It is precisely the limitations of human capacity that make media such a useful tool.

Increasingly, these cognitive capacities and demands are collectively experienced and resolved within digital media culture. A digital cloud capable of storing seemingly limitless information, for example, augments the centrality and ubiquity of memory, just as it makes digital forgetting increasingly impossible.[42] Of course, human memory and digital memory function quite differently, but they can shape each other in both popular imagination and the exchange of responsibility or capacity.[43] Take something like Google Glass, wearable computer tech released in 2013 that some in the media and care organizations blissfully reported might be useful as a "brain prosthetic" for people with Alzheimer's.[44] The glasses' facial recognition software might help a person with dementia to recognize her loved ones, for example, or GPS mapping technology could prevent her from getting lost. The clear challenges of introducing such a prosthetic aside, the discourse reveals the way in which symptom and solution are often tethered through popular media technology.

From this point of view, cognition has a nonhuman, representational presence because cognitive ability exists within material media environments. This is cognition that exceeds human thought and any performance of a self. It may be in the world because of human activity, but it is not necessarily synonymous with human thinking.[45] One of the more important effects of this distributed cognition is the remediation of more situated, human cognition. These nonhuman performances of cognition shape the lived experiences of cognitive disability in everyday life.[46] This is as true of people living with the symptoms of Alzheimer's as it is of anyone. To be clear, I am not making an argument about historical changes to human consciousness or intelligence. I am simply pointing out that cognitive abilities have a life that exceeds individual mental performance or even awareness and that these distributed abilities also help shape human capacities. There seems to be an ongoing insistence, however, that human cognition is somehow discrete. Even the phrase "artificial" intelligence is evidence of the partition we set up between machine learning and human cognition, but also of our fear of its collapse.

Understanding Alzheimer's, then, means exploring a broader ethics of representation and cognition. Key in this cognitive ethics is the paradox that figures representation as both a problem to be solved—representational loss as loss of self is the central crisis of the disease—

and an answer to that crisis, via medical neuroimaging, personal brain training, creative art therapies, and artificial intelligence. Fundamentally, these ethics are tied to the gray zone in the diagnosis of Alzheimer's and more typical experiences of cognitive disability. They describe both the historical importance of cognitive ability for understanding the self and the ways neuroculture permeates diverse aspects of American life. They take into consideration the social, political, and economic insistence on cognitive integration as a conditional armature of personhood. They build off the well-known work of dementia ethicist Stephen Post, who developed the term *hypercognitive* to define a social situation that values foremost the cognitively able.[47] This book advances that ethical principle into the realm of media technology and practice. That means taking the ubiquity of media seriously as it shapes everyday life in the United States and contributing to a genealogy of visuality and media as conditioned by ability, access, and rights.[48] Does representation in fact presuppose cognition? In its social, political realization? Alzheimer's reveals how cognitive value maintains the boundaries of the healthy human just as it defines the limits of the posthuman imagination.

Media's Cognitive Imperative

This book is therefore not simply a collection of media artifacts or images that depict the disease or its constituents; *Mediating Alzheimer's* takes a further step, analyzing how the subject of Alzheimer's is conditioned by cognitively oriented media. By the subject of Alzheimer's, I mean not simply that person diagnosed with the disease but the ongoing field of knowledge that makes up the social experience of the disease in particular contexts. In this book, I qualify that subject within a national context but beyond the boundaries of individual ability. On the other hand, because of its distributed, material nature, cognitive culture far exceeds that subject. Cognition is dispersed within media technologies as capacities, abilities, effects, and intentions. Cognitive value here is not bound to the lived, embodied symptom, nor even to claims of social meaning, but is also qualified and organized by a more dispersed field of media technology.

Far be it from me to isolate what cognition *is* in a comprehensive sense. My goal is not to create a new media formalism, nor is it to rehearse the descriptive work of the cognitive sciences. Given the distributed nature of its effects, defining cognition's limits would be an impossible task. Tracing some of its accretions and values in this limited context should be enough—certainly as a way to understand how Alzheimer's makes itself known and how we model our pathologies and capacities of self. In this sense, the book maps some of the different ways that cognition becomes a cultural fact and thus acquires value as a function of personhood and social belonging.

The link between seeing and knowing is of course an entrenched philosophical debate. While attendant to these philosophical legacies, this book is not so much a philosophical inquiry as it is a political and historical project. It asserts the primacy of memory and recognition within a broader critique of the demands of cognitive culture. I organize this critique within an analysis of what I call *media's cognitive imperative*: a concept that ties the lived symptoms of Alzheimer's to broader relationships with representation. As a rule, it references both the diverse cognitive operations of media and the mandate that we each integrate within those operations as a part of ordinary life. For example, memory is now a ubiquitous media capacity, but it also means humans often rely on media technologies to help them remember.

Why is it still important to reimagine the role of cognition in American culture, if modernity is already overwritten with concern for cognition both as a neurologically, biologically bound ability and as a dispersed cultural symptom? If cognitive science and its disciplinary partners have described cognitive operations in a multitude of environments and processes for at least a half century, why is it worth focusing on the cognitive imperative now?

An obvious answer is the looming crisis of Alzheimer's in an aging population. Another is the dominance of neuroculture in U.S. science, policy, and economic development. Also important is the centrality of artificial intelligence to digital media and its recent emergence as a site of public concern. It is also worth noting that while some people recognize cognition as embodied, distributed, or otherwise complicated, most still maintain traditional cognitive dualisms in their most important values and relationships. And cognition's seeming ubiquity does not erase its imbalanced holds on social life. As media becomes more environmental and prosthetic, it is easy to assume a kind of universal ideology of inclusion, access, and affordability. As I argue in this book, however, the universal promise of media technology belies the abilities and tools required for participation.

This perspective is more in line with the field of disability studies. Though the academic project has been slower to address cognitive disabilities, disability scholars offer useful tools to address the slip between a medical symptom and a social ability.[49] Rather than pathologizing the body, disability scholars emphasize the way that a body can become disabled by virtue of the body's social or physical environment. This is one reason why disability scholars are often at odds with biomedicine—rather than fixing the disability, disability activists and academics have worked to fix the environment, either by addressing the stigma of the disability or by creating access or accommodations.

At the same time, like the neuropathology that accompanies the symptoms of Alzheimer's, biomedicine cannot be shrugged off. Many of the most important advances in helping people with dementia have come from medical professionals, and they arguably share many of the same goals. That Alzheimer's is based on pathological, neurodegenerative processes does not undermine disability's claims as to the value of accommodations, however. Furthermore, disability criticism can help establish Alzheimer's as both social and embodied, an increasingly common part of aging that does not diminish the lived difficulties of the disease. Given cognition's pervasive hold on modern life as well as the lack of a promising therapy, this seems like a more realistic way to locate agency.

Rather than a coincidence, I see the emergence of cognitive culture to be co-constitutive with the contemporary crisis of Alzheimer's. The rise of Alzheimer's as a national concern in the last quarter of the twentieth century roughly coincides with the development of communicative capitalism and a global information economy.[50] The coemergence of the disease and new forms of social and economic participation illuminates cognition's changing roles in American life and labor, changes that echo in transformations in media technologies that foreground particular cognitive values. No longer latent or buried, cognitive abilities increasingly take form through the variable effects and interfaces of these media technologies.

This book thus analyzes how cognition is understood as a site of both pathological loss *and* optimistic productivity in the United States, and it shows how these cognitive values are woven into the media technologies that treat or address Alzheimer's. Consequently, the book is not a polemic against media's cognitive imperative; rather, it describes some of the ways in which this imperative has historically contributed to health care and successful aging in this country. Alzheimer's reveals these ethics as foundational not just to pathological personhood but also to more ordinary modes of living. The universal risk of Alzheimer's harmonizes with a cognitive meritocracy in the United States, underscoring governmentality's claims on both cognitive maintenance and productivity in this conjuncture. Importantly, this meritocracy is dependent not on an individual's "raw intelligence" but on a capacity for media integration. It is in many ways predicated on a myth of media neutrality. While codependent, that meritocracy and its practices of self-optimization stand in direct opposition to ideologies of loss.

Certainly media technologies offer a multitude of benefits that can improve human life, a fact as true of people living with the symptoms of Alzheimer's as it is of anyone else. Media dominates modern living, and it is not going away any time soon, even if we lessen its demands on self and person. Given that fact, it is not my intention to come across as Luddite in my critique or to impose a deterministic argument about media or cognitive effects. Media's cognitive imperative is as much a shared ethic as it is a formal paradigm based on human abilities; as such, we can respond to it and help shape it. One central issue for Alzheimer's where political, historical, and critical efforts can have some effect is in the area of personhood.

If we are to take seriously the implications of a mediated personhood for Alzheimer's, we need to acknowledge media's cognitive imperative as a set of values that remediate the body with pressures to care, to remember, to recognize, and to know. That media technologies can sometimes resolve those pressures only amplifies our dependencies. Just as they extend our cognitive capacities with prosthetic tools and technologies, media help shape the social value of those capacities.

One of Alzheimer's most important lessons is that mediated personhood has little to do with being depicted in a representation, even if it often pretends to exactly that. Mediated personhood is a consequence of media *capacity,* or the promise of media engagement. Media's cognitive imperative is both the rule and the material language for that engagement. I emphasize the term *mediated personhood* instead of *media personhood* because the very potential for personhood is often predetermined by media technologies and practices. This argument does not dismiss human agency, but it does recognize the dominance of media technologies in modern life.

Alzheimer's, then, reveals two intertwined characteristics of mediated personhood, each of which correlates to broader trends in media and society. First, selfhood is increasingly integral to personhood. Arguably, access to personhood even requires a self: having, sharing, curating, performing, fabricating, or otherwise laboring over a self. Whether through email, data mining, social media, art, or some other media practice, that selfhood acquires its social value through its mediation. Second, based in part on that mediation, personhood is cognitively oriented. It requires representational capacities like recognition and memory, capacities that Alzheimer's threatens. A cognitive meritocracy continues to authorize these participatory environments, asserting representational capacity as a central aspect of social belonging.[51]

One of this book's objectives, then, is to take the limited step of describing the cognitive aspects of mediated personhood. However, there are doubtless other aspects left to be described. The effects of mediated personhood can be as diverse as the social or technological environments that shape it. By that same token, mediated personhood is not exclusive to the experience of dementia. This book is ultimately about Alzheimer's, and that limits the scope of my critique. Perhaps these efforts can lead others to explore media's relationship to personhood in different contexts.

Chapter Overview

This book addresses Alzheimer's disease primarily in the context of the United States, but it does so in a way that acknowledges its articulation within global health. Since Alzheimer's discovery, international research collaboration has shaped medical knowledge about the disease. Increasingly, this happens in philanthropic and advocacy circles as well. Certainly a lot of the arguments in this book could apply to other places, and it is not my intention to dismiss any overlaps or exchanges.

The book's national focus, however, is a consequence of the fact that the experience of Alzheimer's in the United States is distinct from other contexts. There are many reasons for this, including widespread embrace of media technologies and representational culture. Just as important, however, is the American myth of individualism and self-determination. The country has a particularly grand claim on individual autonomy that augments the lost-self narrative just as it heightens discourse of personal responsibility.

On the other hand, the homogenizing narrative of a national epidemic can overshadow the uneven experience of Alzheimer's in this country. Baby boomers, in particular, function as the popular figures of an entire generation both under and as threat. They model the future of aging and its burdens, not only because boomers are a large cohort, but because they are expected to live longer than any generation before them. The assumption of a looming crisis of aging—that Alzheimer's threatens an entire generation and thus the stability of the country—obscures the crisis of care already well under way. It also overshadows the pressures put on both cognitive ability and selfhood in the more quotidian pursuit of health and wealth. Each of the book's chapters describes these pressures in different media contexts, exploring the way media's cognitive imperative shapes Alzheimer's and the more broadly held ethic of mediated personhood.

The historical time frame for this account covers roughly the last century of the representational life of the disease in the United States. It begins by describing the importance of Alzheimer's to the professionalization of both psychiatry and neuroimaging at the beginning of the twentieth century. In 1906 the German physician and neuropathologist Alois Alzheimer discovered the pathological characteristics of the disease that would come to bear his name, and he would publish the results of his research soon after. Over the next decade, his research and imaging techniques were translated for an American audience as a small part of the active professionalization of medical sciences of mind and brain.

One imaging method that has remained surprisingly consistent from Alzheimer's research until today is histology, the study of cells and tissues often performed through section, stains, or dyes, and light or electron microscopes. Alzheimer practiced neuropathological histology, which focuses on dead brain tissue. Because it employs staining techniques in addition to microscopic evaluation, histology is always a process of interpretation, recognition, and translation, and thus its relationship to diagnostics can be quite complicated.

The first chapter of the book thus offers a theory of the "histological gaze" as a way to analyze both the scientific labor of the discovery of the disease and the epistemological frames that shaped its description. In addition to Alzheimer, it focuses on Solomon Carter Fuller, the first Black American psychiatrist and one person responsible for importing Alzheimer's research and techniques to the United States. My analysis describes the importance of these imaging techniques to the professionalization of sciences of mind and brain, and in particular, the prioritization of descriptive diagnostics and biologically oriented classification of disease. Rather than focus on the experience of symptom or subjugation of the patient, this chapter addresses the importance of certain media practices to the authority and objectivity of the medical scientist. It situates these psychiatric practices within a narrative of media experimentation and progressive public health in the first two decades of the twentieth century in the United States.

Chapter 2 opens with the peculiar disappearance of Alzheimer's from scientific memory from approximately 1920 to 1960, a four-decade gap explainable in part through the lack of new neuroimaging tools and the rise of psychosocial explanations for dementia.[52] A number of developments in medical research helped return Alzheimer's to biomedical consciousness, including the rise of the electron microscope, the emergence of new techniques for acquiring comparative clinical data, and the gradual realization that senile dementia was far more common than originally thought. As the disease became more scientifically visible in the 1960s and 1970s, national policy makers recognized it as a key threat to an aging population. Because of the way the disease was subsequently linked to transformations in national aging legislation, the disease quickly acquired an identity as a developing public health crisis in the United States.

The chapter, then, describes the role of neuroimaging in the enlistment of a national public as both audience to and eventual subject of U.S. research on Alzheimer's. These trends reveal two complementary investments in this media: first, the promise of neuroimaging technologies to reveal the material basis of the disease, and second, a related investment in an empirically based knowledge economy as a condition of medical progress. Media innovation continued to drive advancement in Alzheimer's research, and key transformations in national health and aging policy were in fact reliant on public acceptance of these neuroimaging practices. While historically, Alzheimer's research relied on dead brain tissue, toward the end of the century, neuroimaging increasingly integrated the living brain as its object of inquiry. The growth of Alzheimer's as a public health threat in the 1980s and 1990s, the inclusion of symptomatic and material imaging biomarkers in research, and the broad Alzheimerization of aging all helped inaugurate Alzheimer's as a defining feature of aging in the United States.

By the beginning of the twenty-first century, the national battle to cure Alzheimer's reinforced a celebratory culture of neuroscience and widespread public awareness of the brain and its agencies. As a way to illustrate this transformation in cognitive value, the chapter describes the history of the NIA's ADNI, a program that began in 2004 and has gone through several stages of renewal. The initiative represents the natural culmination of U.S. prioritization of particular neuroimaging strategies in Alzheimer's research. It has also contributed to the growth of a knowledge economy reliant on media innovation. In other words, as a highly public orientation of technologies of realism, ADNI not only drives material theories of Alzheimer's etiology but in fact underwrites these secondary investments in STEM-based research and professionalization as a national labor priority.

The growing threat of Alzheimer's has incorporated an increasing number of Americans into relationships of self-care and cognitive health. As the Alzheimer's Association urges, "Maintain Your Brain!" The cottage industry that promotes dementia prevention depends on the notion of a threatened self, just as it stigmatizes its loss. Chapter 3 explores a diversity of media that demonstrate these contemporary trends, like popular medical television, self-help discourse, advocacy appeals, and the news media, but it also focuses on the media artifacts that promise to mitigate your risk. I focus in particular on the genre of digital brain games, exercises designed to help people increase their "cognitive reserve," ideally forestalling the onset of the disease. These practices of self-care normalize disease risk within the narrative of successful aging, but they also enforce the promise of a cognitive meritocracy through media technology. The optimistic quest to salvage a threatened brain therefore opens aging to particular forms of governmentality, on one hand, and marketing and commodification, on the other. That culture of threat and agency also helps shape popular understandings of exactly what Alzheimer's is and why it matters.

Chapter 4, then, describes the ways contemporary popular culture that depicts Alzheimer's relies on particular representational logics to communicate collective concerns about the disease. It foregrounds the two documentary aesthetics that dominate the public life of Alzheimer's: the snapshot aesthetic and the neuroscientific aesthetic. The snapshot and the neuroimage each purports to capture, save, or otherwise document the embattled, interior self of the person with dementia, but they depend on collectively held ideas about the media artifact's relationship to time for their legibility in the public eye. In addition to the truth claims that accompany the genre of documentary, these media technologies' material relationships with temporality, durability, and proficiency help structure a social model of cognitive value and anachronistic aspects of Alzheimer's personhood. The snapshot structures personhood through nostalgia and loss, while the neuroimage offers hope for the future. Where does that leave people living with Alzheimer's now?

My argument for a contemporary account of Alzheimer's in the United States thus recognizes the historical embeddedness of disease paradigms, but it also describes these anachronizing media practices. I describe their consequences for Alzheimer's personhood and the way they structure care. A recent trend in memory care, for example, is to re-create the experience of the past so people with Alzheimer's can spend time in environments that may have been normal to them in their youth. Inspired by a so-called dementia village in Amsterdam called Hogeway, this model of care has captured international attention. California's Glenner Town Square, for example, is a nine-thousand-square-foot re-creation of "small-town USA" in the 1950s, complete with era-appropriate films, a barbershop, cars, restaurants, and music.[53] While this kind of reminiscence therapy may help some people with dementia, success is probably due as much to the quality of interpersonal care in those facilities as it is to the virtual time travel. Despite the public appeal of a nostalgia facility like Glenner or Hogeway, caring for people with Alzheimer's still requires a certain presence, and that can be expensive and labor intensive. People with advanced Alzheimer's simply cannot take care of themselves; even people with early symptoms can often use some help.

That is not to say that media have no place in care—quite the opposite—but I argue that they should be used in a way fully reflective of their anachronizing potential. These narratives, ostensibly aimed at rescuing the person with Alzheimer's, can potentially disenfranchise the very people they purport to help. I respond to these anachronistic aesthetics by discussing recent attempts of some people with Alzheimer's to utilize social media as a way to define media engagement on their own terms. Many people who find themselves in the role of caregiver turn to social media for knowledge and support, but it is less common for people who actually have dementia to self-organize in these media spaces. The live-streamed discussions I explore often prohibit participation from anyone not experiencing symptoms of dementia. In addition to sharing resources, they can foster exclusive communities through active media practices.

Building off the last two chapters' discussions of representation and care, chapter 5 focuses on the New York Museum of Modern Art's influential Alzheimer's access program, Meet Me at MoMA. The program is a part of a popular trend in care that promotes art as potentially therapeutic or beneficial to people with dementia as well as to their caregivers. Observations of the sessions, interviews with educators, and analysis of the program's reception reveal broader assumptions about the relationship between modern art, dementia, and personhood. The museum shows an interest in both the capacity and the perceived interiority of *all* participants, an educational perspective that harmonizes with the museum's long-standing focus on temporal and aesthetic modernism.

Whereas chapter 5 focuses on people looking at art, chapter 6 describes the new creative practices of art making increasingly germane to Alzheimer's care. There is little evidence about how art therapy actually works for people with dementia, but nevertheless, its popularity continues to rise. Positivity, art, and creativity are ideological counterpoints to pathologies of loss, and they serve as an optimistic celebration of the power of representational media to authorize personhood. I employ two case studies to demonstrate social attitudes toward creativity and dementia. The first involves William Utermohlen, a contemporary artist with Alzheimer's whose paintings are often described as reflections of a pathologized interiority. The second case study addresses the recent museological reception of Willem de Kooning, one of the more well-known artists with Alzheimer's. Through these examples, I argue that creativity functions as an optimistic coordination of human capacity: a medical tool celebrated precisely for its mythmaking abilities. Seemingly pure categories like creativity and art can be refreshingly hopeful in a situation without a cure. Though attentive to the viability of this kind of practice, I argue that we ought to reconsider the unmarked positivity of Alzheimer's care, especially given the way it harmonizes with ideologies of creative self-management in a communicative economy.

Following that critique, chapter 7 unites several themes of the book by orienting the national crisis of caregiving as a problem of representation and recognition. In particular, I investigate the slippage between love and care in the popular culture of Alzheimer's in the United States from 1994 to 2020. This period saw caregiving rise as a new national concern in narratives of Alzheimer's, a trend primarily represented in the media as a crisis of familial and romantic love. As a person with Alzheimer's loses the ability to recognize friends and family, nostalgia for a lost love is what fuels the possibility for good care in the present. This narrative of loss collapses love and representation, disenfranchising those who may have access to neither. I show how love is often disguised as cognition's other, but I argue that love might also be recognized *as* cognition in our current conjuncture, especially within representational culture. Love is disguised as noncognitive affect, but it is actually a central logic of media's cognitive imperative.

This chapter, then, charts how love functions ironically to strip personhood from the very individuals upon whom it is bestowed, introducing an interpersonal politics of representation and recognition often unavailable to the cognitively disabled person. This trend articulates love into neoliberal models of health, aging, and labor, and the autonomy of the family unit is framed as instrumental to later-life health care in the United States. This trend contributes to traditional mind–body dualisms whereby science is offered as the solution to the future with love maintained as the answer to an incurable present. Evidence here—including a seemingly disparate range of popular, scientific, and public media—demonstrates how the affective capacities of individual citizens are systematically harnessed to the national interest, but to the detriment of their own.

It may seem cynical to disparage the tools of positivity, and at the outset my position is not likely to be popular to members of an already embattled care industry, nor perhaps to caregivers themselves. I hope it is clear that my aim is not to disparage those tools unequivocally. Optimism and hope are important to care, just as caregiving relationships can often be positive and rewarding for all parties involved. I also believe that cultural fixtures like human rights, art, creativity, love, and hope will continue to do important work even if we operate with a better understanding of their ideological and social operations. Rather than working against positivity itself, I argue that it is often deployed in ways antithetical to the interests of people living with Alzheimer's. By showing how positivity pretends to erase the pathologies of the present, perhaps we can live more honestly with the truth of the symptoms.

1

Origin Myths

*History, Histology,
and Representational Value*

> It is one of the paradoxes of astronomy that we can best
> study the constitution of the sun when that orb is in
> eclipse; it is one of the paradoxes of psychology, that we
> can best study the mysteries of the mind when that
> function is eclipsed by disease. Of old, men regarded an
> eclipse of the sun as a proof of the wrath of some hateful
> Deity, and they ran from it in horror; in these days men
> run to an eclipse as to a glad and special messenger of
> science, and cross oceans and continents, and ascend high
> mountains, that through the clearer air they may the more
> distinctly see the glories of the corona and wait for the
> appearing of unknown stars.
>
> —George M. Beard, *The Problems of Insanity,* 1880

On November 3, 1906, Alois Alzheimer delivered a lecture to a group
of colleagues at the thirty-seventh meeting of the Southwest German
Psychiatrists. Indicative of his acclaimed skills as an image maker, he
made use of a range of projected slides in his presentation. These
included images of brain tissue drawn with the aid of a camera lucida
and microscope. The object of his gaze was a fifty-one-year-old German
woman named "Auguste D.," admitted to the Frankfurt mental asylum
in 1901 by her husband. Her hospitalization had allowed Alzheimer

an opportunity to observe her behavior and perform a series of clinical interviews, during which he found evidence of hallucinations, memory loss, aphasia, helplessness, disorientation, focal signs, and "general dementia."[1]

After she died in 1906, Alzheimer's examination of her brain tissue identified what would later become known as the amyloid plaques and neurofibrillary tangles that still constitute a central mystery of the disease today. His lecture, then, synthesized these observations into what he called a "peculiar disease of the cerebral cortex," a disease entity united by microscopic evidence and the clinical symptomatology of senile dementia in a subject who was relatively young. The substance and contentiousness of his discovery framed the scientific debates that would condition research on Alzheimer's disease for the next century.

But for whatever reason, Alzheimer's presentation met with relative silence at that conference. Instead, the discussion that finished the day's colloquium echoed the rift that populated psychiatry at the time between the neurobiological and the psychoanalytic perspectives. The first group, composed of psychiatrists like Alzheimer and his colleagues from his Munich laboratory, occupied the position that mental disorders originate organically in the brain. According to this perspective, good science makes connections between microscopic or macroscopic evidence in the brain and a patient's clinical behavior. This research was bolstered by active conversations on brain localization and specialization; new neuronal theory; and developing histological technologies in microscopy, staining, and fixing.

A different psychiatry was also represented at the meeting, the psychoanalytic perspective, developed by another trained neurologist, Sigmund Freud. This stance attributed mental disorders not to lesions in the brain but to past experience and psychic defenses against trauma. While not against the principle of neurological degeneration per se (atrophy, for example), psychoanalysis did take an active stance against biological determinism, the deeper premise of Alzheimer's argument. One psychiatrist in the biological camp gave a paper at the conference attacking Freud and psychoanalysis: local press reported that a youthful Carl Jung vigorously defended Freud and his theories in response to the criticism.² Part of Jung's defense was based on the fact that none of the present attendees could prove Freud wrong.

One way of differentiating between these psychiatric perspectives is to examine the way each approaches the challenge of representing an illness with no manifestations on the outside of the body. How to comprehend a symptom? Where does it come from? How to image the unseen? How does the notion of an "interiority" manifest as evidence? Through dissection or analysis? Through narrative, behavior, or microscopic lesion? And given these questions, what is the role of the psychiatrist as observer? This battle in the history of psychiatry is well rehearsed from a range of disciplinary perspectives. Indeed, the very popularity of the history of the professional schism is revealing of some debates that continue to circulate around Alzheimer's disease today.

Certainly neither side won the debate on that auspicious day in 1906. Alzheimer would publish the results of his research soon after. A few years later, Alzheimer's supervisor, Emil Kraepelin, would include Alzheimer's findings in his highly influential textbook, dubbing it "Alzheimer's disease." From 1908 until a few years after his death in 1916, Alzheimer's research and imaging techniques were translated for an American audience as a small part of the active professionalization of medical sciences of mind and brain. His specific discovery, however, was dubiously received in both Germany and the United States.

The operative problem for these doctors was the relationship of the cerebral "plaques and tangles" and atrophy that Alzheimer ascribed to presenile dementia. To begin with, these plaques and tangles were material artifacts also found in the brains of people who displayed no symptoms of dementia. Did they actually cause Alzheimer's? Did they in fact constitute a unique disease entity? Also a problem was the younger age of the patient. Was there a difference between senile and presenile dementia? These issues were never fully sorted out, and scientists still ask these kinds of questions of the disease today.

Consequently, historians of psychiatry, aging, and dementia have spent a great deal of effort analyzing Alzheimer and his purported discovery, so much so that this historical narrative has acquired special validity as a way to organize knowledge about the disease. Contemporary rehearsals of the origin myth have generally followed two distinct paths, each of which, I argue, reinforces the very bioethical dilemmas it ostensibly seeks to disturb.

The first reason for this sustained interest in Alzheimer's discovery is the continued importance of plaques and tangles as a way to understand the disease and concordant disagreement about their etiological relevance.[3] More directly, Alzheimer's efforts to visualize or represent this pathology echo in contemporary battles to do the same thing.[4] The plaques and tangles that Alzheimer discovered with his microscope are still actively researched, analyzed, and described, albeit with much more sophisticated imaging technology and far greater knowledge and symptomatic context.[5]

The second reason for rehearsals of the origin myth can be attributed to that tradition in the history of science that focuses on great doctors, innovations, and discoveries.[6] Historians frequently debate who exactly is responsible for discovering Alzheimer's disease, often arguing for the recognition of Alzheimer's many contemporaries, students, and competitors, such as Oskar Fischer, Solomon Carter Fuller, Francesco Bonfiglio, Gaetano Perusini, Paul Blocq, and Georges Marinesco.[7] Beyond the name itself, Alois Alzheimer is a popular touchstone for the narration of the ongoing mystery of the disease, perhaps because his biography offers a kind of historical materiality that contributes to the disease's ontological potential. One could even argue that those invested in the material nature of the disease hold a similar investment in the narrative of the man and his work. For example, the American pharmaceutical company Eli Lilly recently purchased the house in Marktbreit, Germany, where Alzheimer was born so that it could be turned into a museum. Alzheimer's microscope and Auguste D.'s brain tissue were brought from Munich to the museum for display. It is now run as a tourist memorial and conference site.[8] In this way, the histories of both the man and his labor are synthesized in a kind of celebratory hagiography.[9]

These two historical traditions are important to understanding the disease's claims on representational culture, but they leave out or at the very least devalue another critical perspective, and that is the importance of the everyday technologies, labor, and techniques of representation— all of which are fundamental to understanding the story of Alzheimer's disease in the United States. In other words, to understand Alzheimer's origins, we must understand how it mattered to the people who were studying it.

Alzheimer was foremost a champion of the German microscope and histological technique. His American counterparts actively appropriated and learned those techniques via their own processes of medical professionalization in the United States. It was through these optical techniques and visually oriented practices of psychiatry that Alzheimer's was discovered, created, and charged in the first two decades of the twentieth century.

My hope with this early chapter is to underscore those two earlier historical positions as regards representation but also to stress the importance of cognition to these imaging practices. It offers a historical narrative that covers the first two decades of Alzheimer's research in the twentieth century in Germany and the United States. What this narrative draws out is the historical codependence of cognition and visual media and the ways that those relationships were ideologically maintained. In particular, this chapter offers a theory of the *histological gaze,* a set of historical viewing practices, techniques, and neuroscientific knowledge that asserted a highly particular mode of visuality as the foundational logic of Alzheimer's. It arises from those practices of histology used to discover the disease: fixing, staining, and imaging dead brain tissue. It is similar, perhaps, to Michel Foucault's well-known concept of the medical gaze, whereby practices of medical perception both penetrated and prefigured the body of the patient. But more clearly, it arises as a legacy of Foucault's more particular anatomo-clinical gaze, whereby the patient's death allowed for the visualization of the pathological fact through anatomical dissection; as Foucault provides, "the living night is dissipated in the brightness of death."[10]

The concept of the histological gaze draws on this historical tension between life and death in Alzheimer's research. This is because the neuropathological practices that defined and shaped Alzheimer's disease through the localization of biological plaques and tangles required the death of the patient. These researchers needed to cut, fix, stain, and microscopically analyze brain tissue to correlate symptom and disease. Indeed, this fact remained true for most of the twentieth-century research on Alzheimer's.

Given my focus on medical practice, readers may wonder where everyday patients fit into this narrative. Fully aware of the complicated status of representation within discourses of dementia, I am careful not to map these cognitive ethics onto a mythical community of patients in this early chapter. I avoid description of an imagined interiority or its concurrent lack on behalf of symptomatic individuals. This isn't to say I do not engage with the patient; rather, I do so, like these scientists, at the level of the brain tissue and the economy of knowledge making that revolved around it. The patient's living body acquired secondary status under the histological gaze. This is despite clear, methodological concern for clinical symptomatology. That secondary status was systematically maintained in three ways: institutionally, through the separation of pedagogically oriented laboratory research from asylum care; methodologically, through nosology or classification that privileged material disease description over etiology or cure; and epistemologically, through an optical objectivity distrustful of the isolated symptom and deeply invested in inclusive medical intellect and reproducible histological technique. The histological gaze, of which Alzheimer's disease was a part, thus helped shape professional, cognitive engagement with public health and an international optimism in sciences of mind.

Psychiatric Professionalization

Thus far, I have spoken about the history of Alzheimer's disease in a kind of universal sense, without any sustained recourse to race, class, gender, or other forms of difference.[11] I do this in part because the disease is consistently framed that way: as something either antagonistic toward or reflecting on what it means to be human. It unites the pathologies of aging to the freedoms of intellect and purported meritocracies of science. But it also stems from the way the early representations of

the disease shared in practices of transatlantic modernization and progressive health and social reform at the turn of the century.

Early neuroscience was engaged in practices of discovering and making the human: diagnosing its problems and mapping its powers. And
it did so in an optimistic tense. Michael Hagner and Cornelius Borck
clarify that "since linking the mind to the head, brain research has frequently operated in an outspokenly futuristic mode."[12] These authors
attribute this, in part, to the "proleptic" structure of the neurosciences,
whereby the objects of interest consistently exceed the inquiries of their
investigators. The brain, a century ago, as today, is understood as a generative mystery. As research accumulates, the scientist leaves definitive conclusions to the future because too much is still unanswered.
The brain is simply too complex. With regard to neuropathology, this
model can be associated with the uneasy relationship between mental
symptom and material pathology; this is the historically conditioned
paradox of psychiatry: the discipline claims organic, material causes of
mental illness, but generally speaking, those causes have not always
been distinctly articulated.[13] The brain's complexity encourages description and classification but prohibits etiological clarity.

A proleptic theory of neuroscientific practice has ramifications for
the visual study of Alzheimer's, particularly regarding the issues of
classification and representation. The ability to image the brain using
increasingly diversified techniques has often led to just that: diversified practices of imaging. These representations are then used either
to address a priori structures of difference or to offer new categories
of difference to be comprehended at a later date. Asserting the differences as rooted in biological proof does not necessarily mean anything
apart from that assertion. But it does say quite a lot about the scientist's orientation with truth *making*. As Lisa Cartwright has argued
about imaging practices of the early twentieth century, "distinguish-
ing between organic, psychogenic, and social causes of behavior has
been as much a matter of divvying up bodies among professional ter-
ritories as uncovering the 'true' source of pathological behavior."[14] Key
to recognize in this rhetoric is precisely how professionalizing this truth
making can be. The early study of Alzheimer's in the United States is

associated in particular with two brain-oriented disciplines still finding their footing at the end of the nineteenth century: neurology and
psychiatry. But those disciplinary arrangements were far from secure,
and territorial divides were shaped by a variety of practical and epistemological concerns like geography, technique, and the proper roles of
scientist and caregiver. But neurology and psychiatry would eventually
cohere in the Progressive Era in the United States through their shared
interest in the neuropathological origin of mental illnesses, the medicalization of psychiatry, and the desire to reform a corrupted asylum
system.[15]

Another uniting factor was these professions' shared interest in
European research on mental illness. Of course, Americans developed
some of their own technologies of care and diagnosis, but neuroscience was still dominated by increasingly partitioned European expertise. Indeed, it is important to understand how the technologization
of neuroscience at the end of the nineteenth century was necessarily
linked to the specialization of its focus.[16] The complexity of the brain
required that one develop specific research techniques that could answer
increasingly divergent research questions.

What some refer to as the imposition of science onto medicine in
the latter part of the nineteenth century was in fact a more complex
set of transformations in American and European medical practice
and education. As medicine became more specialized in research and
practice, new disciplinary engagements diversified the techniques and
technologies of medical professionals. This led to a new focus on medical education as a process of specialization. Additionally, the laboratory
and the lecture hall increasingly vied for validity as explicitly opposed
to bedside instruction. An array of technological developments in medicine required physicians to learn new techniques and reconsider traditional epistemological stances.

Beginning in the 1870s, neuroscientific research in Britain and
Germany began to dominate this new laboratory science while the
French clinical model, most famously represented by Jean-Martin
Charcot at the Salpêtrière Hospital in Paris, lost some of its rele-
vance. The French were committed to the model of the clinic and their

observations of lesions and pathology, but the Germans in particular increasingly developed more specialized and sophisticated laboratory research combined with large teaching lectures.[17] American physicians were by and large convinced by the technical expertise of German laboratories, despite some uneasiness with this gradual departure from the patient's bedside.[18]

The rise of histology is an excellent example of increased laboratory specialization and technological proficiency in the field of medical optics. Though histology had been around arguably since the seventeenth century, it truly flourished at the end of the nineteenth, largely because of new developments in cutting, fixing, staining, and microscopy, but also because of the shifting nature of medical research toward smaller scales.[19] These developments in histology paved the way for the identification of the plaques and tangles on Auguste D.'s brain. They arrived as a part of a wave of German experimental medicine intent on taxonomic clarity rooted in biologically oriented representation.

Practice and Pedagogy at the Munich Clinic

Alois Alzheimer's supervisor and mentor, Emil Kraepelin, was a German neurologist known as a champion of the classification movement and the father of modern psychiatry. His research methods are a good example of this German approach more popular with U.S. researchers at the end of the twentieth century. Kraepelin maintained a positivist stance toward diagnostics and eagerly pursued classification of mental illness. His classificatory system attributed mental illness to biological causes and also attempted to describe discrete categories of sickness and health. This taxonomy helped him achieve a primary goal: the medicalization of psychiatry and the elevation of the discipline's authority and recognizance.[20] Kraepelin utilized the two-stage approach of clinical observation and neuropathological analysis when possible. He was a progenitor of the contemporary science of neuropharmacology, experimenting with the effects of various drugs on patient behavior. Kraepelin was a positivist in that he distrusted descriptions of causality—insofar as they were speculative—but he did still address causality in his textbooks. He generally privileged empirical observation, but he did also still recognize the idea of a psyche, eventually pursuing theories of psychology, hypnotism, and genetics.

These epistemological tensions are indicative of broader professional battles in German neuroscience.[21] Diagnostic uncertainty was essentially built into structures of labor in the neurosciences.[22] The stakes for professional advancement were based on a nosological and classificatory primacy, and many of Kraepelin's efforts were targeted to that end. Regardless of professional intention, Kraepelin's taxonomy of mental disorders has remained influential throughout the twentieth and twenty-first centuries.[23]

Kraepelin's overwhelming emphasis on diagnostics and classification of disease may seem odd to contemporary readers, given that these were practices of medicine and therefore ostensibly driven toward therapy or cure. But this was germane to the practices of most European teaching hospitals at the turn of the century, where it was believed that letting diseases "run their course" enabled a better opportunity to illustrate the full scope of the medical condition.[24] Furthermore, given the radical emphasis placed on postmortem brain histology, it would be neither heartless nor Whiggish to assume these physicians treated their patients less as patients than as experiments or agents in the extension of medical knowledge. In other words, the greater cause here was not just public health but professional knowledge. Indeed, Kraepelin was a great teacher and disseminator of information. His scientific practice was not necessarily isolated from his teaching.[25] Kraepelin managed the clinic, performed research, and also remained involved in the publication and oversight of his and his colleagues' material.

In 1903 Kraepelin was offered the position of director of the Psychiatric Clinic at the University of Munich, Germany. He invited Alzheimer, who had recently begun to work with Kraepelin in Heidelburg, to join him and participate in the redevelopment and reconstruction of the clinic. Alzheimer was only six years younger than Kraepelin, but he was far junior in reputation, and this move was good for his career. Alzheimer was in charge of setting up the anatomic laboratories, and he helped Kraepelin with the procurement and arrangement of almost all of the research equipment and furnishings in the labs in the clinic. That equipment included a range of sophisticated technology, all arranged according to their direction.[26]

At the ceremonial opening of the clinic in 1904, the local newspaper made special note of the clinic's equipment. In particular, it commented on how well it was set up for observation, carefully noting advancements in microscopy, photomicrography, histology, and clinical analysis.[27] The celebration of the optical technology in the popular press is not incidental.[28] Although the lab's technology had already passed several hurdles of legitimation in European scientific networks by 1904, the public celebration of the laboratory via discourse of the prestigious "observer" enforces a social dimension to technologies of sight we might otherwise relegate simply to professional reception.

Indeed, this technology was part of a pattern of public and professional relations at the clinic that included publishing, textbooks, classes, and mentorships. The clinic not only included state-of-the-art technology and laboratories to this end but was also set up to accommodate professional collaboration and teaching for visiting scholars.[29] Aside from his lectures, Kraepelin also published textbooks. In fact, it was precisely because of his textbook publications that Kraepelin was so widely known in Europe and the United States, and scientists made a special point to come study with him to learn his techniques. Kraepelin and his colleagues even ran a special, intensive continuing education course covering recent research developments that was largely populated by international scholars.

This engagement was not specific to Kraepelin's lab; many European countries had begun to pool neuroscientific knowledge and histological resources as a process of new international cooperation in neuroscience. In 1903, some of the most dominant laboratories in Europe formed the International Brain Commission. These included brain research centers from, among other countries, Spain, England, Switzerland, and Germany. In 1906 the United States would join via the Neurological Department of Philadelphia's Wistar Institute. The Commission would be responsible for the standardization of publications, sharing of information, and general organization of neurological study according to common principles. Other important goals included the

creation of "brain banks" of cerebral tissue, the free exchange of techniques of staining and imaging, and other kinds of histological collaboration.[30] This cooperation would ostensibly save time and money in
the production of slides and neuroanatomical description.[31]

Kraepelin and Alzheimer both participated actively in this international cooperative spirit by virtue of their teaching and clinical collaboration. The international group of scholars who learned from
Alzheimer in particular at the Munich clinic include Ugo Cerletti,
Gaetano Perusini, Frederic Lewy, Nicolas Achucarro, Hans Gerhardt
Creutzfeldt, and Alfons Jakob, recognized scholars representing a diversity of European laboratory talent. U.S. psychiatrists and neurologists
also came to study with Kraepelin and Alzheimer, including Solomon
Carter Fuller (Figure 1), who would go on to translate Alzheimer's
research and techniques in the United States; Louis Casamajor, the

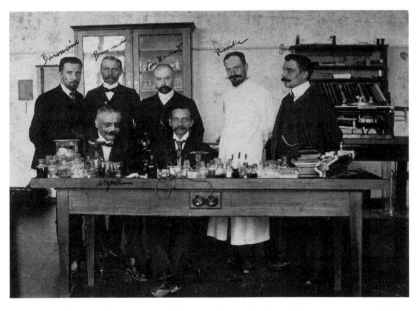

FIGURE 1. Alois Alzheimer and Solomon Carter Fuller sitting at the lower left
on either side of the microscope, 1905. Courtesy of the Boston University
Alumni Medical Library Archives.

first director of the American Board of Psychiatry and Neurology; and Smith Ely Jelliffe, an early American proponent of psychoanalysis and one of the more dominant figures in psychiatric publishing in the first half of the twentieth century. Each of these scholars studied at the Munich clinic as a part of his formal training in German histology, anatomy, and laboratory optics.

It could be argued that teaching histology was Alzheimer's primary labor. Despite his relatively young age, he was invited on numerous speaking engagements around Germany to demonstrate his techniques and research. He even developed his own special projection system to show his slides. According to Kraepelin and his colleagues, Alzheimer took great pride in his scientific communication.[32] His instruction in the classes at the clinic was filled with visual demonstrations, and he generally handled the slide presentations himself. When not giving a presentation, he could be found with his students at the microscope table, carefully teaching them how to read the details of the microscopic image.[33] Solomon Carter Fuller remarked in his memoirs that individualized instruction with the microscope was Alzheimer's true forte.[34]

By 1906 Alzheimer had achieved the position of chief physician of the clinic, and his exacting standards and hard labor were widely recognized and appreciated in the laboratories. Like Kraepelin, Alzheimer believed in the importance of making connections between anatomical, histological analysis and clinical, behavioral evidence. Despite criticisms, Alzheimer and his colleagues at the Munich lab defended the organic thesis as a way of approaching a set of ideal or universal disease categories.

The actual practice of clinical analysis, to which Alzheimer was also dedicated, was a complicated component of the histological gaze. For Alzheimer to gain access to a patient, she had to be diagnosed—at least informally—by someone else as a condition to her admittance. This socially oriented diagnosis is an important pre-empirical step to the organization of mental illness. Furthermore, Alzheimer did not have free access to whichever patients or illnesses he wanted to analyze because of the bureaucratic division in the kinds of patients treated in German university clinics versus those in asylums.[35] The urban clinics generally housed short-term, acute illnesses, and they were overseen by a psychiatrist in the general pursuit of education, teaching, and greater knowledge. They were designed to help alleviate the overcrowding that plagued the much larger asylums, which were generally responsible for longer-term care.

Alzheimer worked at both kinds of institutes, and his original interviews of Auguste D. occurred when he worked at an asylum before his move to the Munich clinic. He was arguably dedicated to clinical observations, if not to the patients themselves, and his attention to Auguste D.'s behavior can be seen in his careful, handwritten notes, many of which still survive.[36] After Auguste D.'s death, her brain was shipped to Alzheimer at the Munich clinic for his examination. It was only because of a contractual relationship with the asylum that he had access to that brain, and it was only because he had previously worked at the asylum that he could have performed his original interviews with the patient. Thus it was somewhat fortuitous that Alzheimer was able to view Auguste D.'s brain and make the necessary correlative conclusions about a "peculiar disease process."

For clinical neuropathologists, brains were very useful.[37] The economy of their use, their circulation, and their contractual exchange impacted both the research questions and techniques of neuroscience. But the lack of ongoing, sustained contact with patients also contributed toward a paucity of clinical data when it came to senile dementia, something often noted in contemporary histories of the nosological genesis of Alzheimer's. So although the clinical interviews and observations were important to Alzheimer, those patients were more important to him, because, as Kraepelin offered in his obituary of Alzheimer, of the "rich collection of brains" they afforded.[38]

The Histological Gaze

In addition to pedagogy, Alzheimer was deeply invested in the advancement of histological technology and technique. He obtained his doctorate from the microscopy department at the Wurzburg Anatomical Institute, learning his practice from two of the most acclaimed histologists of the time, Carl Weigert and Ludwig Edinger.[39] He completed his

early postdoctoral research in an environment of intense histological experimentation around staining, microscopy, and camera lucida.
It was there that Alzheimer met the man who would become his best
friend, mentor, and collaborator, Franz Nissl. Nissl would later become famous for his staining techniques, but he developed them with
Alzheimer's help. Nissl and Alzheimer would go on together, under
Kraepelin's advisement, to add photomicrography to their arsenal of
optical techniques. Photomicrography is the practice of taking photographs through a microscope, and it required careful coordination of
the variables of camera, light, stain, microscope, and magnification.

However, Alzheimer possessed widely admired skills in draftsman-
ship with the aid of camera lucida and microscope, and he clearly favored
that technique over the photomicrograph. Not to be confused with the
more well-known camera obscura, the camera lucida is a tool for drawing images. It allowed Alzheimer to look through the lens of his microscope and draw onto a surface at the same time, seeing the microscopic
image and his own marks together. His ability to articulate clearly that
which he saw through the lens was a significant component of his professional reputation and arguably a reason he was brought to the Munich
clinic.[40] John Hammond, a historian of the camera lucida, argues that
the drawing aid was in fact very difficult to master; it required a "knack"
only achieved through special training.[41] It is important to understand
that the camera lucida does not strictly conform to mimetic principles;
the camera lucida assists an observer. One can make points of emphasis, articulate evidence practically, and render clear what is murky. It
required not only careful training but also good judgment within the
context of specific research design.

Because of these subjective relationships, the camera lucida technique caused consternation among some of Alzheimer's colleagues.
A true positivist, Nissl preferred using photomicrography over camera
lucida drawings because he believed photomicrography removed the
subjective element from his analysis. He distrusted the camera lucida
because, as he said, "one sees in a rather unpleasant and persistent
way that which one believes oneself to have understood intellectually."[42]
Of course, their use was not mutually exclusive. It was not uncommon

for biological scientists to provide photomicrographs alongside camera lucida drawings to demonstrate some key features in the image.[43]

The choice in imaging technology was not made simply because of the danger of subjective infringement; there were other considerations as well, such as cost, ease of use, speed of production, and ease of translation. Indeed, the personal relationships these scientists fostered with their technologies are also important: Alzheimer was described by his colleagues as appearing "happiest when he was looking into his microscope."[44] Rather than dismiss that relationship as idiosyncratic, it is perhaps more productive to foreground the ways in which that excitement might be contagious or shared with his colleagues.

Indeed, that affective relationship was buoyed by broad public and professional excitement about visual technologies in Germany. The two decades between 1890 and 1910 saw the fruition of the collaborative efforts of two Germans in particular, the physicist Ernst Abbe and the optical manufacturer Carl Zeiss.[45] Abbe camera lucidas and Zeiss microscopes were some of the most popular and reputable optical technologies available to these histologists, and their development coincided with Germany's domination of laboratory optics at the turn of the century.

Alzheimer's histological technique, however, was not practiced simply by looking through a microscope and camera lucida; there are many other important histological techniques. Once the brain arrived at the lab, the brain tissue of interest needed to be grossed, or cut out.[46] It was then fixed and preserved in some sort of stabilizing treatment. Formaldehyde dominated this practice for a long time, but multiple techniques were available to histologists. The fixed sections could then be frozen or stabilized in paraffin. Then the tissue was thinly sliced for application to a slide.

Perhaps the most important optical technology was neuronal staining. In this stage, chemical dyes were applied to the fixed brain tissue. Certain dyes demonstrated an affinity for the chemical makeup of certain parts of the neuron. The idea was to use the stain to provide a contrast that could be recognized under the microscope in a differential manner. Different dyes revealed different neuronal structures and

changes to those structures. However, they also naturalized pathological or morphological difference precisely because that color contrast
appeared natural. Staining thus naturalized difference in morphology
that reverberated into nosology.

Over the last decades of the nineteenth century, staining experimentation was rampant in German labs. The rush to find the best
stains led scientists to experiment with just about every colored substance available.[47] Much of this experimentation led to advances in
neuroanatomy. This is, in part, how Santiago Ramón y Cajal won the
Nobel Prize in 1906 with Camillo Golgi: for his research in histology
and his descriptions of the neuronal structure.

The stain that Alzheimer used to identify the plaques and tangles
on Auguste D.'s brain tissue is called Bielschowsky silver stain, and it
is still in use in dementia research today. It was invented just a few
years before Alzheimer's discovery, and researchers were still figuring
it out. Crucially, the Bielschowsky method is different from a traditional
dye stain in that it requires a secondary step of chemical transformation
to work. While the traditional histological staining process is relatively
stable, silver staining as a chemical transformation is highly amenable
to the working conditions and techniques of the histologist, and it can
be difficult to replicate the results of other histologists.[48]

The techniques of silver staining, called "impregnation," are even
described with the vocabulary of photographic development: the use
of "physical developers," for example. In fact, many of the obstacles in
photographic development at that time were related to those in silver
staining for histology. Not by accident, many of the people experimenting with histology were also amateur photographers. Santiago Ramón
y Cajal, for example, was an avid photographer. So was Solomon Carter
Fuller. It is safe to say that the histological technique that described
Alzheimer's plaques and tangles is deeply indebted to experiments in
photography, except in this kind of histological practice, scientists did
not develop chemicals on paper or a plate; they were developing brain
tissue.

Once the silver stain has bound to the proteins in the neuron that
the scientist wishes to detect, the neuron can then be imaged, and it is

here that the histologist uses the camera lucida or photomicrograph. The variability of the staining technique, however, impinges on the empirical status of the image before that step, so it is no surprise that Alzheimer preferred to use the camera lucida over the photomicrograph. His techniques could help correct the image relationship, to develop it further. He was fully aware of the subjective nature of the techniques and the capriciousness of their material production. This is arguably why he put such emphasis on technique and pedagogy, and it is a key component of the histological gaze.

The relationship these neuropathologists maintained with their professional practices employed modes of objective visualization that Lorraine Daston and Peter Galison call "mechanical objectivity" and "trained judgment." An older mode of scientific visualization, mechanical objectivity was "the insistent drive to repress the willful intervention of the artist-author, and to put in its stead a set of procedures that would, as it were, move nature to the page through a strict protocol, if not automatically."[49] Key to understand here is the faith these scientists had in their imaging technologies and their simultaneous awareness of the need for a protocol of imaging technique.

Daston and Galison, however, point out a historically oriented epistemological shift at the turn of the century, whereby scientists increasingly began to realize the problems of mechanical objectivity under increased proficiency. The images produced under its regime were simply prone to too much variability in their creation, and no amount of professional protocol could alleviate that variability. Given that problem, at the beginning of the twentieth century, scientists increasingly chose to embrace a mode of trained judgment, which required training and intellectual prowess with the mechanically produced image. So trained judgment in this model does not sacrifice truth, but it deals with the threat of subjective influence in a different manner because of the givenness of fallibility.[50]

To understand how trained judgment fits into the histological gaze, one must understand exactly how these visual techniques were being used. Psychiatrists like Alzheimer did not simply describe the neural architecture as a neuroanatomist might. They recognized, identified, and then incorporated the object of inquiry into a broader symptomatic pattern. The silver stain is therefore an exercise in inclusion, and identification is often a means of building quantitative data.[51] From the perspective of pedagogy, this means the scientist is teaching techniques of recognition; it should be no surprise that histological pedagogy is historically framed through recourse to repetition, memorization, and a library of slides for the aid of the histologist.[52]

The techniques of histology, then, weigh heavily on the status of the clinical symptom and the professionalization of psychiatry. Because of Alzheimer's insistence on material, biological description, a clinical symptom was not useful without brain tissue to provide empirical evidence. For scientists in the neurobiological camp, the clinical symptom is only legitimated by the histological practice. The brain tissue existed to be seen, examined, and compared to other tissue. And that brain tissue could only be harvested after a patient's death. This is a clinical abstraction perhaps not possible in an asylum setting where patients became individuals in the eyes of their caretakers, individuals with long-standing personalities and relationships.[53]

This is the quandary of the case study style of evidence that Alzheimer privileged. The presumed anonymity of the patient Auguste D. made her part of a nosological system, rendering her "individuality" systemic. A good example of this process is the photographic portrait of Auguste D. The photograph was taken of the patient sitting, staring down off camera. This is one of four photographs of the patient that were found in Alzheimer's files, and the discovery raised some excitement among Alzheimer's historians.[54] Her photo, however, maintained dubious utility for Alzheimer because of the way in which it betrays her privacy and indexically marks her as an individual. Her photograph often accompanies biographies of Alzheimer and histories of the disease, but that deployment testifies more to a biographical impulse than psychiatric relevance.[55] Individual bodies (or asylum bodies) get in the way of the reproducibility of science and hence its authority. The reproducibility of objective observation is what ostensibly legitimates medicine and what brings it into the realm of science. Of course, curing or fixing bodies might help establish medical authority as well, but only if the saving or curing can be done at a reproducible level.[56] In this case, reproducibility only arrives in the professional, histological labor (whatever you practice you get good at), not in the case studies of senile dementia.

Look at how Alzheimer describes the symptoms of Auguste D.: "clinically, this case presented an unusual picture that did not fit any known disease."[57] Those symptoms were understood to be associated somehow with senile dementia—the symptoms were similar but the age was wrong: Auguste D. was younger than she should have been if she had had that illness. That is why it is distinct. It is important to remember that the categories of senile and presenile dementia *prefigure* their empirical, neuropathological display in these studies. Both categories of dementia were associated with the images of plaques and tangles, even if the association was vague. Was there a difference between senile and presenile dementia? Was this symptom pattern distinct? For Kraepelin and Alzheimer, the answer was a resounding "unsure," but pressures toward an ideal that had yet to be invented demanded the ideation of an ontological possibility, a possibility that irrevocably entered into a complex economy of psychiatric discourse.

The goal with Alzheimer's disease, as with all of this psychiatric research, was diagnostic and classificatory representation, not etiology or cure. Auguste D. became valuable at the moment of death and at the moment of inscription into psychiatric classification. The live body of the patient and the performance of recognizable symptoms entered her into a nosological possibility, but the dead brain tissue was required for any useful analysis. So despite Alzheimer's stated interest in clinical behavior in his method, and despite his careful notations of Auguste D.'s individual symptoms, the live symptom was only made legible and useful through death. Institutionally, methodologically, and epistemologically, the experience of the patient was defined and overdetermined by the techniques of the image and the histological gaze.

The image of the plaques and tangles has since been deeply legitimated as a site of inquiry. And it is an inclusive image that still contributes to the confusion over the relationship between senile and non-senile dementia. Then, as now, Kraepelinian diagnostics are attacked as fundamentally error-prone, a methodological equivalent to what one of Kraepelin's critics called hunting "phantoms."[58] The image stands in for the symptom in terms of its circulation, in that it references both the possibility of senile dementia and presenile dementia. What it indexes is not simply a biological state or disease pathology, but also the labor of its scientific creation. This is what Foucault refers to as the "whole hermeneutics of the pathological fact."[59] And with regard to the history of the Kraepelinian teaching clinic, the labor of the image is the dominant practice that is taught, practiced, and valued. As Jelliffe wrote in Alzheimer's obituary, "his microscope, as he stated it, stood at the service of psychiatric advance."[60] The techniques of image making are validated precisely by the clinically observed symptom, but no necessary causal relationship is claimed. The image is enough.

One of the standard questions for historians of Alzheimer's disease is who exactly is responsible for the discovery of the disease. Rather than establishing a decisive founder, this book takes the position that the commingling labor of these histologists is the defining condition of the genesis of the disease category rather than results of one man's study. The profound overlap of Kraepelinian nosology with Alzheimer's images abstracts the symptom within descriptive, inclusive histological technique. It is at that level that the disease category is learned, translated, and incorporated into the practices of U.S. psychiatry in the early twentieth century.

American Image Makers

The man largely cited as responsible for importing Alzheimer's discoveries and histological techniques for an American practice is Solomon Carter Fuller, the country's first Black psychiatrist and an early student of Alzheimer's at the Munich clinic in 1904. Also a neuropathologist, Fuller was part of a larger group of American physicians trying to corroborate the somatic or material model of mental illness. Just as Kraepelin faced challenges securing the professional reputation of German psychiatry, American psychiatrists like Fuller were attempting to bolster their profession via recourse to laboratory research and disease pathology.

Fuller was born in Liberia, the son of Black missionary immigrants from New York, but he moved to the United States to pursue his education at Livingston College and then medical school at Boston University. He took his first job as the pathologist at the Westborough State Hospital for the Insane in Massachusetts in 1897 and then also as an instructor of pathology at Boston University Medical School in 1899. At the time, the prospect of working with dead bodies made pathology somewhat undesirable as a career, but it was a job that a young Black man could pursue even while institutionally disenfranchised in other ways. Searching out better laboratory training, Fuller spent a year abroad in Munich at Kraepelin's clinic. Under Alzheimer's direction, Fuller studied neurofibrillary degeneration, leading him to publish on that research in 1907.

After his year in Munich, Fuller returned to Westborough, where he redoubled his efforts in the neuropathology lab. His international training, knowledge of the German language, and total devotion to technique made him an important figure in the development of American psychiatry. In many ways, Fuller's approach to his subject was similar to Alzheimer's. He was devoted to innovative histological practice, and his laboratory would become a destination for young medical students.[61] Just like his colleague in Munich, his professional relationships with both Westborough and Boston Medical School allowed him to split his time between laboratory research and pedagogy. And like Alzheimer, he believed clinical symptoms ultimately found value in neuropathological correlation. His official pathologist records betray the clear value of cadavers to his research; in them, he would list the number of brains the hospital had obtained based on diagnosis. Each of those brains would be cut out, fixed, imaged, and then stored for future research. His 1911 report to the hospital's trustees even details the sectioning of the brain of a person with Alzheimer's, what he described as only the eighth recorded case of the disease.[62]

Fuller clearly recognized the limitations of contemporary medical knowledge and image technology. He frequently experimented with both the camera lucida and the photomicrograph, even going so far as to publish recommendations for technological design and practice. In 1901, shortly out of medical school, he wrote an article designed for medical students instructing them how to build their own photomicrograph apparatus.[63] For Fuller, histology was often a collaborative affair. For example, he sometimes relied on others to create camera lucida drawings for him. But he also helped his colleagues with their photomicrographs, sometimes authoring images in support of their clinical research (Figure 2). This kind of collaborative experimentation may be one reason why Fuller is sometimes credited for inventing the photomicrograph. In truth, William Henry Fox Talbot, an early inventor of photographic technology, was probably the first person to take photomicrographs successfully, as early as the 1830s.[64]

Fuller's interest in imaging technologies was not limited to histology. He was also an avid amateur photographer. Inspired by his wife, the well-known sculptor Meta Vaux Warrick, Fuller specialized in photographic portraits. He saw no concrete separation between the imaging practices, suggesting that knowledge of the limitations and strengths of photographic technology could only aid in understanding its implications for medical research.[65] Unfortunately, his interest in visual technology and aesthetics would be compromised by blindness later in life.

In 1911 Fuller seemed to validate Alzheimer's disease as a nosological category, pointing out the "convincing illustrations . . . of the histological composition of the plaques which relieve these structures of their former mystery."[66] The next year, he would further validate the research by translating Alzheimer's first case study of Auguste D. (which Alzheimer had published in German himself in 1907). In 1912 he published a case study of a person with Alzheimer's at Westborough alongside a comparative review of other published cases related to Alzheimer's. But in another study published that same year with Henry Klopp, he cast doubt on the value of the disease category, citing inconsistencies and lack of proper evidence.[67]

Indeed, Alzheimer's disease never really caught on as a widely useful diagnostic category in the United States until much later in the

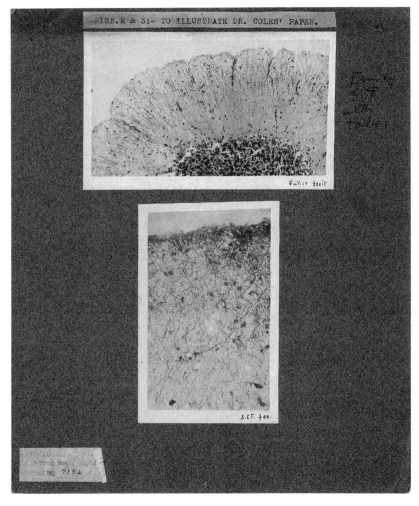

FIGURE 2. Photomicrographs created, mounted, and displayed by Solomon Carter Fuller for a colleague at Westborough (date unknown). Courtesy of the Francis A. Countway Center for the History of Medicine.

century, in part because the plaques and tangles could be imaged in both presenile and senile cases. And while that problem was never ultimately solved, it was certainly argued upon at length as a part of psychiatric professionalization. In the first two decades of the twentieth century, a great deal of journal space was taken up with the subject of senile dementia's difference from presenile dementia and that difference's relationship to the plaques and tangles.[68] Even Alzheimer and his colleagues in Munich went on to publish further research on the subject.[69] This research never fully confirmed the validity of the category, despite Kraepelin's inclusion of the disease in his textbook. Theories of arteriosclerosis continued to confuse the situation.[70] As one American researcher lamented in 1910, the category of senile dementia was often used as a "dumping ground" for all things misunderstood in aging, a situation from which psychiatrists found it difficult to extricate themselves.[71] So while Alzheimer's discoveries did not necessarily convince an American audience of the legitimacy of the diagnostic category, and Kraepelin's diagnostic schemas were not entirely appropriated, the research certainly informed professional debate.

American psychiatrists were probably more interested in learning Alzheimer's techniques for other kinds of neurological research. The paucity of adequate local histological resources was limiting, and American neuropathologists faced an uphill battle acquiring the highly variable techniques of fixing, staining, and microscopy. If a researcher could not travel abroad, he had to rely on often poorly translated textbooks to learn his trade.[72] But this also led to collective advancement of the discipline in the form of collaborative learning. For example, at a meeting of the New England Society of Psychiatry in 1908, which Fuller attended, the group attempted to teach each other Alzheimer's staining techniques for cerebrospinal fluid, which they claimed were better than other techniques.[73] Another attendee of that meeting, the head of the Trenton State Hospital, Henry Cotton, had also spent time studying in Alzheimer's Munich laboratory from 1905 to 1907.[74] Cotton appreciated Alzheimer's work enough that he also translated Alzheimer's research, an important consideration in the spread of both doctrine and technique.[75]

In addition to the kinds of educational values these physicians fostered, they helped to condition a broader set of epistemological assumptions about their trade. As histologists, they demonstrated a keen awareness of the subjective nature of the image, but they also understood the importance of good training to deliver better scientific medicine.[76] The future of the American neurosciences was based on the very separation of technology and technique and at the variability of the histological interpretation. Of course, recognition of the inadequacies of imaging technologies and the skills at hand does not necessarily translate into a diminished epistemological value for those technologies. As Jutta Schickore has argued with regard to nineteenth-century microscopy, recognition of an instrument's limitations can have powerful positive results for future research.[77] Interest in better future skills and techniques was in fact a fundamental part of these doctors' approach to truth.

Look, for example, at the way Fuller described his mode of objectivity in his 1907 paper on neurofibrillary degeneration. He chose to use only the Bielschowsky stains on neurofibrils because, as he wrote, "in our hands this method provides the most uniform results."[78] He is careful to cite the authors of his images as well as mechanical technique. One image in his study was made by E. B. Smith and M. E. Dickinson, "drawn with the aid of an Abbe camera lucida. Zeiss 2 mm. apochromatic obj., No. 8 comp. oc."[79] Central to these descriptions is Fuller's awareness of the difficulty in repeating this work and his wariness about drawing any final conclusions from his images. This does not prevent him from making conclusions; rather, he does so increasingly as a part of collective professionalization and with full awareness and reflection on his training and resources.

It is important to see the kind of self-awareness these physicians had of their own labor as a part of that mode of objectivity. This manifests in the respect for colleagues' labors and insecurity about the validity of their own contributions. Some of these papers are notable for their treatment of fellow colleagues as "workers," whose "work" and intellect are definable by virtue of the labor of production, research, and laboratory technique. There is great optimism and respect for the industry in Fuller's work, for example, or for the leaders of psychiatry: Kraepelin's "masterful" diagnostic skills are called "genius" by a Cincinnati psychiatrist, but he adds, "genius being here, as usual, simply a synonym for a high order of painstaking work."[80]

Another way of understanding the self-awareness these scientists shared is through their own forms of collective, professional representation. For example, medical history at the turn of the century was still a nascent profession. In the United States especially, writing medical history had generally been an amateur activity, despite the inclusion of the subject in some medical training. But this changed, as self-awareness gradually became important to the processes of professionalization. This model of medical history mostly cited the cutting-edge discoveries of well-known doctors.[81] The narratives of Kraepelin, Alzheimer, and Fuller echo in these new traditions of historical awareness, as do the debates over their labor.[82]

An Audience to Intellect

The introduction of Alzheimer's disease into the United States thus occurred as a part of a significant transformation of American medicine and its relationship to truth, intellect, and visual technology. This transformation depended on the optimism of an American public regarding the role and education of the medical scientist. This was part of what is often called the Flexnerian revolution in American medicine, marked by an extensive report published in 1910 by Abraham Flexner that called for stricter scientific regulation and oversight of both medical practice and education.[83] The Flexner report marked a major turning point in American medical training, as the American research institution began to develop more prominence and credibility. Critically, however, developments in research and education did not necessarily translate into public health practice. Health care itself took longer to develop in the United States, and what was being sold did not instantaneously transform the American experience of medicine.

By the first decades of the twentieth century, U.S. physicians were beginning to incorporate a more German style of laboratory science as a means to add authority to their American enterprise. But that mode of inquiry still required better training because of its specialization. When Flexner argued in his influential report that "scientific medicine has its eyes open," he was in fact working against empiricist traditions in medicine and arguing for a more honest appraisal of the intellectual requirements of laboratory medicine.[84] American physicians realized that laboratory science could help explain disease pathology, but it required better technique. This was an intellectually oriented scientific medicine of which the intricacies of histopathology were a part.[85]

In sum, science would do for American medicine what the lay observer could not understand, so the public had to trust those medical specialists with the best knowledge. American optimism with regard to the new laboratory science was in part guided by the cultural authority and status that science provided. During the Progressive Era, Americans increasingly placed their trust in intellectual enterprise and in specialized knowledge and learning. Laboratory medicine and its special techniques benefited from this model of trust. As John Harley Warner argues, "the laboratory provided the material and cognitive basis for an elitist epistemology and a regrounding of medicine on a decidedly privileged body of knowledge accessible only to a small proportion of Americans."[86] The transformation, then, of neuroscientific research practice cannot be separated from the public enthusiasm for those practices.

This celebration of medical research was also reliant on public fascination with the visual technologies that formed its practices and missionary armature. The turn of the century was an era of massive transformation of visual technology in the service of public health and medicine, and it is easy to understand popular and medical interests as overlapping. For example, Wilhelm Konrad Roentgen discovered x-rays in 1895, and his new techniques for imaging the insides of living bodies catapulted him into public stardom and earned him the Nobel Prize. Soon the x-ray was a popular public technology for spectacle and social subversion, perceived as illustrative of a deep individual and social interiority.[87] The magic lantern was also wildly popular at this time, used in households and traveling shows for a range of purposes, from education to spectacle. The cinema played a key role in the development of sciences of physiology, physics, and eugenics even as it delighted and shocked audiences with the spectacle of a kiss, the electrocution of an elephant, or a trip to the moon. Lisa Cartwright has argued that the rise of cinema as a popular medium needs to be understood not as distinct from the development of imaging technologies generally accorded as "scientific" but instead as part of broader interest in visual cultures of health, the body, science, and nature on the one hand, and notions of interiority and the mind on the other.[88] The paradox of this overlap in scientific and popular visual technologies, however, is that the elevation of the public audience for medicine had the reverse effect of giving authority to the elite idiosyncrasies and potential of Science.

That visual technology played an important role in the development of ideologies of public health at the beginning of the twentieth century. In the decades leading up to 1900, public health outreach was more limited to educating the public about the importance of good hygiene and sanitary living in increasingly crowded urban situations. But this representation became more complex in the Progressive Era, leading to the celebration of medical technologies and educated practitioners as the future of public well-being. For example, photographers were actively invited into hospitals to document the patients' experiences, sanitary conditions, hospital training, wondrous new machines, efficient and impressive surgeries, and overall medical progress.[89] Americans were thus asked to take an active role in developing their own health as both audiences to and consumers of engaging spectacles of modern health and medicine.[90]

Public health was also articulated visually by way of major international exhibitions held in the United States. The 1904 Louisiana Purchase Exhibition in St. Louis, for example, was almost a city unto itself, offering seventy thousand distinct exhibits to an estimated 19.5 million attendees.[91] Exhibitors had to learn how to develop specific styles of display and modes of information visualization to help communicate complex medical topics and data to an interested public. Medical professionals spread awareness of new developments in bacteriology and sanitary science, helping visitors understand the dangers of tuberculosis and other diseases. Anatomical model manufacturers demonstrated the inner workings of the human body. Pathology exhibits displayed not only an array of specimens, slides, and samples but also full-blown replicas of pathology laboratories. Military medical practitioners took on the role of public educators with demonstrations of military field hospitals. New York State even sponsored a full-size diorama of an asylum room of the Utica State Asylum, showing the past, antiquated technologies of mental health on one side and the newer, more current facilities with modern and comfortable care on the other.[92]

This time period also marked a significant transformation in the appeals of health-oriented advertising, and Americans increasingly became the arbiters of their own health through direct appeals to their wallets. While medical advertising had in fact been a cornerstone of the early U.S. advertising industry (most notably through the marketing of patent medicines), ads increasingly advocated for consumer responsibility by building anxiety around mysterious new ailments, on one hand, and more general ideologies of self-improvement, on the other.[93] This tension represents a novel model of individual responsibility toward one's health. Increasingly, the patient was asked to buy in to the authority of the medical professional while also understanding health as something to be consumed in a responsible, active manner.[94] Advertising and other forms of consumerist visual culture, while still underregulated at this point, helped popularize health care's technological and institutional developments while orienting its practice within the realm of everyday consumption. The transformation of the patient into a consumer not only restructured health care as a commodity in the United States but fundamentally reoriented the debate over public health into haves and have-nots as a part of the progressive dialogue over population management.

It may seem as if this book makes a sizable leap between Alzheimer's laboratory and Progressive Era public health in America, but the professional visual labor of that lab directly and indirectly informed medical practice. Progressive Era medical visualization, taken as a part of a broader conjunctural shift, helped articulate the public within a consumerist promise of medical practice as intellectual, moral, and ideal.

It is in this sense that the histological gaze also directly contributed to the professionalization of American medicine at the turn of the century, as it helped organize knowledge of health and mind.[95] It should be noted that other practices inform the early visuality of Alzheimer's in the United States—surveillance as a way to manage aging bodies in a vastly overcrowded asylum system, for example—and those practices could certainly inform my theory of the histological gaze. A comprehensive genealogy of that visuality is perhaps beyond the purview of this book.

This chapter has aimed to shift representational critique from questions of medical othering and instead introduce critical representational paradigms based on ability, access, productivity, and value. This, of course, is not new; it contributes to an active body of literature that investigates the legibility of the medical image as a practice of making the self, a deeply Foucaultian consideration that could be written with his vocabulary of paradigmatic medical optics in mind.[96]

The historical social construction of Alzheimer's is already well tended in other, more dedicated works, and arguably by gerontology as a discipline.[97] It is no accident that geriatrics and gerontology have their own origins in the turn-of-the-century management of populations, but an assertion of the primacy of the intellect as a mode of civic participation in that discourse is perhaps underemphasized.

A good example of this is doctor and legal philosopher George M. Beard's theories of aging and the law. His philosophies are often cited as indicative of a social stigma that sutures symptoms of dementia to civic exclusion. As the historian Thomas Cole argues, "Beard deserves the dubious distinction of being the first to scientifically legitimate the reduction of human beings to their productive capacities."[98] Indeed, many gerontologists attribute Beard's rhetoric as a foundation of ageism in this country. It also provides a hegemonic buttress that supports the reorganization of senility—previously understood as a simple definition of the elderly—into operable categories of normal and abnormal aging. And, crucially, it does so under the model of an optimistic science of mind.

What makes Beard even more important to this account, however, is the way in which he attaches morality to questions of cognitive ability.

Conversant with popular eugenic philosophies of the time, Beard's highly influential vocabulary of age-oriented productivity and value help to construct dementia as a symptomatology obstructive to functional personhood. In one of his more well-known lectures, Beard detailed the moral decline that accompanies aging; this moral decline directly relates to an individual's status as a legitimate member of society.[99] In another lecture, "Legal Responsibility in Old Age," he advocates for the elevation and social advancement of what he calls "brain workers."[100] In this talk, he maps the young ages at which "great men" in history achieved various intellectual milestones. Understanding Beard as someone who contributed to dementia-oriented stigma is certainly a common and valid interpretation of his work.[101] Limiting scholarship to that interpretation, however, would also exclude a key ethic for which this work found an eager audience. "Legal Responsibility" is every bit an optimistic piece, a public, loud, scientific celebration of intellectual labor. While his work predates the Flexnerian revolution by at least thirty years, scientific intelligence, loosely defined, is here already a medicalized marker of social potential and the mirror of a stigmatized personhood. And it promised to serve as a cornerstone of modern social advance. As Beard argued, "the intellect is the eye of conscience."[102]

The desire to image and understand the plaques and tangles continues to organize much of the research on Alzheimer's across cause, cure, and diagnosis.[103] Whether plaques and tangles are considered anomalous or normal, biologically central or inconsequential, their representational presence is heavily operative.[104] And this dilemma over the status of the plaques and tangles underwrites the history of the disease, despite efforts to get beyond it.[105] Scientists cannot escape the plaques and tangles inasmuch as they cannot entirely dismiss their own history; it is thus more helpful to think of the plaques and tangles less as an ontological problem to be solved and more as a plurality of articulations of scientific practice, mind, and brain.[106]

In other words, if there is an ontological eureka in the origin myth, it is to be found in a particular mode of visuality based on histological insight, international education, and cognitive productivity. The viability of selfhood—both scientific and symptomatic—was increasingly located in the biological primacy of brain and mind, but visual techniques and media technologies made it so. That blend of contradictory, desirous visuality is precisely what was imported to the United States as part of the processes of professionalization, social transformation, and progressive medical reform.

2

New Media Pioneers

Neuroimaging a National Crisis

An ongoing dilemma for historians of Alzheimer's regards the perceived absence in scientific research on the disease after it was named and recognized as a disease entity. Popular accounts of the disease's history often acknowledge Alzheimer's work with Kraepelin as a kind of touchstone for the research and descriptive paradigms that would sediment much later in the century, but they leave out the important research done in the early to midcentury. Jesse Ballenger, for example, argues that the decades following Alzheimer's discovery were in fact a productive time period in dementia research; after the discovery, however, he says that many historians "jump to the research of the 1970s—implying that most of the twentieth century was essentially a dark age."[1] What explains the gap, this "dark age" in the research, or was there one? Clearly scientists in the first half of the century were frustrated by the lack of a good etiological explanation and the paucity of dependable data, and that led many to seek alternate explanations for clinical behavior.

Solomon Carter Fuller, for example, quit his position as pathologist at Westborough State Hospital in 1919. While he continued to teach psychiatry at Boston University School of Medicine, he also took on private psychoanalytic practice. Probably because he was Black, Fuller was never paid an adequate salary at Westborough, and he could make more money in private practice and teaching.[2] Perhaps as important to Fuller, however, was the fact that even though his research was widely admired by other psychiatrists, and even though he worked at Westborough for more than two decades, he was never offered the chance at promotion within the hospital administration.[3]

This issue of Fuller's race was not incidental to his labor; rather, it was integral to debates in psychiatry at the time. More directly, many of Fuller's contemporaries actively promoted eugenics, a science that promoted racist beliefs and practices. After he quit Westborough, one of the people who took over his pathologist duties at the hospital was Myrtelle Canavan. Canavan was also a proficient image maker, but in addition to microscopic images, she created hundreds of large-scale postmortem photographs of brains.[4] Like Fuller, she published neuropathological research, but she was more interested in promoting eugenic science. Her mentor (whose brain she also photographed after he died) was Ernest Southard, who would go on to run the influential Eugenics Record Office at Cold Spring Harbor.

Eugenics' relationship with neuropathology makes sense, given that eugenics privileged an explanatory model of illness based on inherited, biological predisposition. Canavan's and Southard's interests in eugenics were certainly more directed at eradicating mental illness than at enforcing racial disparity. The fact remains, however, that eugenic science did not offer any solutions to disease other than sterilization. In 1921, Canavan received recognition from the International Congress of Eugenics for her photographs of the brains of men deemed feebleminded and criminal. The official commendation cited her work done on behalf of "the improvement of racial qualities in man."[5] A few years later, Canavan was appointed to the faculty at Boston University medical school, where Fuller himself taught, and she would go on to run the medical museum there. Given the location, focus, and success of Canavan's research, that Fuller withdrew from his clinical research and began to embrace other models of psychiatry is not surprising. Because of its divisive emphasis and narrow view on the discipline of psychiatry, eugenics was not a science that Fuller could endorse. Psychoanalysis, on the other hand, offered a more optimistic, socially oriented model of illness and cure.[6]

Fuller's interest in psychoanalysis also echoes in the widespread incorporation of nonbiological explanations for mental conditions more generally and the symptoms of dementia more specifically. Even though its early investigators were unsure about Alzheimer's as a useful disease category, in fact a great number of articles were published on presenile and senile dementia in the ensuing decades. This rise of diverse explanations for the condition might be attributed simply to the new diversity in psychiatric perspectives, if not the need for a better understanding of cause and classification.

If this is true, then why exactly is there a more contemporary historiographic gap in the story of Alzheimer's from 1915 to the 1960s, as Ballenger points out? The simple explanation may be that because biological explanations for the disease are so common now, the history of other kinds of research on Alzheimer's is not always acknowledged. In other words, if it is understood that, during this time, there were no significant research advances in the field of Alzheimer's disease, it is because, from a historical perspective, the disease is largely associated with the plaques and tangles Alzheimer, Fischer, Fuller, and others had already described. While research into the nature of that pathology continued, the plaques and tangles offered disagreement rather than consensus.[7] Because research on those plaques and tangles did not play a significant role in resolving debates about clinical symptoms, some adopted a more psychosocial perspective on causality. Ultimately, psychosocial explanations were not central to Alzheimer's research later in the twentieth century, when the disease became more widely known.[8] Thus they play no real role in the popular and scientific history of the disease.

I would argue, however, that this historiographic gap can also be explained by recognizing the importance of neuroimaging innovation in scientific narratives of Alzheimer's. Ballenger's reference to the popular characterization of midcentury science as a "dark age" is apt; darkness here indicates a perceived lack of knowledge but also the difficulty in seeing or representing the disease. One of the more influential Alzheimer's researchers of the last sixty years, Robert Terry, labeled midcentury science "primitive" precisely because of its lack of sophisticated images.[9] According to this view, advances in histology, microscopy, and related clinical advances presumably led to better research.

Indeed, there were only modest advances in histology and microscopy from 1915 to 1960 in the United States that would play a key role in Alzheimer's research. What little progress was made did relatively little to solve the research problems that had confounded Alzheimer and his contemporaries. Some advances in staining, for example, helped detail the morphology of the plaques and tangles.[10] In 1927 the Belgian neurologist Paul Divry successfully stained the core of senile plaques with Congo red stain, showing their amyloid character.[11] This stain would go on to become important in successive morphological studies. New silver impregnation methods like those derived by A. Von Braunmuhl and David Bodian were increasingly deployed alongside the Bielschowsky method used by Alzheimer.[12] But generally speaking, after the high point of stain experimentation at the turn of the century, new discovery fell progressively until the 1940s.[13] During World War I, American histologists found that inconsistently produced stains were compromising their research. The introduction of the Commission on the Standardization of Biological Stains in the 1920s allowed for the coordination of standards among stain manufacturers and various U.S. scientific organizations.[14] While this strengthened transatlantic collaboration in histology, psychiatrists continued to discuss the limitations of their practice.[15] And any histological advances only reinforced the key dilemmas that haunted research on Alzheimer's: the questionable etiology of the plaques and tangles and the problem of age-oriented classification.

The question of the difference between senile and presenile dementia, in fact, shaped a lot of the clinical and laboratory research on Alzheimer's in the United States through the 1950s.[16] The discordance in objective standards for disease description naturally led to debates as to the disease's frequency or incidence.[17] The category of "Alzheimer's disease" was generally used in this research to designate the presenile condition or the neurofibrillary tangles Alzheimer was understood to have discovered. This was underscored by new research in the 1930s that showed inconsistent familial connections to presenile dementia.[18]

Sporadic predisposition to the disease only muddied the water further. There was simply no consensus as to the clinical definition of the disease, its pathogenesis, or even the biological trajectory of the normal aging brain.[19]

Disciplinary rifts in psychiatry echoed in these debates. Many psychiatrists, for example, discounted biology as causal. Chief among them was David Rothschild, who published a series of articles in the 1930s and 1940s that acknowledged and described material pathology but attributed symptoms to social, emotional, or behavioral causes.[20] Other psychiatrists and gerontologists discounted pathology entirely. While some have argued that subsequent advances in disease description helped erase these insecurities, the debates continued throughout subsequent decades, both in the United States and in Europe.[21]

As the last chapter pointed out, the "prehistory" of Alzheimer's disease has largely been understood through the Alzheimer's discovery narrative. That narrative is deemed "pre-" because it was not until the late 1970s that Alzheimer's disease became a recognized disease category in the public eye and until the 1980s that it became known as a viable public health threat. So while Alzheimer's was certainly studied in scientific research for much of the twentieth century, it did not always figure prominently in public discourse of aging or dementia. Several major developments in the 1960s and 1970s helped to suture representations of Alzheimer's pathology to the representation of older Americans, effectively communicating the disease as a risk to all. These included an interest in obtaining objective and comparative clinical data, an insecure scientific consensus that Alzheimer's was common in elderly populations, and the founding of the NIA. Each of these shifts in disease regulation and research, however, also depended on related developments in media technologies and neuroimaging.

To understand the relationship between these areas, the remainder of this chapter explores the history of the scientific mediation of Alzheimer's in the United States from approximately 1960 to 2020. Neuroimaging would become the dominant tool for researching cause, diagnosis, treatment, and cure, but it also served as the primary way the public learned about those efforts. More recently, new technology able to image the brains of living people made that public more than just an audience, setting up significant recruitment efforts designed to facilitate the description and diagnosis of symptomatic and asymptomatic populations alike. Even though these neuroimaging technologies differed in the ways they represented the brain, the target of their inquiry—the amyloid plaques and neurofibrillary tangles—remained remarkably consistent. This chapter, then, is most concerned with the authorization of Alzheimer's research paradigms under the rubric of media progress and expertise. These scientists—for all their medical training—were *new media pioneers.* Public investments in Alzheimer's research were shaped as much by trust in those media technologies as by growing concern that the disease was a threat to national health and welfare.

Technologies of Visibility:
Electron Microscopes and Assessment Scales

In the early 1960s, Robert Terry, a neuropathologist at Albert Einstein College of Medicine in New York, used a Siemens electron microscope to revisit the plaques and tangles of Alzheimer's disease. An electron microscope uses a beam of electrons as a source of description or illumination rather than light, creating images at a far higher resolution than is possible with light microscopy. These microscopes were relatively new in American labs at the time, so researchers were busy applying the technology to a range of different materials.[22] Terry and his research partner, Saul Korey, were able to more carefully and complexly describe the ultrastructural morphology of Alzheimer's pathology, publishing first on the nature of the neurofibrillary tangles and then on the plaques. Whether they were the first to do so with the electron microscope was the source of some debate. Michael Kidd, a researcher in England, published similar results at about the same time, describing in particular the paired helical filament composition of the tangles.[23] The debate over who did what first illustrates the professional pressures to master the latest representational technologies.

The electron microscope's ability to show the ultrastructure of the plaques and tangles incited significant research in the 1960s and 1970s from other neuroanatomists and neuropathologists, sparking what some refer to as the "modern era of Alzheimer's disease research."[24] Much of the relevant research was descriptive and comparative. Far more anatomical details were accessible with this technology, which then afforded a more complex understanding of the ultrastructure of the brain. In addition to more careful description of the plaques and tangles, for example, researchers discovered the presence of accompanying characteristics, such as Hirano bodies.[25] Of course, optical technology is never entirely determinant, and Terry's research was not instantly transformative. The focus of much of the research advanced by the electron microscope was in fact similar to the older research that employed the light microscope. Both the objective focus of that research, Alzheimer's plaques and tangles, and its mode of inquiry, clinical and laboratory-based neuropathology, helped solidify the technology and the research questions as an enduringly effective "scene of inquiry."[26]

It is perhaps somewhat surprising that after half a century, the research focus for Alzheimer's was so little changed, even with the electron microscope. One reason for the consistency is that the representational technology was actually designed to *mimic* its predecessors. Nicholas Rasmussen has shown that the scientists who helped to develop the techniques of electron microscopy in the 1940s and 1950s struggled to align its pictorial techniques with the conventions of older practices of scientific representation. This included the techniques of both histology and the light microscope.[27] Rasmussen argued that this pictorial strategy aided the technology's acceptance by both public and scientific audiences. From its early production by RCA in the 1940s, the electron microscope was hailed by the public as a new kind of "super-eye," capable of imaging the unseen to a remarkable degree.[28] The optical principle of magnification, however, was already quite familiar to an American public, which helped them relate to the new technology with few reservations as to its legitimacy.

This is also true of those scientists experimenting with the electron microscope for their research. Robert Terry admits to looking at Alzheimer's and his colleagues' "recognizably beautiful silver impregnations," but he saw himself as doing a more sophisticated mode of research.[29]

As he later argued, "the electron microscope offered opportunities in chiaroscuro, in lights and shadow composition."[30] The cutting-edge optical equipment allowed for a creative and corrective understanding of the biochemical makeup and morphology of the proteins that formed the plaques and tangles that Alzheimer had rudimentarily identified. While knowledge of disease etiology had not advanced significantly, the new technology helped scientists confront the obstacles of the older research, providing just enough descriptive insight that the plaques and tangles remained central to scientific inquiry.

In addition to the electron microscope, there were some important midcentury advances in histochemistry, that branch of histology that explores the chemical transformations of biological tissue.[31] Rather than understand the brain as a static artifact, neurochemistry reveals morphology as a relational process. Terry's collaboration with Korey, a neurochemist, echoed the rapid expansion of collaborative histochemistry in the 1950s and 1960s. The electron microscope may have been an exciting new tool in brain research, but it required collaboration and different kinds of expertise to produce useful results. Along with those collaborations, advanced tissue processors, new fixatives, automatic stainers, new tissue cutters, new stains, and a host of other new preparation and development techniques were popularized in labs around the United States. The epistemological range of histotechnology would expand again dramatically in the 1970s and 1980s with the rise of immunohistochemistry. Rather than using a stain to match a cellular component, the practice relies on antibodies that bind to antigens in the cell, thereby acting as a tracer for some kind of stain or marker.[32] Immunohistochemistry allowed for more targeted description, and the field continues to add techniques to the histological arsenal even today.

Thus the histological gaze so crucial to the origins of Alzheimer's disease was still flourishing half a century later in the descriptive work of the electron microscope. Korey provided the neurochemistry background, and Terry provided the expertise in crafting images. Just like Fuller and Ramón y Cajal a half century before, Terry was an amateur photographer, a hobby he dates to his own youth. Terry's dedication to image technology was probably helpful to his efforts to incorporate the new technology into disease research. Electron microscopy did not just automatically provide a better image; it required some experimentation to produce the desired results. It could be very difficult to create a good electron micrograph, especially because different techniques could reveal different structural aspects of the tissue. Just like the camera lucida, the electron microscope allowed histologists to make an argument, to prove, recognize, or diagnose the presence of some chemical process or structural characteristic. Terry was proficient, but he was also a pioneer, which is likely why his work is celebrated as transformational to Alzheimer's research. One of his electron micrographs of Tay Sachs pathology was even shown at the New York Museum of Modern Art as part of a 1967 exhibition called *Once Invisible*.[33]

Generally speaking, the electron microscope was still a rudimentary technology when researchers like Terry and Kidd refocused their gaze on the plaques and tangles, and it served more as a jump start to research than as an indication of a paradigm shift. In fact, after the introduction of the electron microscope, many researchers continued to work with a light microscope.[34] Light and electron microscopes were also used in tandem and in comparative research, just as they are today. The more researchers looked, the more questions arose. As two scientists in the 1960s put it, "the literature is abundant and . . . senile dementia finds itself in the center, it is as it were the angular stone of it. However, it would be false to believe that this puts us on sure ground. . . . The contrary is true. When we form a clear idea of our present knowledge of senile dementia, we perceive gaps everywhere. What contradictions and open discussions!"[35]

Beyond simply describing the biological characteristics of the plaques and tangles, the electron microscope would contribute to the realization of quantified measures of that pathology.[36] The historical standardization of clinical data was an essential stepping-stone on the path to understanding Alzheimer's as a disease of the elderly. By the late 1960s, new clinical dementia assessments were developed specifically as quantified correlates to microscopically described plaque counts and brain atrophy. In particular, a group of researchers led by Martin

Roth in Newcastle, England, published a series of studies that demonstrated the clear prevalence of Alzheimer's pathology among aging populations.[37] They were working with large hospital populations that allowed for comparative clinical research. The clinical tool that emerged from those studies, the Blessed Dementia Scale, allowed a researcher to ascertain the severity of dementia by attaching a number or score to a particular symptom. That dementia score could then be correlated with postmortem plaque counts and brain atrophy as an objective measure of the disease. Of course, recognition of the symptoms of Alzheimer's was not purely objective, nor even were the symptoms themselves based on any consensus criteria.[38]

The availability of these kinds of clinical data on Alzheimer's has been described variously through shifts in institutional, political, and caregiving priorities, but an important ideological and epistemological influence can be located in the broader importance of representation to contemporary sciences of mind and related appeals to the connection between brain localization and mental behavior. The historical rise of cognitivism and its attendant practices in psychology, computer science, artificial intelligence, linguistics, and neuroscience marked the broad-based externalization of mental processes vis-à-vis representation. Cognitive science itself reaches disciplinary status at the same time that the clinical scales for describing dementia begin to appear. It is not simply that cognitive abilities are increasingly given shape by scientific discourse; it is their objective status within that discourse that matters. As objective, they are imminently recognizable and comparative.

Whether by clinical scale or pathological lesion, the carefully trained authority of the objective observer could now articulate the symptom within a representational frame. That a cognitive symptom had objective status was easily as important to disease description as the objective fact of material pathology. Each was externalized through formal representation and then legitimated through its inclusion within a nosological system. Their shared status as objective, systemic, and comparative made causality entirely secondary; correlation is all that was necessary. And as a kind of universal biological process, aging was an ideal correlative frame.

Without claiming causality, the Newcastle research maintained bio-logical primacy within the explanation of clinical symptomatology, re-invigorating the older, material arguments for a new social audience and a new generation of researchers.[39] The proviso of objectivity helped inspire more research into Alzheimer's disease as well as a range of other clinical, correlative scales,[40] but it also helped authorize the bio-logically oriented cognitive symptom for broader, public organization of the disease. Most central to that effort, it helped solidify aging as a key risk factor for Alzheimer's while at the same time reasserting Alz-heimer's as a disease of the aged rather than a normal part of aging. The claim that Alzheimer's was a disease that primarily affected older people would become a crucial component of its narration for a public audience.

By the mid-1970s, despite all this new laboratory and clinical research on Alzheimer's, the disease was still relatively unknown in America outside of a few psychiatric circles. That changed with the publication of the much-heralded 1976 editorial in the journal *Archives of Neurology* written by Richard Katzman.[41] Katzman sounded the warning alarms to the scientific community, arguing that Alzheimer's disease was the fourth or fifth most common cause of death in the United States. While it had been increasingly apparent to many that Alzheimer's was a big-ger problem than originally imagined, the editorial created quite a stir. Accepted or not, his epidemiological argument galvanized researchers in more diverse scientific arenas to begin research on the disease. It also formed the bedrock for a broader organization of researchers, govern-ment, advocacy groups, and the public, what Patrick Fox has described as the "rise of the Alzheimer's disease movement."[42]

Enlisting Support: From Advocacy to Awareness

Katzman, Terry, and their colleague Katherine Bick organized a 1977 workshop conference at the NIH to help coordinate the rising interest in Alzheimer's. Cosponsored by the National Institute of Neurological Communicative Diseases and Stroke, the National Institute of Mental Health, and the NIA, the workshop brought together scientists from a range of fields to clarify research approaches and educate both the medical and research communities. The workshop was successful in focusing perhaps disparate research strands into a more coordinated plan. One notable outcome was that the commission recommended the disorder be called "Alzheimer's disease" for younger people and "senile dementia of the Alzheimer's type" for the older population, reflecting continued insecurity around the issue of age but a certain resolve that aging be integral to the disease narrative.[43]

At about the same time as the NIH workshop, a highly visible gerontologist, Robert Butler, was helping to found the NIA. The NIA was struggling for recognition in an already fractured NIH, and the Alzheimer's disease category became important to that effort.[44] In his arguments to Congress seeking funding, Butler pointed toward Alzheimer's as a massive threat to a rapidly aging population and a key focus for future research. The disease-specific appeal that Butler utilized in his lobbying was in fact a common tactic for dealing with the NIH. Butler says that he specifically chose to build the NIA on the foundation of a "'health politics of anguish,' that is, public concern about a specific disease, expressed by families who have suffered and by advocacy groups."[45] This tactic was useful because a war on a disease was something that the federal government could sell to a fearful public as dollars well spent.[46]

In that same spirit, the end of the 1970s saw the development of the Alzheimer's Disease and Related Disorders Association (ADRDA), which would eventually become the powerful Alzheimer's Association so active today. The ADRDA united several disparate organizations on the divisive perspective that research into Alzheimer's disease in particular was the best way to bring public attention to—and eventually cure—the full spectrum of related disorders.[47] This conglomerative move was divisive because Alzheimer's was not yet a placeholder for senile dementia in the public eye. The proposal to insert Alzheimer's as the dominant logic for philanthropic and political lobbying was seen as an obstacle to the recognition of other kinds of dementia. After some contentious debate, the member groups settled on the ADRDA, helping to insert Alzheimer's as a proxy for all manner of dementia in scientific, philanthropic, and public culture.[48] The advocacy group would go on to become instrumental to building public awareness for the disease in the early 1980s. The primary strategy they used to enlist government support for research was the same as Butler's. They built public awareness around the incidence of the disease as well as excitement about scientific advances; this public interest would then compel the government to fund more research, as politicians were often keenly attendant to the voices of their constituents.[49]

That the threat of Alzheimer's was used to draw awareness to problems around aging more broadly is key to the visible magnification of its threat more concretely. In each of these venues—scientific, civic, and philanthropic—imaging technologies were celebrated and encouraged, but they also became part of the rhetorical bridge for public communication about aging and dementia. In a 1980 joint Senate subcommittee meeting called "Impact of Alzheimer's Disease on the Nation's Elderly," references to instrumentation and technology were sprinkled throughout testimony and supporting documents. Diagnostics and description were the twin logics of research advance advocated by the research and advocacy organizations in attendance.[50] Neuroimaging technologies like computed tomography (CAT or CT), PET, and electric electroencephalography (EEG) were offered as helpful diagnostic tools just as the electron microscope was reinforced as the arbiter of morphological truth claims.

Included in the testimony, for example, was a new pamphlet published by the NIA called *Alzheimer's Disease Q&A*. The first page, titled "What Is Alzheimer's?," used the history of neuroimaging technology to tell the story of the disease. After describing the basic light microscope research Alois Alzheimer performed in 1906, it described the new advances in image science: "new and highly sophisticated instruments and techniques—such as the *electron microscope* which can magnify cells more than a hundred thousand times—have revealed other changes in the brain that are characteristic of the disease."[51] The document went on to insist that persons suspected of having Alzheimer's should undergo a series of tests, including EEGs and CT scans. That the document suggested neuroimaging as a useful diagnostic tool would not be all that remarkable if neuroimaging were not linked so clearly to advances in disease description made by the introduction of the electron microscope. As ever, the instability of clinical and morpholog-ical connections was masked through the technological ability to peer into the brain.

Thus the end of the 1970s fostered the epidemic of Alzheimer's visibility: cautious progress in imaging technologies and clinical descrip-tion, the development of the NIA and concordant national prioritization of the well-being of the elderly, and, as a uniting factor, the prioritiza-tion of Alzheimer's disease as a nosological descriptor. Important to recognize about this narrative, however, is that none of these develop-ments happened alone. Each was interdependent, each helped shape the others, all under the dominant ethic of descriptive visibility: symp-tom, pathology, and patient. The visibility of the disease was a major step for biomedical progress. Someday the medical community might have a better understanding of cause and cure, but visualization as progress was best practice in light of the absence of actual solutions to those objectives.

In order to understand the development of Alzheimer's research over the last forty years, one must recognize neuroimaging's role in the enlistment of a national public as both audience to and eventual subject of U.S. research on the disease. The 1980s saw an explosive rise in the use of imaging technologies to describe not just the plaques and tan-gles but increasingly detailed morphology that drew on broad research expertise. But concurrent with that expansion in research was the rise in public awareness and disease visibility. The ADRDA played the key role in educating the public, but popular culture and its spokespeople were central to the effort.

A 1980 Dear Abby letter sparked one of the first public conversa-tions about Alzheimer's.[52] A caregiver, identified as "Desperate in N.Y.," wrote the advice column about her husband's recent diagnosis, asking how to manage the disease. "Have you ever heard of Alzheimer's dis-ease?" she wrote. "I feel so helpless. How do others cope with this afflic-tion?"[53] In response, the author of Dear Abby, Pauline Phillips, provided her with the address of the ADRDA. In the two weeks following the publication of that column, the national headquarters received twenty-two thousand letters asking for more information. Phillips eventually

became a significant advocate for Alzheimer's awareness, in part because she would go on to develop Alzheimer's herself. Lonnie Wollin,
who ran the national headquarters of the ADRDA when the letter was
written, says that 1980 column "put Alzheimer's disease in the public
spotlight and put the Alzheimer's Association on the map."[54]

The first major figure in the United States to reveal her diagnosis of
Alzheimer's disease was the film star Rita Hayworth. She had exhib-
ited erratic behavior for years, and many people thought she was an
alcoholic.[55] She revealed her diagnosis to the public in 1981 in part as
a way to correct that misinformation but also to spread awareness of
the disease. As a highly visible celebrity, Hayworth not only brought
instant attention to Alzheimer's but also communicated a useful narrative for understanding the symptoms of the disease. The public was
attached to the collective memory of her performances as a younger
actress, so the symptom of memory loss became particularly poignant
as a symbolic threat to that past. Her experience helped authorize the
disease as a narrative of decline. The same argument can be made for
any celebrity with dementia, but Hayworth was particularly important
because of the way her experience helped teach the public about this
new disease and its symptoms.[56]

With Hayworth's public diagnosis, senile dementia and Alzheimer's
had become more widely visible in the media.[57] The ADRDA welcomed
Hayworth's participation in awareness efforts, but it was her daughter Yasmin Aga Khan who would become her public voice. In 1982 a
small group of advocates including ADRDA president Jerome Stone
and Aga Khan secured a private meeting with President Ronald Reagan to make a case for government support. Reagan expressed surprising interest in the disease at the meeting, and his advocacy would
eventually become a boon for government interventions. Stone would
later describe how Reagan brought up his own mother, Nelle Reagan,
after hearing about some of the symptoms. Stone postulated it was
because Reagan realized that Alzheimer's might have had something
to do with his mother's own dementia.[58] The president, who would of
course eventually develop Alzheimer's disease himself, became a key
supporter in the enlistment of federal research funding.

Shortly thereafter, Congress passed a joint resolution officially designating November as National Alzheimer's Disease Month. The specific rationale was public awareness. The proclamation states that "an increase in the national awareness of the problem of Alzheimer's disease may stimulate the interest and concern of the American people, which may lead, in turn, to increased research and eventually to the discovery of a cure for Alzheimer's disease."[59] In other words, Congress needed public endorsement before putting tax dollars into research.

From a medical researcher's perspective, however, public participation was not just a matter of money. Better research design was dependent on the availability of people to study, and the rise in public interest promised higher rates of diagnosis and an entirely new approach to research design. Gradual advances in neuroimaging technology helped foster two interdependent clinical paradigms that were an important component of that transformation: description and diagnostics. Effective diagnosis gave people dealing with the symptoms of Alzheimer's a name for their condition, and descriptive research offered a possible cure. Alzheimer's disease's arrival as a newly visible public threat began to articulate the disease as a powerful social nexus predicated on these new modes of visibility. In the early 1980s, however, everyday deployment of neuroimaging—clinical or laboratory—was still far from realistic.

When Alzheimer's researchers and advocates convened in Washington, D.C., in 1983 to advocate for Senate appropriations, image technology and instrumentation were central to their vision for the future. Nancy Mace, author of the first popular guide to caring for someone with Alzheimer's, *The 36 Hour Day,* urged funding for research above all.[60] Heads of various medical centers made direct appeals for neuroimaging and clinical infrastructure.[61] Oleg Jardetzky, director of the Stanford Magnetic Resonance Laboratory, argued for better funding for imaging technology, especially given the expense of the machines. He complained in particular that the allocations for instrumentation were "not adequate to meet the new needs generated by recent explosive technological developments."[62] Of particular concern was the easy obsolescence of the technology and the need for sustained funding to keep up to date with the advances. Eventually Congress passed legislation to help streamline funding for Alzheimer's and to orient research priorities around diagnostics, description, and care.[63] The law gave the NIA the responsibility to distribute funds and ergo the opportunity to help structure Alzheimer's research.

Despite the growing attention to technology and focused research paradigms, the medical community was still missing strong clinical procedures to coordinate and validate that research. Furthermore, an unfortunate side effect of the rush to inclusion was improper diagnosis. These early obstacles were all part of the public image of the disease. The *New York Times*, reporting from an Alzheimer's conference, cited several experts who complained that Alzheimer's had become a "'garbage pail' diagnosis, a catch-all term to describe any elderly patient whose mind is deteriorating for reasons that are not immediately obvious."[64]

In 1984 an Alzheimer's task force for the Department of Health and Human Services published clinical criteria for the diagnosis of Alzheimer's disease to help fix the situation. The publication specifically highlighted the importance of CT, PET, and MRI, describing the ways in which neuroimaging might be useful for longitudinal studies for disease description and monitoring therapeutic interventions. The authors of the study were careful to note that the criteria "were not yet fully operational because of insufficient knowledge of the disease."[65] The primary strategy for diagnosing Alzheimer's was still exclusion. Any diagnosis was far from secure, not just because it required a battery of clinical tests for other conditions, but also because a secure diagnosis was predicated on postmortem autopsy of the plaques and tangles. This narrative was an important disclaimer that also helped secure the importance of material pathology. Postmortem plaques and tangles maintained the "last word" on Alzheimer's.

The public visibility of neuroimaging practices was central to their eventual acceptance within a diagnostic frame. Neuroimaging technology was beginning to seep into popular culture, and its authority was brought to bear in some highly public venues. For example, after John Hinckley Jr. attempted to assassinate Reagan in 1981, the defense team introduced CT scans of Hinckley's brain as evidence in court. Several medical experts testified that the "brain shrinkage" the images revealed was indicative of schizophrenia.[66] Along with the brain images, the defense introduced into evidence the movie *Taxi Driver,* arguing that Hinckley's obsession with the movie had motivated the assassination attempt. The jury actually watched the movie in court.[67] That argument closed the defense's case, and they won—Hinckley was found not guilty by reason of insanity. Public opinion widely derided the outcome, and it inspired a movement to challenge the validity of an insanity defense.[68] That derision, however, does not reveal distrust in the evidence itself; rather, it shows a discomfort with the issue of responsibility and mental illness. While an x-ray of a brain and a Hollywood movie might seem like very different artifacts, their use in the case relies on a broader belief in media effects. The film and the CT scan each betrays public interest in the power of the image to reveal some essential truth about human behavior, just as public dissatisfaction with the trial's outcome explains public insecurity with mental health.

Indeed, despite public interest in neuroimaging technology, the challenges to accurately diagnosing Alzheimer's were part of the disease's early public identity. The first feature to directly address Alzheimer's, the 1985 Emmy Award–winning *Do You Remember Love,* foregrounds this uncertainty in a diagnosis montage early in the narrative. After dealing with classic symptoms of Alzheimer's, the main character undergoes a visibly exhausting barrage of tests at the hospital. She has her blood drawn, she has several different brain scans, and doctors gaze at screens with careful scrutiny. There are more tests and more scans to analyze. All of this is designed to appear strenuous and exhausting, as she becomes increasingly agitated and upset. The diagnosis montage culminates with her finding her husband asleep in a chair in the hospital hallway. Leaving a pile of spent coffee cups on the chair, it is time to go home. Her doctor, meeting with them later, says, "I have to preface this by saying it is extremely difficult to make a diagnosis" but that he can in fact make a "tentative" diagnosis of Alzheimer's disease.

The film's diagnosis montage shows not only a growing interest in the disease but also the important role of neuroimaging in a clinical setting. The film is indicative of a broader discursive trend that framed advances in imaging technology as synonymous with a certain order of progress. In a surprisingly astute 1986 *Washington Post* article describing the state of Alzheimer's research titled "Scientists Can Explain What Happens to the Brain, but Not Why," the author wrote, "With each advance in imaging technology—from X-ray to PET—and with comparable progress in neuroscience, biochemistry and cell biology, researchers have learned more about how normal brain cells work and what happens when something interferes."[69] Neuroimaging, both in the film and in public discourse more generally, bore the rhetorical weight of both diagnosis and description, but it was clearly a work in progress. Diagnostic uncertainty, in other words, was underwritten by descriptive advance.

One of the other ways diagnosis and description merged in the 1980s was through the rise of clinical research collaboration. On one hand, this happened with the national coordination of cognitive assessment measures. Zaven Khachaturian, former director at the NIH's Office of Alzheimer's Disease Research and editor of the Alzheimer's Association journal *Alzheimer's and Dementia,* claims that the "availability of standardized, well-validated quantitative assessment instruments were indispensable prerequisites for NIA's subsequent initiatives."[70] Just as important as those instruments was the coordination of clinical infrastructure. The "subsequent initiatives" Khachaturian describes provided for a series of Alzheimer's Disease Centers and cooperative studies around the United States that helped to coordinate research. A new Alzheimer's Patient Registry led to further clinical coordination and standardization. Streamlined funding and resource management led to sharing of space and collaborative research design.

These structural shifts led to a range of new descriptive research on possible causes and biomedical interventions. The protein tau was associated with the neurofibrillary tangles in the mid-1980s, and that discovery would go on to become the basis of a massive new paradigm in disease research.[71] Discoveries of neurotransmitter imbalances in the brains of people with dementia would fuel the cholinergic hypothesis of Alzheimer's, eventually leading to the development of drugs like rivastigmine (Exelon) and donepezil (Aricept). These drugs, still in use today, can be used to lessen cognitive symptoms for some people with Alzheimer's. Other research discovered gene mutations correlated with early-onset Alzheimer's, and by the 1990s, genetic markers had been found in some late-onset populations.[72] These are just a few of the many research paths that emerged from the national orchestration of resources, infrastructure, and awareness.

In Vivo: Coordinating Diagnostics and Description

Eventually the histological gaze, originally predicated on specific relationships between scientific expertise and neuropathology, disappeared into a more complicated organization of research and the public. That is not to say that the histological gaze became irrelevant; to the contrary, certain aspects remained quite viable. For example, the proleptic structure of the neurosciences continues to this day, where significant work is performed strictly in the service of better future research.[73] Broad public embrace of the practice of neuroscience also continues to drive the circulation of research dollars and expertise. Even histology itself, an entrenched practice of description and recognition, continues to be an important part of intersectional disease research. These practices are deeply wedded to biologically oriented theories of cause and cure. However, the volume of actors that informed research on Alzheimer's exploded in the 1980s and 1990s, outstripping the comparatively diminutive research corpus of the previous century.

More importantly, researchers no longer focused their inquiry simply on clinically supportive, dead brain tissue, as they had for much of the twentieth century. As public awareness of Alzheimer's grew, the experience of everyday aging people became a key aspect of the search for cause and cure. Public health relationships and clinical transformations helped researchers access those people, but a more exact in vivo approach to neuroimaging also became a driving goal in disease research. No longer satisfied with looking at postmortem brain tissue, scientists began actively to pursue technologies that captured images of the living brain.

As noted in the previous chapter, the traditional approach was to monitor and care for people with dementia until they were dead so that they could be autopsied and their brain tissue inspected. It was largely agreed that Alzheimer's could only be diagnosed through postmortem analysis, and doctors had to cut open the skull and brain to verify the presence of neurofibrillary tangles and amyloid plaques or brain atrophy. Any attempt to render the brain useful functioned—in the last instance—at the level of histology and neuropathology.[74] In fact, the line between life and death was extremely important for these researchers. Neuropathologists were keenly interested in the "freshness" of their tissue samples. A key site of variability in histological analysis is the proximity to death—after which cutting, staining, and imaging took place.

This was evident from the very beginning of Alzheimer's research; look, for example, at Solomon Fuller's careful comparative research of brain tissues twelve and then forty-eight hours after death.[75] Histologists like Fuller and Alzheimer understood that the proximity to death altered the viability of the specimen. No technology could microscopically analyze living brain tissue, so the biosociality of the disease was limited to the objective techniques and technologies of the researcher, on one hand, and asylum control over people with dementia, on the other. This early system was not sustainable. The primary way in which those living bodies "mattered" in a social sense was the tremendous strain they imposed on this country's asylum system. After the first few decades of the twentieth century, asylums in America were overflowing with newly classified, aberrant bodies. This is another reason for the shift from neuropathological explanations to psychosocial ones,[76] a shift that was itself a step in orienting Alzheimer's and dementia within biopolitical governance. Psychosocial methods, however, could not satisfactorily explain disease etiology, which ultimately led the theories to fall from favor.

This trend, however, led to a range of different attempts to validate the living person with dementia. The standardization of clinical scales and the quantification of symptoms in the 1970s were important steps in that integration. A related shift in histology can be located in the occasional use of live tissue biopsies to create more effective images with the electron microscope. The freshness of the tissue sample continued to be operative in midcentury histology, but this was particularly true with electron microscopy. A neurosurgeon performed the surgery while the histologist waited in the wings to fix the tissue. In an interview, Terry said that one of the main reasons he decided to do research on Alzheimer's was simply because of his access to live tissue samples. Researchers like Terry were only able to gain access to biopsies when the disease condition was understood to be fatal.[77] Many of the live tissue biopsies for this kind of research came from people dying with Alzheimer's. Aside from being ethically dubious, these aggressive methods were inherently limited by logistic access, as an increasing number of researchers turned their focus to Alzheimer's. Clearly needed was a technology to safely image the brain while the person experiencing symptoms was still alive.

One precursor to modern in vivo neuroimaging of Alzheimer's was an x-ray technology called pneumoencephalography. *Encephalography* simply denotes the practice of creating a representation of the brain, and there are different strategies that have proved historically popular (EEG, for example, is electroencephalography). Pneumoencephalography was a common diagnostic or descriptive practice from the 1930s to the 1970s, until PET and CT made it irrelevant. It involved extracting cerebrospinal fluid and replacing it with air or gas. An x-ray of the head could then reveal visual contrast around the brain. Investigators confronted with the symptoms of dementia could use these images to rule out brain tumors and to describe and localize cerebral atrophy. William Menninger was the first to advise its application to diagnosing Alzheimer's in 1934, and it was consequently used to rule out tumors or other conditions, such as Pick's disease.[78] In a clinical situation, it was occasionally used to diagnose Alzheimer's in vivo, but it was neither a safe nor a pleasant activity.[79] In fact, that this procedure was done to living patients likely had much to do with its eventual fall from fashion. Patients could endure vomiting, pain, and disorientation, not to mention possible infection, brain damage, or death.

CT, PET, and EEG brain scans offered a safer promise of in vivo description of brain atrophy. Although some of these technologies had been in development since midcentury or earlier, it wasn't until the mid- to late 1970s that researchers began to apply them more actively to people experiencing symptoms of dementia.[80] These technologies, however, were by no means available for widespread clinical use. This was true not just because of the limited availability of the machines but because of the difficulty in objective standardization of the data. CT and PET, for example, allowed for the early quantification of cerebral atrophy, but there was disagreement about how exactly to measure that atrophy, not to mention the lack of clear correlation between atrophy and clinical symptom.[81] Regardless of clinical value, the new availability of brain-scanning technology set up a horizon of research potential crucial to the imagination of diagnosis and description. In other words, disagreement about how to use the technology did not eliminate the consensus that it be adopted and advanced.

The 1977 NIH workshop on Alzheimer's was particularly notable in that the committee described the need for better clinical data and a cautious optimism in brain-scanning technologies for delivering that data.[82] This endorsement of neuroimaging was largely associated with the value of longitudinal research. Several workshop members stressed the importance of research on younger people at earlier stages in life: "the improvement in the overall diagnostic accuracy and the identification of very early cases of persons at risk would be achieved if a clinical method for identifying the presence of tangles and plaques or a biochemical change . . . could be found."[83]

This formal interest in studying people not in advanced stages of the disease marks a key transformation in research on Alzheimer's, and it was in many ways only made possible by promising transformations in imaging technology. The dream of in vivo imaging asserts the viability of the living person as an object of study. Furthermore, changes in the tradition of cross-sectional studies to longitudinal studies show the importance of research of brain change over time.[84] The validity of the living body is that it can serve as a longitudinal control for the study of Alzheimer's even if it has no observable symptoms or disease. The principle of in vivo imaging represents a shift in what kinds of bodies are important to Alzheimer's research. Clinical research found itself increasingly able to integrate people with moderate symptoms or even no symptoms at all. Changes to diagnostic categories have mirrored that interest, most notably with the introduction of MCI as a risk category for Alzheimer's.

MRI and, eventually, functional MRI (fMRI) grew to become the dominant neuroimaging tools by the turn of the century because they provided better contrast of brains than any other neuroimaging technology but also because of their safe, noninvasive, in vivo capacities.[85] As a clinical practice, a technology that uses a magnet is preferable to one that uses radiation in that it is presumably less harmful to the subject. That allows the easy inclusion of healthy human adults in research studies. Over the last two decades, a range of functional neuroimaging strategies have been put to use for in vivo imaging, such as PET and single photon emission computed tomography (SPECT).

As a part of the drive to in vivo diagnostics and description, functional neuroimaging also introduced the principle of time or duration to neurostructure. Rather than generating a static image, fMRI or PET can foreground the brain as a process, as a living agent both responsive to outside stimuli and correspondent to the rest of the body's activities. Functional neuroimaging is not like a snapshot of the brain. Generally speaking, functional neuroimaging models brain activity through a "coupling" of metabolism or blood flow measurement with a cognitively oriented theory of neuronal activity.[86] Functional imaging can indicate brain activity, which allows for localization of symptoms as well as longitudinal tracking of changes. What exactly is being tracked, of course, is not always easy to ascertain, and functional technologies represent morphology and change differently.

Another key development in contemporary Alzheimer's research has been the development of molecular imaging, which allows researchers to introduce an element into the body and track its effects. This has been especially important to drug research. If a pharmaceutical company can develop an agent that binds to amyloid plaques, for example, then changes to those plaques can be tracked; in theory, one could then monitor therapeutic interventions. The gradual incorporation of "effects"-based research into long-standing pathological determination is partially based on the newfound ability to image the brain in vivo, and it is a remarkable shift from simple pathological description.[87] It allows for a more careful and targeted description of microlevel changes happening in the brain.

However, discovering and regulating imaging agents that can cross the blood–brain barrier posed quite an obstacle to researchers. It has been perhaps the single greatest hurdle in modern neuroimaging of Alzheimer's, and it is only just now beginning to be surmounted. The blood–brain barrier is a natural barrier in the body that keeps the "wrong" substances from entering the brain through the bloodstream. It is a regulatory and protective mechanism that also inhibits researchers from introducing any sort of functional imaging agent into the brain. Different imaging technologies offer different solutions to crossing the barrier, generally by way of a tracer or surrogate marker.

Broadly speaking, a surrogate marker or biomarker is an indication of a biological process, and biomarkers of Alzheimer's can indicate the presence of the disease or its progression. One way to think about biomarkers is as a kind of code or shorthand. High blood pressure might be a biomarker for heart disease, for example. Neuroimaging biomarkers, however, are somewhat more complicated in that they serve as a vehicle for the introduction of some other element that can itself be harmful (radioactivity, for example). As such, they require approval and active regulation by the U.S. Food and Drug Administration (FDA) in their use, itself a controversial process.[88] In PET imaging of Alzheimer's, for example, a radiotracer can be injected into the blood, where it circulates into the brain and, ideally, interacts with the neurological tissue under scrutiny. One of the first commonly used techniques was fluorodeoxyglucose-PET (FDG-PET), which can measure glucose metabolism.[89] In 2002 Pittsburgh compound B (PiB) became the first radiotracer to be able functionally to detect beta-amyloid plaques in the brain. Since then, other advances in PET imaging have allowed for targeted, effects-based research on amyloid—most notably florbetapir, which became the first radiotracer to be approved by the FDA in 2012, but also other compounds, such as florbetaben and flutemetamol.[90]

Developments in live neuroimaging like PET radiotracers were met with celebration and optimism at the turn of the century by scientists, politicians, and journalists alike, but they still face regulatory hurdles even today. One of the key regulatory roadblocks is the same one medical researchers have encountered for more than a century: the difficulty in making conclusive arguments about the relationship between amyloid plaques and clinical symptoms.[91] In other words, diagnostic neuroimaging continues to be a process only of exclusion, despite the many advances in neuroimaging technology. A 2013 joint task force on amyloid imaging sponsored by the Society of Nuclear Medicine and Molecular Imaging and the Alzheimer's Association recommended that amyloid PET technology not be a substitute for careful clinical evaluation. Beyond the issue of the "high prevalence of amyloid positivity in normal older individuals," the task force also concluded that "the clinical value of amyloid PET imaging is entirely dependent on the quality of the images and accuracy of interpretation."[92]

In other words, imaging technology is not a substitute for the skilled diagnostic expertise of the clinicians who are deploying the technology. Despite significant advances in neuroimaging technology, diagnostics and description continue to dominate the logic of neuroimaging. Scientists are fully aware of the tenuous nature of their results, but that instability is understood as an important stepping-stone to better research in the future.[93] Training, experimentation, and innovation are the keywords of the present, each crucial to public endorsement of research strategies.

Note, for example, the proleptic slippage between description and cure in the following sequence from the Emmy Award–winning PBS documentary *The Forgetting: A Portrait of Alzheimer's*. The narrator of the film and an Alzheimer's researcher who helped develop PiB, William Klunk, describe the importance of in vivo imaging:

NARRATOR: The small group of chemists at the University of Pittsburgh tested hundreds of compounds, and one after the other, they failed. But Dekosky's team was determined because they knew the only way to stop the coming epidemic is to speed up the process of finding effective drugs. And the only way to do that is to be able to see what's really happening inside the brain.

KLUNK: If you can see the enemy and you know what it's doing, you can
begin to see how your war against it is working. I'm hoping that this
will lead to a much more successful era in treatment, of early diagnosis, of learning how to prevent the disease, which as we know in all of
medicine, is a much better place to be than treating the disease.

Scientific authority situates proleptic success precisely in the representation of the living brain ("what's really happening"). While no cure or
cause is found, temporary successes in imaging the early presence of
the disease can help articulate the ongoing progress toward those goals.

Bringing It All Together:
The Alzheimer's Disease Neuroimaging Initiative

Scientists and clinicians currently employ a diversity of neuroimaging technologies in Alzheimer's research. Although economic restrictions might once have kept them out of all but the wealthiest of labs,
an increasingly specialized array of technologies have become more
common in both university and private research centers. Research
approaches are generally divided between structural and functional
techniques, and they often embrace molecular, effects-based research.[94]
Some also focus on the macro level of the brain, describing holistic
or localized theories of activity or progression. Microscopy has continued to be an important technique, though it has gone through patterns
of popularity in different fields. Electron microscopy, which experienced its heyday from the late 1950s until the early 1980s, fell out of
fashion for a time, only to be replaced by advancements in light microscopy, new fluorescent microscopy, and a truly expansive array of imaging strategies.[95]

In fact, the boundaries between something like microscopy and brain
scans are blurring as imaging platforms increasingly draw on a range
of different techniques for more targeted representational objectives.
No one technique or image paradigm dominates research, despite the
way in which public attention often focuses on specific studies or technologies.[96] These new neuroimaging techniques demand collaboration
because of complex research design and the specializations required

of neuroscience and its technologies of inquiry. Collaborative experimentation allows researchers to address specific representational challenges endemic to the research focus. Brain imaging should not and really cannot be practiced by one scientist any longer; instead, it requires the collaboration of a range of researchers in neuroscience but also clinicians, imaging professionals, and the technical and administrative staff required to operate these research centers. Furthermore, new knowledge around the brain emerges daily, and increasingly, interdisciplinary research requires an approach to sharing not just resources, but also data sets and subjects. Collaboration is often the logic of new approaches to Alzheimer's.[97] This growth also means that in theory, no single research center, no single disease, and no single discipline can claim research or funding priority.

The brain now functions as a kind of integrative backdrop for an emergent national neuroculture that embraces a broad spectrum of health, economics, and education. Celebrity health advocate Atul Gawande, speaking with President Barack Obama at the White House Frontiers Conference on innovation and the brain, offered his vision of a dynamic, neural research network:

> The last century was the century of the molecule. We were trying to—the power of reductionism—boil it down to the most small possible part: the atom, the gene, the neuron. Give me the drug, the device, the super-specialist. And that provided enormous good. But in this century . . . now we're trying to figure out: how do they all fit together? How do the neurons fit together to create the kinds of behaviors that you're trying to solve in mental illness? How do the genes network and fit together in genetics and epigenetics to account for the health and disease of the future that we all may face . . . trying to make a system that can actually bring it all together really is a completely different kind of science than the last century . . . surrounding these problems with people who come from incredibly different perspectives. . . . It really isn't the age of the hero scientist anymore.[98]

Gawande's vision was remarkable in that it described a synthesis of scientific labor and a model of brain function. The entire purpose of the conference, of course, was to generate optimism and excitement around brain innovation and research, part of the Obama administration's wider celebration of neuroscience and health care. Gawande's rhetorical model was ultimately about the historical integration of parts into a whole, from neurons to research questions to a national public. Successful science depends on the public's participation and endorsement, just as it requires public and private research collaboration.

In 2004 the NIA launched the ADNI as a means to coordinate neuroimaging research from diverse research centers under one collaborative umbrella. The initial five-year program was developed and funded with the aid of $67 million in funding provided by the NIA and partner organizations and the support of the Alzheimer's Association, the Institute for the Study of Aging, numerous pharmaceutical companies, the National Institute for Biomedical Imaging and Bioengineering, and the NIH. After the original study, another $91 million extended the study for an additional five years as ADNI 2, with a two-year interim bridge. ADNI 3, which began in 2016, was scheduled to run for another five years.[99] ADNI prides itself on remaining flexible through its staged progression, and it is able to incorporate innovation and advance into each of its different grant cycles.[100] The initiative draws together research institutions primarily from around the United States, but in recent years it has allowed the participation of international partners. The program is committed to the open ethic of advance, and any data generated by an ADNI study are freely available to researchers who qualify. Control over ADNI participation helps with the broader goal of standardization, a crucial prerequisite for interdisciplinary and collaborative work. According to the Foundation for the National Institutes of Health, there were more than 115 million downloads of ADNI data as of 2020, and that data has led to the publication of more than eighteen hundred papers.[101]

According to the principal investigator of the program, Michael Weiner, the primary goals of ADNI were "to determine the relationships among the clinical, cognitive, imaging, genetic, and biochemical biomarker characteristics of the entire spectrum of Alzheimer's disease as the pathology evolves from normal aging through very mild symptoms, to MCI, to dementia, and to establish standardized methods for imaging/biomarker collection and analysis for ultimate use in clinical trials."[102] Biomarkers can include anything from amyloid PET imaging to the measurement of cerebral atrophy to memory loss measured in a clinical exam.[103]

Crucial to the appeal for early diagnosis with a biomarker is the idea that neuroimaging can anticipate the disease before symptoms appear. Biomarkers are not reliant, therefore, on the recognition of symptom or behavior. This is a sign of a bigger trend in American psychiatry: translational neuroscience focused on biomarkers like genes and proteins dominates clinical research.[104] Even though assessment scales have advanced considerably since the pioneering work at Newcastle, they present a range of limitations that neuroimaging is thought by many to help solve. The surrogate biomarkers ADNI currently investigates are deemed a helpful replacement to cognitive testing for subject recruitment.[105]

Whether they are described naturally in the body (atrophy or genes) or introduced as a molecular tracer (PiB or florbetapir), biomarkers participate in the proleptic ethic of neuroscience. This is because biomarkers cannot entirely account for the presence of a disease; rather, they translate or indicate risk and incorporate or exclude bodies in the service of future research. As both an ideal and a material process, a biomarker can mediate and thus incorporate Alzheimer's earlier and earlier in life, offering value long before the appearance of any symptom. To study neurological change over time or develop prevention strategies, one must involve participants as early as possible, and early subject recruitment is a primary objective for Alzheimer's research.

From its inception, ADNI has recruited participants from the full spectrum of disease onset as well as presumably healthy controls. The director of ADNI actually appeared in a recruitment video on an early version of its website telling viewers that even he was participating in the study because he wanted to demonstrate that it was enjoyable and that the risks were low. The Alzheimer's Association has also helped enlist research participation; it is firmly committed to ADNI advance, claiming responsibility for the inclusion of amyloid PET studies.[106] It can be difficult, however, to enlist the public's support in medical research when they are not themselves dealing with the full-blown symptoms of dementia. A 2011 study found that while 89 percent of Americans would want a doctor to tell them if their symptoms of dementia were due to Alzheimer's disease, only 29 percent would want a diagnostic test before the appearance of any symptoms.[107] In this sense, enlisting healthy volunteers is more akin to a blood drive than a medical procedure. Symptomatic individuals, on the other hand, might be more eager to enlist in trials that could lead to a cure.

ADNI's broad descriptive goal of locating and describing biomarkers is of course fundamentally tied to therapy, and one central goal is drug and treatment development. Only a limited number of FDA-approved drugs are available for people with Alzheimer's, most of them cholinesterase inhibitors, which slow or prevent the breakdown of acetylcholine in the brain. This ostensibly aids cognitive function. While sales and prescriptions for these drugs are strong, their effects are limited. Also, some of the drugs are now available in a generic form, which lessens the value of the original brand. Those facts and the lack of a cure mean the pharmaceutical industry has seen the market for new medications as a "tremendous opportunity."[108] Biomarkers are often seen as essential to new drug research, as the employment of biomarkers in clinical trials can reduce sample sizes and observation time, which can speed new drugs through the pipeline.[109]

In 2021 the FDA approved the first drug to directly target amyloid in the brain, an intravenous therapy made by Biogen called aducanumab (or ADUHELM). Critics attacked the move on the very basis that Biogen's trials did not show a valid clinical benefit. Instead, approval was based on the biomarker-promise of amyloid reduction. There was widespread denunciation of the move. Several scientists even resigned from the committee that was tasked with advising the FDA in protest of the approval. One of them said, "This might be the worst approval decision the FDA has made that I can remember." Another wrote, "Biomarker justification for approval in the absence of consistent clinical benefit after 18 months of treatment is indefensible."[110]

Therapeutics aside, biomarkers seem to many to offer great promise for making Alzheimer's research more efficient. In 2011 the NIA and

Alzheimer's Association released a jointly sponsored update on the criteria for the diagnosis of Alzheimer's that echoed the new era of research priorities. This—the first major update since the 1984 clinical recommendations—was perhaps most notable for the new diagnostic categories, including a preclinical stage and MCI. These new categories were designed to allow for people to participate in studies even if they have minor symptoms or even no symptoms at all; instead biomarkers are a sufficient standard of inclusion. However, the working group charged with the use of biomarkers in diagnostic criteria indicated that there was very little consensus as to clinical applicability. Given ADNI prioritization of subject recruitment as well as early disease intervention or prevention, the separation of clinical viability from biomarkers employed for "pure research purposes" seems like a necessary compromise.[111] ADNI continues to support increasingly diverse interventions into biomarker research, from new tau radiotracers to home computer diagnostics. As more organizations both contribute to and utilize ADNI data, the opportunities for biomarker research continue to expand.[112]

Since the late 1970s, then, the U.S. government has been central to coordinating imaging technologies within Alzheimer's research. As clinical data grew in importance and interest in in vivo neuroimaging began to translate into viable technology, the histological gaze faded into a broader constellation of neuroimaging practice. Instead of just focusing on people with advanced symptoms, researchers seek to enlist a significantly broader population that may or may not one day get Alzheimer's. The inclusion of a presymptomatic body is underwritten both empirically and ideologically by government-led neuroimaging projects performed specifically in the interest of national welfare. While caregiving continues to be a key interest for funding, it is overwhelmed both financially and ideologically by the now entrenched tradition of biomedical research, ever emboldened by the promise of a cure.

ADNI marks the natural culmination of U.S. prioritization of particular neuroimaging strategies in Alzheimer's research, just as the incorporation of an aging American public within the diagnostic gaze marks the realization of Alzheimer's disease as a national crisis. While the initiative organizes some research not related to "visual technologies" per se (blood or cerebrospinal biomarkers, bioinformatics, etc.), ADNI frames neuroimaging as epistemologically and rhetorically primary. Along with the 2013 BRAIN Initiative,[113] the other large public–private partnership in neurorepresentation, ADNI rides a trend of descriptive and translational neuroscience in the service of national innovation and expertise. Though ADNI is gradually becoming more global in reach, funding and collaboration clearly orient the initiative as a national priority. For example, the $24 million of funding required for the interim years between ADNI 1 and ADNI 2 (what was called ADNI GO) actually came from stimulus funds from the American Recovery Act. Outside of national policy, funding, and organization organized around the search for cause and cure, the federal government has invested in imaging technologies through an emphasis on innovation, deregulation, and insurance reimbursement practices.[114] As former secretary of health and human services Kathleen Sebelius described about the plan to fight Alzheimer's, "this is a national plan—not a federal one, because reducing the burden of Alzheimer's will require the active engagement of both the public and private sectors."[115]

Despite transnational research partnerships, collaborative advocacy, and the discourse of a universal threat, the disease takes on a uniquely American status in its public life. I will continue to address the dialectic of the disease's local and universal characteristics throughout the remainder of this book, but it is worth pointing out now that the broad visibility of Alzheimer's as a viable threat marks the emergence of its national character. This is not simply because Americans see Alzheimer's as a threat to their families and communities but also because the cure is articulated through a vision of American advance through economic investment, STEM education, and technological innovation.

In 2013 President Obama announced the Brain Research through Advancing Innovative Technologies (BRAIN) Initiative, a national, public–private research collaboration in neuroscience and technology. Its basic goal was anything but simple: to comprehensively describe how the brain works at the micro and macro scales—essentially to map

the activity of the human brain. The initiative promised "to help unlock the mysteries of the brain, to improve our treatment of conditions like Alzheimer's and autism and to deepen our understanding of
how we think, learn and remember."[116] Linked ideologically to national
ambitions like the human genome project, Obama described the initiative as much as a way to secure jobs and promote education as
an investment in health and technology. While some of the research
attached to the initiative specifically addressed Alzheimer's, the participants were in fact quite diverse, from Google to the National Football
League. It received support from obvious interests, such as the NIH,
FDA, NSF, and several philanthropic and private organizations, but also
from perhaps more unlikely contributors, such as the Defense Advanced
Research Projects Agency and the Intelligence Advanced Research Projects Activity.

The BRAIN Initiative readily adopts the proleptic stance common to
neuroscientific research through its mapping and descriptive efforts.
However, it is unclear precisely how researchers will eventually be able
to make use of the data that is currently being generated. Because of
that fact, the BRAIN Initiative has been controversial since its inception. Many see the challenge of mapping the brain as a hopeless waste
of money and warn that we lack the analytic tools to deal with such
a mass of data.[117] However, others see national investments in STEM
education and media technology as a hopeful correlative to the preliminary stages of data collection.

For example, at the 2016 White House Frontiers Conference, the
neuroscientist Kafui Dzirasa described new research within the BRAIN
Initiative that could one day help with Alzheimer's. He addressed the
need for more expertise to eventually help coordinate the data, but he
did so within a narrative of generational, media advance:

Within twenty-four hours, he's pulling in about twenty terabytes of data,
alright? So I'm not that old, I remember when I was in high school and
my hard drive had a hundred megabytes of data. So we're at a place now
where we're gonna have to bring in other disciplines to know how to
handle that data. I sat with a high school kid last night, Gabe, and it was

pretty clear to me that the people who are gonna solve this challenge of the brain are probably in seventh or eighth grade right now, right? So how do we create an ecosystem where all those different perspectives can come in?[118]

What are the consequences of such a deferral? What does it mean to endow such a media ecosystem with a national narrative of capacity, progress, and promise, and then to live amid that dream? As the nation orchestrates economic and educational goals through brain innovation and brain expertise, it seems a solution to the brain's ills can only be discovered through a national embrace of neuroculture in all its manifestations.[119]

3

Use It or Lose It

Affirming the Self, Defining the Person

The proleptic industry of Alzheimer's neuroimaging—the diagnostic, descriptive, and mapping efforts of a seemingly ever more complex brain—serves as the leading force of a much broader, national fight against Alzheimer's. Investments in neuroscience like the BRAIN Initiative and the Decade of the Brain have overlapped with the prioritization of dementia research, making the cure for Alzheimer's a challenge for science akin to the moon landing. But instead of outward to space, we look inward, to our own living selves. In the public life of the neuroimaginary, science fights a war against an enemy potentially hiding inside us all, a battle with a national threat for the sake of a collective future.

A century ago, that battle was fought by just a few psychiatrists in a laboratory, peering into a microscope, but over the last forty years, Alzheimer's has developed into one of the defining problems of aging in the United States. In 2012, in the wake of the National Alzheimer's Project Act (NAPA), President Obama mandated the delivery of an effective treatment for the disease by 2025. That mandate now looks like a stretch. Despite several new drugs in the pipeline, the daily drumbeat of pharmaceutical promise has met with an unfortunate litany of failures.[1] Pharmaceutical treatments for symptoms of dementia have been found to be modest or ineffective at best (and lethal or harmful at worst).[2] Cure aside, the estimated costs to develop a single treatment for Alzheimer's are $5.6 billion spread over thirteen years, and the success rate of trials for disease-modifying agents is 0.4 percent.[3] Globally, there were more than fifty thousand different scientific publications related to Alzheimer's disease from 2014 to 2018 alone, with roughly one-third of those authored in the United States.[4] The NIH tripled its funding for Alzheimer's research over that same time period.[5] But despite all of the money and effort put into research, there is still no known cause, and there is no cure.

The public visibility of the disease increases daily just as the diagnostic net grows wider. The coexistence of that public culture and a relatively high prevalence helps situate the disease as an epidemic in the public eye. Alzheimer's is now the most feared disease in the country.[6] Medical and media professionals continue to describe, detect, and diagnose in a kind of representational holding pattern, mapping ever wider circles of incidence; ever more detailed pictures of pathology; and increasing narratives of sustenance, love, and pain. It takes an immense affective engagement, a national optimism articulated over the labor of sustaining care, to keep that representational initiative aloft.

Because the disease has no known cause or cure, the space of description and diagnosis is immensely broad. As Paula Treichler points out in her analysis of AIDS, an epidemic will always supersede the boundaries of scientific discourse, producing "a parallel epidemic of meanings, definitions, and attributions . . . an epidemic of signification."[7] The same might be said of Alzheimer's, but this signifying epidemic is reductive and collusive, orienting the disease within supposed universals like aging and threatened memory. Unlike AIDS or other well-publicized conditions for which that discourse often enforces the minoritarian or disenfranchised status of those affected, Alzheimer's seems to be situated as if it is in everyone's future. Despite higher incidence in the Unites States in communities of color, among women, and among people without money, education, and other resources, and despite the pervasive, othering stigma of lost selfhood, Alzheimer's erases most discourse of difference under narratives of aging, risk, and loss. As I have argued earlier in this book, whether Alzheimer's disease is actually an inevitable or normal part of aging is a controversial debate, and groups like the Alzheimer's Association have worked very hard to articulate it as an abnormal disease that can and must be cured. Regardless of etiology, however, the risk of Alzheimer's is increasingly a fact that all Americans are asked to live with as a part of everyday aging and modern life.

Indeed, Alzheimer's threatens not only the fiscal, emotional, and social welfare of individual aging people but also the nation at large. Awareness campaigns from the Alzheimer's Association and the NIA and language and initiatives from NAPA share a mutual focus on the burgeoning epidemic, offering risk data linked to arbitrary dates that U.S. citizens can map onto their own futures. For example, the Alzheimer's Association's dire warnings are now a rote element of its outreach: "The graying of America means the bankrupting of America—and Alzheimer's is a major reason why. . . . Unless something is done, the costs of Alzheimer's in 2050 are estimated to total $1.1 trillion (in today's dollars). Costs to Medicare and Medicaid will increase nearly 500 percent."[8] In other words, the universal threat of Alzheimer's is also a threat to national economic welfare. This kind of discourse is quite common. The "graying of America" is usually oriented as a generational claim, foregrounding the experience of U.S. baby boomers in particular. Alzheimer's is an unknowable and incurable epidemic that is futuristically, functionally equivalent to aging itself, and it needs to be stopped or the country will not survive.

Despite the nationalizing discourse around disease threat, the war on Alzheimer's has moved forward since the late 1970s because of a variety of independent and private actors, often working together, but each trying to address the disease in its own way. Of course, this collaborative, all-hands-on-deck approach is common to disease research, and significant funding has in fact come from various federal agencies, but the U.S. government has largely taken its cues for disease management and research from independent interests. As a consequence, the entire Alzheimer's public health apparatus now depends on a network of different corporate, academic, and philanthropic agencies for progress. This is arguably a positive development in the history of the disease. As I explained in the last chapter, one of the greatest success stories in the war on Alzheimer's has been the collaboration and data pooling afforded by the ADNI.

Beyond disease research, however, a different kind of privatization shapes health care at the level of the individual citizen. In the absence of a cure, Alzheimer's is very much a disease for which aging Americans are asked to take responsibility as a part of successful aging. A public health industry of proactive self-care now caters to individuals who live with cautious fear of the disease, an industry primarily dedicated to cognitive health and wellness. This public investment in private agencies is what is sometimes called "governmentality." Governmentality refers to the idea that we are governed by the exercise of our freedoms and agencies and, in particular, through our self-awareness and self-improvement: what Foucault called technologies of the self.[9] Agencies of the self are also directed to the stability of society, as the maintenance of a healthy self is useful for a great many social and economic interests.[10]

Alzheimer's complicates self-care, however, because what is understood to be at risk is the self itself: one's identity, values, and mind and the cognitive powers that help shape and empower that self. In this case, practices of self-management and optimization ironically *reinforce* the power or threat of Alzheimer's, just as they ostensibly help mitigate disease risk.[11] In the fight against Alzheimer's, as you work to preserve or improve a self, you raise the importance of that self in the economy of everyday living, making the disease that much more impactful. As Nikolas Rose explains, "on the one hand our very personhood is increasingly being defined by others, and by ourselves, in terms of our contemporary understandings of the possibilities and limits of our corporeality. On the other hand, our somatic individuality has become opened up to choice, prudence, and responsibility, to experimentation, to contestation. This, then, is the problem space that defines the biopolitics of our contemporary emergent form of life."[12] That biopolitical formation is actively conditioned by Alzheimer's because the perceived self that Alzheimer's attacks forms the very rationally, responsibly, and cognitively oriented somatic individuality that the biopolitical formation requires as the condition of membership.[13] This paradox of Alzheimer's personhood is a kind of limit case for the "problem space" that Rose describes. It indicates a complex biopolitics of self-care germane to Alzheimer's risk culture, made even more complex by the ways "our corporeality" is increasingly fashioned, tracked, and imagined through media technology.

This chapter explores the contemporary risk culture of Alzheimer's in the United States and its relationship to media and cognitive health. Public health and advocacy campaigns have been quite successful in spreading disease awareness over the last forty years, but a confusing mixture of fear, promise, and agency now occupies the space created by the absence of a cure or successful treatment. I first show how different forms of media have shaped the universal threat of the disease, putting pressure on all aging Americans to care for themselves. I then explore different technologies used for self-empowerment and cognitive health, paying particular attention to "brain games" marketed by companies like Lumosity. It is precisely through cultures and technologies of media that aging Americans are sold agency in the fight against Alzheimer's. This risk culture also has an interesting side effect—a burgeoning genre of interactive media that simulate the symptoms of dementia. The chapter concludes by describing these virtual reality technologies designed to create empathy for people with Alzheimer's.

Take a Walk, Eat a Pistachio: Self-Affirmation and Risk

The historical biomedicalization of aging is probably most responsible for the expansion of the threat of Alzheimer's.[14] Age is understood as a primary risk factor for Alzheimer's. In fact, every major national organization focused on Alzheimer's, from the Centers for Disease Control and Prevention to the NIH to the Alzheimer's Association, now lists age as *the* main risk factor. This means anyone who expects to grow older could potentially get this disease. A significant component of public health outreach is making people aware of that risk, especially because there is no cure or effective therapy.[15] Whether the message is demonstrating the urgency of the epidemic, helping people get an earlier diagnosis to prepare for care, or urging citizens to commit to a better national policy and research agenda, the primary public health

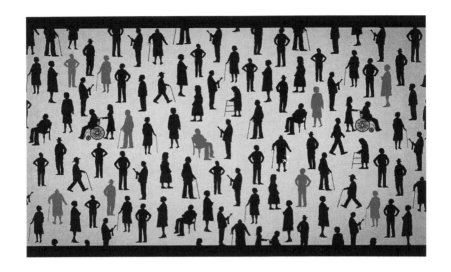

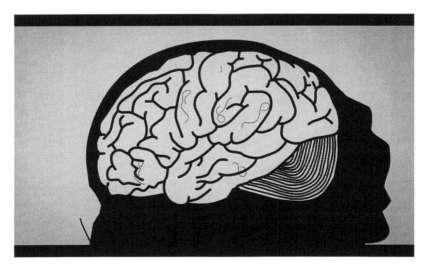

FIGURE 3. Stills from *What Is Alzheimer's?*, a film sponsored by the MetLife Foundation and the Alliance for Aging Research. http://aboutalz.org/.

message of the last forty years has been at the diagnostic and informational level. Get tested, know the signs, and spread the message, because the disease can affect anyone.

A good example of the scale of this kind of messaging can be seen in a series of Alzheimer's awareness videos sponsored by the MetLife Foundation and the Alliance for Aging Research.[16] Dubbed "pocket films," the animated series covers a range of topics, including caregiving, new developments in scientific research, and the genetics of Alzheimer's. The first film, *What Is Alzheimer's?*, relies on a graphic composition that alternates between a picture of a single brain and a picture of several small stick figures indicating the general population. The brain sections depict how Alzheimer's affects the brain, while the population sections show who can be affected. Illustrations of wheelchairs, canes, and walkers orient this threatened population as old and physically disabled, as these are the only defining characteristics in an otherwise simple graphic composition. The video renders the possibility of difference moot, focusing instead on the way in which the disease can seemingly attack any older person. Some of the bodies turn from black to blue, symbolizing that those people now have the disease. Then the video zooms in on the brain of one blue figure with Alzheimer's and shows how the disease progressively damages its brain. The effect of this animation strategy is to give all viewers the best chance to identify with the threat because it avoids any biological characteristics constitutive of difference other than aging brains and bodies.

The paradox of this kind of normalization is that it manages to articulate Alzheimer's as both insidiously aggressive as a disease condition and also truly banal in the way it can affect anyone. Because of the focus on age, other risk factors of Alzheimer's, such as gender, race, and class, are largely occluded from public discourse, even if that diversity is a representational focus. In other words, despite public health campaigns that target some of these different groups, they only augment the narrative of universal risk rather than detracting from it.[17] Narratives of people with Alzheimer's generally follow rules of racial, class, and gender harmony: they're just normal, middle-class old people behaving oddly. These normal people could be any person anywhere: they could be you, your friend, or someone in your family.

Given widespread fear of the disease, Americans increasingly live out their lives in cautious relationships with Alzheimer's, whether or not it directly impacts them. Risk management is an important aspect of healthy living. As the philanthropic organization Alzheimer's Foundation of America (AFA) suggests, "being proactive is a vital step on your journey towards successful aging."[18] Joseph Dumit has argued that health messaging like this encourages people to reconfigure their personal relationships to disease such that "rather than illness punctuating ordinary life, the everyday conceals illness."[19] Furthermore, the use of the goal-oriented language of gerontology in this context (successful aging) indicates that there are good and bad ways of dealing with that risk.[20] This naturalization of disease risk within normal aging invokes a kind of inevitability to Alzheimer's, but it also imposes responsibility on a person to monitor herself in the right manner to prevent it.[21]

Popular medical culture interprets the risk of Alzheimer's in a variety of ways, but it is most active in medically themed talk shows. For example, the daytime television program *The Dr. Oz Show* aired a special on Alzheimer's called "What's Your Risk?" that strongly advocated for diagnostics as a form of social responsibility.[22] Standing in front of a giant model of a brain, host Dr. Mehmet Oz claimed, "Incredible new advances are allowing us to detect Alzheimer's years before you show symptoms. Could you have Alzheimer's right now and not even know it? Well today I'll tell you what you need to know to find out if you're at risk." The show introduced Dr. P. Murali Doraiswamy, author of the 2008 self-help manual *The Alzheimer's Action Plan,* head of Duke University's biological psychiatry division, and a senior fellow at Duke's Center for the Study of Aging. Dr. Doraiswamy and Dr. Oz sat on either side of a large television monitor that showed PET images of "control" brains and "Alzheimer's" brains, and they discussed the various risk factors for Alzheimer's. The message in the television show was that early diagnosis is the best practice for individuals but also for science. In response to Dr. Oz's question about the significance of a PET scan diagnosis, Doraiswamy cited two primary benefits: first, your contribution helps doctors make more accurate diagnoses because you enhance the data pool, and second, your diagnosis helps you, because early detection can lead to earlier intervention and therapy. What is not made clear in this conversation is the fact that therapy is also still in development, so the latter benefit is tabled, while research science is the beneficiary of the diagnostic contract.[23]

Like the ADNI recruitment language described in chapter 2, the message in "What's Your Risk?" belongs to a trend in diagnostic citizenship where individual participation is encouraged for the betterment of science and national health. It is especially important in the context of recent developments in precision medicine, where genetic recruitment is understood to be central to success. The public face of the NIH's Precision Medicine Initiative—a.k.a. All of Us—is entirely focused on recruitment: "The All of Us Research Program is a historic effort to gather data from one million or more people living in the United States to accelerate research and improve health."[24] Convincing people, especially those people who have been historically disenfranchised by biomedicine, to forfeit their health privacy can be tricky,[25] but this individual choice is framed as a civic virtue: "we are actively partnering with others to create a groundbreaking national research resource platform." All of Us is a part of a broad effort to shape health civics, where Americans are urged to "Sync for Science" or "Sync for Genes" regardless of their illness status.[26] Taken in this context, understanding your own risk for Alzheimer's is a form of self-care but is also a way to take part in the national fight against Alzheimer's. In both senses, risk culture creates a kind of agency.

Given the long odds on a cure for Alzheimer's, however, participatory diagnostics requires an optimistic if not celebratory relationship with biomedicine. Alzheimer's author, activist, and advocate Richard Taylor, who was diagnosed with "dementia of the Alzheimer's type," is worth quoting at length on this subject. Before his death in 2015, Taylor was one of the more outspoken proponents of nonmedical interventions into dementia care and a vocal opponent of the way funding is consistently funneled into biomedical research. His frustration with biomedicine is evident in the following paragraph, taken from one of his monthly e-newsletters:

> If we were able to image and predict dementia early enough we could try to sell Mom's new vitamins, pills, treatments which would /might/ perhaps avoid/postpone/eliminate the chance that their embryo would grow into someone living with the symptoms of dementia? Of course, this rush to the brain photo machines at the end of the Mall ignores the fact that for 25 plus years we have been spending time, effort, and money trying to find treatments, and so far the best we can offer people is "maybes, some people seem," a dozen nude mice living in stage 1–11 of dementia, maybe/probably of the maybe/probably Alzheimer's type benefited from early identification found some subjectively based (but they do have numbers attached to them) evidence of some form of help, some part of the time, but not everyone, every time.[27]

Taylor attacks the promise of biomedicine precisely because it is (still) only a promise. As someone living with dementia, Taylor was understandably far more interested in prioritizing research on care. His argument, however, points toward an important crisis in the establishment logic of diagnosis: because of limitations on resources, it can disenfranchise the very people it is designed to support, and it shows how biomedical optimism might actually be at odds with best-care practices. Instead of focusing on the needs of people with dementia now, this kind of research prioritizes the future, bringing whole populations into anticipatory relationships with Alzheimer's. Many would argue that early diagnosis is in fact a form of preemptive care or that the research–care relationship is not a zero-sum game the way Taylor suggests. Regardless, his argument is evidence of an active debate on the prioritization of proactive screenings and early diagnosis.

While the neuroimaging industry is still the authority in diagnostic culture, many screenings for Alzheimer's can be performed more informally (if not cheaply). For example, the AFA used to sponsor a "national screening day," but now it offers year-round, free, virtual screenings for anyone who wants one. The organization recommends these screenings for anyone worried about her memory but also for anyone concerned about successful aging more generally. These kinds of screenings are performed by medical professionals with a combination of questions and tests. And while not as common, screenings can also be completed by a physician as a part of simple wellness checkups, as many instruments that test for Alzheimer's can be finished in fewer than ten minutes.[28]

Initial neuropsychological assessment may include questions about personal history or popular culture interspersed with interference tasks. They often include tests of visuospatial abilities. For example, the well-known clock-drawing test is one of the older screening tools still in use.[29] Participants are asked to draw a clock with all of the numbers on it, and then draw hands that designate certain times on the face of the clock. Another common test, the Montreal Cognitive Assessment (MoCA), differentiates between normal cognitive health, MCI, and more serious dementia.[30] Along with short-term memory and visuospatial abilities, it tests attention, concentration, and language use. Sometimes family members or caregivers are asked about a person's abilities and behaviors as a part of these tests.

MoCA fell under public scrutiny during the 2020 presidential campaign when President Trump celebrated his performance on the test as evidence of his mental capacities. This came during a time when both presidential candidates were frequently accused of having Alzheimer's. But rather than as a simple screening test used to exclude dementia, Trump seemed to interpret his MoCA score as an indication of his formidable intelligence, a topic that had long been a point of interest to him. In a series of interviews, he boasted about his ability to remember five words in order: person, woman, man, camera, and TV. This string of words became something of a comedic cultural meme, and many mocked him for bragging about passing an Alzheimer's test.[31] Even the conservative Fox News reporter Chris Wallace challenged Trump, telling him in an interview, "Well, it's not the hardest test. They have a picture and it says 'What's that?' And it's an elephant."[32] Because this was such a well-publicized moment, a relatively unknown cognitive test to diagnose Alzheimer's became part of a broader public conversation about cognitive health. Regardless of political affiliation, the U.S. public was asked to evaluate the specific diagnostic value of a test like MoCA as part of the voting process.

A 2014 U.S. Preventive Services Task Force found that while these kinds of screenings can detect dementia in moderate cases, their perceived benefits are offset by lack of standardization and reproducibility. There is also little evidence as to how the screenings themselves affect those being tested.[33] While cognitive tests and interviews have dominated the history of clinical evaluation—often in tandem with neuroimaging—most physicians would complete a more thorough evaluation of a person's overall health before making any kind of diagnosis.

A more infrequent form of screening for Alzheimer's is accomplished through genetic tests. There are genetic links to both early- and late-onset Alzheimer's, but genetic testing has historically been associated with early-onset familial Alzheimer's. One might imagine that the aura of determinacy that accompanies genetics would elevate its importance in Alzheimer's risk culture. That can sometimes be true. One study of children of parents diagnosed with Alzheimer's actually found that genetics was *de-emphasized* as a theme in clinical settings. Respondents were more concerned with the everyday difficulties of caregiving than with their own future diagnoses.[34] Rather than definitively excluding genetics as a source of fear of Alzheimer's, this study points toward the ways familial risk can be folded into everyday disease management and successful aging.

While familial Alzheimer's figures actively in the news media, it does not often merit outsized status in the public reception of Alzheimer's risk. This is especially true now that genetic links have been identified to both early- and late-onset Alzheimer's, muddying the narrative of early-onset determinacy.[35] One of the more well-known genetic research narratives regards an extended family living near Medellín, Colombia. Because a high proportion of the family has had dementia at an early age, as the *New York Times* puts it, they are "center stage in a potentially groundbreaking assault on Alzheimer's."[36] The large scale of the study offers promise for research into both early- and late-onset Alzheimer's. While the Colombia research study is a special case

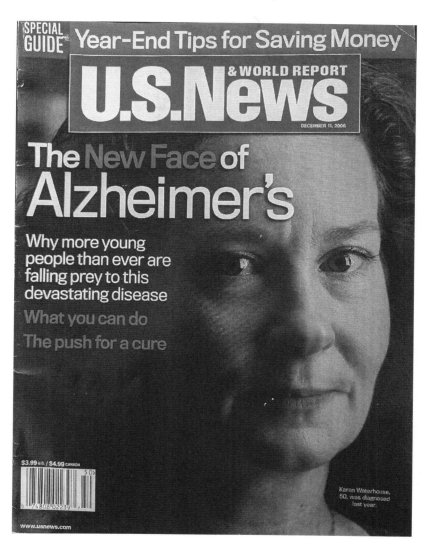

SPECIAL GUIDE Year-End Tips for Saving Money

U.S.News & WORLD REPORT

DECEMBER 11, 2006

The New Face of Alzheimer's

Why more young people than ever are falling prey to this devastating disease

What you can do

The push for a cure

$3.99 U.S. / $4.99 CANADA

Karen Waterhouse, 50, was diagnosed last year.

www.usnews.com

FIGURE 4. "The New Face of Alzheimer's," cover of *U.S. News and World Report*, December 11, 2006.

that may lead to new therapies, it does not shift the more powerful narrative of Alzheimer's in the United States as a disease of older adults. Historically, news media reports like these have often balanced warnings of disease threat with hype around promising new research. For example, *U.S. News and World Report* published a cover story in 2006 with the headline "The New Face of Alzheimer's: Why More Young People than Ever Are Falling Prey to This Devastating Disease."[37] The ominous cover depicted a fifty-year-old woman staring directly into the camera, but the story inside the magazine described promising new research on genetic links to the disease.

Stories about genetics are only one way the news media plays a central role in shaping Alzheimer's risk culture. Another common theme in the news is pharmaceutical research and the promise and failures of drug trials. Given the ongoing problems with these trials, however, the more dominant trend in the news of the last two decades has been stories about ways to prevent disease onset.[38] Given the instability of disease etiology, the message is overwhelmingly broad. What follows is a partial list of purported risk factors for Alzheimer's, along with a list of ways to mitigate those risks. Despite their length, these lists are in no way comprehensive; rather, they simply suggest the vast and contradictory territory of risk management. I gathered the data for these lists from a range of reports in the popular U.S. media and from books in the genre of Alzheimer's prevention.[39]

Purported Causes/Risk Factors

> age
> sex
> genes
> hard hits to the head
> football, sports in general
> physical inactivity
> smoking
> depression
> low education
> hypertension

obesity
poor diet (high fat, low vegetable intake)
diabetes
alcohol consumption
gingivitis
poor balance
iron
copper
zinc
aluminum
tap water
infections
inflammation
poor sleep habits or bad sleep
sleep apnea
cities
stress
solitude

Prevention Claims

DIET

folic acid
vitamin B_{12}
omega-3 fatty acids
vitamin E
ginkgo biloba
niacin
coenzyme Q10
turmeric
Mediterranean diet
berries
dark chocolate
cinnamon
curry

fish

whole grains

yeast

peanuts

pistachios

pecans

cashews

almonds

green, yellow, red vegetables

spinach

brussels sprouts

cauliflower

meats

low-fat diary

green, white, and oolong teas

coffee

coconut oil

anti-inflammatories

asprin

Motrin

statins

wine, beer, liquor

resveratrol

ACTIVITIES

cooking

reading

needlepoint, knitting

flossing

treadmills

brain exercises

puzzles

riddles

board games

cards
bridge
crossword puzzles
sudoku
sleep
friends
aerobic exercise
gardening
cleaning
chores
strength training
yoga
tai chi
walking
biking
hiking
swimming
volunteer work
religious services
donating blood
marriage
nature
anything new or novel
sense of purpose in life
being a boss
hard work
being sensitive, aware of your surroundings

These self-help lists are quite broad and at times even contradictory. They seem to include almost any aspect of modern life. None of these activities includes any of the regulated treatments, such as FDA-approved pharmaceuticals or biologics (like estrogen replacement therapy) or technological implants (such as electric brain stimulation). Indeed, what is central about these lists is that they are steps that can be taken without professional medical assistance, but they are still medicalized.

Prevention discourse like this promotes consumerism as a form of agency, foremost through references to preventive tactics that one can purchase but also because these strategies are actively marketed to readers in the form of self-help books, news stories, and talk shows. What makes this form of marketing all the more insidious is that in 2010, the NIH published the results of a special study, widely reported in the national news, that made clear that there is no evidence that anything can prevent, delay, or deter the onset of Alzheimer's disease.[40] This language was retained explicitly in the NIA website through the next decade, even as the NIA also expressed optimism about research trials in various stages of completion.[41] Because no one wants to give up hope, and because many prevention strategies are otherwise understood as healthy, this kind of optimism against evidence is normalized.

But given the vagaries of the claims, the responsibility to decide which of these steps to take is up to you, the consumer. The choices about which behaviors to adopt can be difficult, even contradictory. Take, for example, the following advice offered by Oprah.com:

Q: What about caffeine—good or bad?
A: A 2009 study done in Finland found that subjects who drank three to five cups of coffee a day had a 65 percent lower risk of dementia and Alzheimer's. But too much coffee makes it hard to sleep, and sleep is important for brain health. Moderation is key.[42]

Should we all start drinking three to five cups of coffee a day? Or is this advice simply affirming coffee as a lifestyle choice? How is a person to decide? Websites like CognitiveVitality.org and CognitiveTraining Data.org offer users tools to make better choices about cognitive consumerism, "empowering you to make informed decisions about your brain health."[43] Websites like these do not debate that cognitive health is important but rather more simply advise that consumers might need help deciding how best to optimize their brain health strategy. It is unclear how much consumers actually rely on these tools. Both websites operate under the guise of consumer responsibility, but each also directs users to its own research on brain health. CognitiveTraining Data.org, for example, is run by Michael Merzenich, author of the self-help manual *Soft-Wired: How the New Science of Brain Plasticity Can Change Your Life.* CognitiveVitality.org is run by the Alzheimer's Drug Discovery Foundation. So while hope is still lodged in the promise of the pharmaceutical miracle, that hope is increasingly integrated into the practices of responsible, healthy living.

An enormous number of tools are now available to cognitive consumers, all marketed as simple ways to take charge of your own future. As the Alzheimer's Association quips, "Maintain Your Brain!" What has changed most dramatically in the last decade of Alzheimer's outreach is the *you*. "You"—the patient, the individual, and the citizen—are increasingly responsible for a healthy brain in the face and fear of an epidemic. "You" are charged doubly in this pastoral model of biopolitics. "You" can be lodged in the brain's claims on selfhood—this is an identitarian claim. And "you" are responsible for maintaining and taking care of that brain—this is an orientation of social responsibility. The enfoldment of these neuroselves creates an ambiguous regulatory space where Alzheimer's, still a medical mystery, lurks in the background of everyday life. Given the diversity and ubiquity of risk mitigators, the central question then becomes not simply how much choice consumers have, but how much their own cognitive capacities are integrated into that pastoral responsibility.

Despite the warnings that nothing has been shown to prevent Alzheimer's, cognitive enhancement theories proliferate, and the media continues to report them, marketing optimism and responsibility in the face of an epidemic: optimism because the situation is perceived to be so dire, and responsibility because we are obliged to maintain our own threatened selfhood. As Dr. Oz affirms, "this is a disease that we all fear . . . but you actually have a ton more control than you think you do through the lifestyle we keep talking about."[44] In other words, we can live with or even thrive under conditions of risk—rather than defeating or fatalistic, risk culture can actually be empowering, even enjoyable.[45]

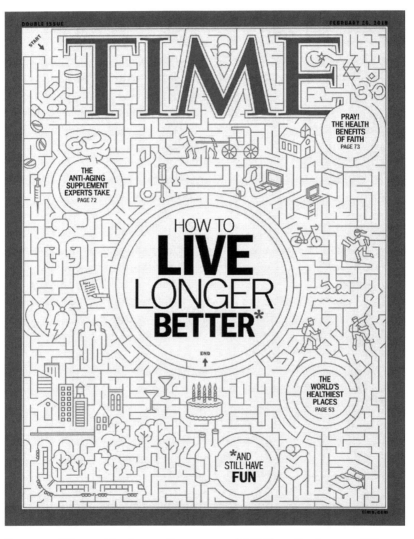

Figure 5. "How to Live Longer Better . . . and Still Have Fun," cover of *Time*, February 26, 2018.

In 2018, *Time* magazine published a special issue on aging with a maze on the front cover, titled "How to Live Longer Better . . . and Still Have Fun."[46] Reflecting on the burgeoning culture of cognitive health, various icons are sprinkled throughout the maze, including pictures of a brain, pills, outdoor activities, religious icons, relationships, and so on. The editors literalize "successful aging" and the idea that risk management can be entertaining: "for this week's cover on how to live a longer, fuller life, we created an actual puzzle: the first interactive cover in TIME's 94-year history. By solving it, you'll discover some of the many healthy-aging secrets that are tucked inside this double issue." Inside the magazine, articles on dying and a promising new Alzheimer's drug are surrounded by articles on lifestyle changes and the "good life." Perspectives like these show how the risk of Alzheimer's can be oddly affirming of everyday modern life—to someone who, say, likes to play video games, socialize, or do crossword puzzles. That claim does not dismiss the fear or horror of Alzheimer's; rather, it is dependent on it. In the culture of risk management, cognitive consumerism is often a process of self-affirmation, a redoubling of cognitive value that does not put an undue burden on your own cognitive capacities. If it's good for you, why not?

Brain Training: The Promise of Cognitive Reserve

One of the more popular forms of Alzheimer's prevention is cognitive training, popularly known as brain training. There is a lack of evidence that it actually prevents disease onset, but in 2017 the National Academies of Sciences, Engineering, and Medicine issued a report identifying cognitive training as one of three prevention areas with "encouraging but inconclusive evidence."[47] A member of the committee that issued the report warned, "Many people assume that cognitive training means computer based brain games. It's a much more complicated intervention than just sitting at the computer by yourself." Despite admonitions like this, digital brain training has harnessed significant public interest in the past decade. And exactly because the evidence on how they work is so "complicated," all manner of digital interventions are marketed as tools for cognitive health.

Popular online media apps include Mindfit, CogniFit, LearningRx, Peak, or AARP's Staying Sharp, but the most well-known and perhaps controversial brain-training program of the last two decades is Lumosity.[48] Lumosity is an internet-based platform that runs on a laptop, tablet, or other screen device. It offers users the chance to interact in daily puzzles, games, or other exercises based on specific cognitive improvements they wish to make. Lumosity emerged out of Silicon Valley techno-utopias around 2005, so its emphasis on improving productivity in a digital environment should not be surprising. As of 2020, it claimed more than one hundred million registered users and that it was collaborating with more than one hundred "leading researchers, clinicians, and teachers" in the improvement of its techniques.[49] Access is free for basic use, but paid memberships allow better tracking of results and more diverse training tools. The tracking is key to its membership structure, as Lumosity claims to tailor its games specifically to your own needs and desires. This tracking also allows you to see how you measure up against other scores. The specificity of "you" within a competitive marketplace of "yous" is central to its success.

This leads to another important rationale for brain-training companies like Lumosity: the brain's plasticity. Neuroscientists used to assume that the brain was basically a fixed tool, but now they understand it as evolving, adaptive, and ever malleable in reaction to contextual stimuli. Hence it can be exercised and optimized. The relatively new science of neuroplasticity increasingly shapes everyday cognitive governance by virtue of its entrance into popular culture. The fact that brains are now popularly understood to be "plastic"—that they can change to accommodate experiences in life—means you can theoretically have some agency over your own brain power. Media technology is the vehicle for that agency. Lumosity also uses the concept of brain plasticity to help authorize its interventions, foregrounding plasticity research in its marketing and educational information. The general hope behind the program is that improvements in Lumosity brain exercises will lead to improvements in everyday non-Lumosity cognitive activity. The company doesn't promise those improvements to users, but it does actively promote research that might allow users to come to their own optimistic conclusions.

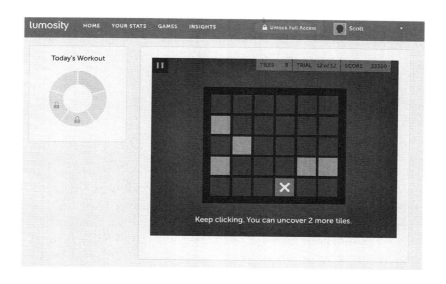

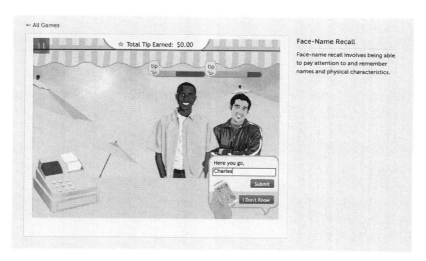

FIGURE 6. Cognitive workout from Lumosity. Each of these games focuses on memory.

Complicating matters, critics argue that programs like Lumosity don't work, or that they don't work any better than playing a video game or surfing the internet.[50] In 2014, seventy-five researchers at the Stanford Center for Longevity released a consensus letter objecting to the digital brain games industry, arguing that the "promise of a magic bullet detracts from the best evidence to date, which is that cognitive health in old age reflects the long-term effects of healthy, engaged lifestyles."[51] More than one hundred different brain researchers responded with their own open letter, providing research and data supporting their claims that brain training was in fact effective.[52] Of course, the very idea of "effective" is complicated by the individualized promise of the programs, where one is often competing against one's own performances and those of other users in a shared media ecosystem. Any number of factors might set the benchmark for improvement. Furthermore, the kinds of cognitive abilities that brain training purports to improve— something like memory or flexibility—are themselves quite complex areas and highly dependent on context. Demonstrating that Lumosity can improve performance on a memory test does not necessarily translate to memory improvements in other life tasks, even if that is part of the program's ideal.

But this is the key: the instability of Lumosity's tools is part and parcel of its success. User performance is actually used to make better tools, and no absolute knowledge is claimed. The science of the brain is always evolving, and Lumosity is contributing to new and ongoing research. In addition to the basic training it offers users, Lumosity curates something called the Human Cognition Project, what it calls a "collaborative research platform."[53] Basically, it gives its results to researchers, but it also claims to base its products on relevant, cutting-edge neuroscience. Of course, one doesn't need to be diagnosed with Alzheimer's to participate. Just as asymptomatic or healthy people are essential to the success of many current Alzheimer's research studies, everyone's performance on Lumosity is essential to the future of brain health. Just like the rest of neuroscience, it has a proleptic, optimistic tense. Precisely because we do not yet understand the brain, we need to contribute to its study for the sake of future knowledge and welfare.

This relationship with the future is based not simply on fear but also on desire—not just for a cure for something like Alzheimer's but for better knowledge, better performance, and a better you. But the stakes are also maintained within the present via discourses of exercise, fun, and social comparison.

The primary way this happens is through the goal-oriented practices of gamification. While a broad concept, gamification basically refers to the use of gaming principles in nongaming contexts. Gamification as a concept is not new, but its pervasiveness certainly is. Increasingly, it functions within online communicative capitalism as a part of the erasure of the old boundaries between entertainment and labor.[54] The basic skills required for these Lumosity games are understood to be the same skills needed in everyday social or career success.[55] Lumosity users can select from a number of areas of brain improvement, such as attention, memory, speed, flexibility, and problem solving. In fact, the idea that these are fun and practical "health" games helps authorize the company's interventions, while there is no clear evidence that they actually work to prevent cognitive decline.

The risk of Alzheimer's may drive users to sign up for brain training, but it is not a central part of Lumosity's marketing. The company may very well want to advertise brain games as a treatment of or prevention for Alzheimer's, but the government prohibits that kind of marketing. In 2016, the company that owns Lumosity actually paid $2 million to settle charges that "they deceived consumers with unfounded claims that Lumosity games can help users perform better at work and in school, and reduce or delay cognitive impairment associated with age and other serious health conditions."[56]

In the meantime, a neurological concept like cognitive reserve is an effective work-around for a company like Lumosity. For Alzheimer's, the theory of cognitive reserve basically means that those who have used their cognitive abilities more at younger ages express symptoms of dementia at later ages. A person's cognitive reserve may come from education, employment, or other forms of social engagement. The theory helps explain the wide variety of individual experiences of Alzheimer's under the same pathological changes. There are different ideas of how cognitive reserve correlates to pathology, but the general argument is that cognitive reserve can mitigate the pathological effects of brain changes due to Alzheimer's—at least for a while.[57] In other words, even if you are predisposed to Alzheimer's, cognitive reserve can help postpone the inevitable decline to a later point in life. Lumosity offers exactly the kinds of tools one might need for building up such a reserve. Direct claims about preventing Alzheimer's are unnecessary.

Of course, like any kind of insurance, cognitive reserve is only available to those who have the resources to invest. People who have access to advanced cognitive training, better education, more leisure time, or other social resources are better situated for the future. Unfortunately, cognitive capacity is marketed as universally attainable with the right kinds of efforts. The presumed universality of access overwrites these other social variables, offering a cognitive meritocracy in their place. Furthermore, the way in which this cognitive meritocracy overlaps with other social investments in the brain helps to authorize a broader ethics of cognitive agency.

In addition to social or economic barriers to access, another problem is that cognitive enhancement technologies do not simply free you up for a better life. They reinforce dependencies and create new cognitive demands, demands often disguised as freedoms. Joseph Le Doux describes these kinds of demands in his book *Synaptic Self:* "That the self is synaptic can be a curse—it doesn't take much to break it apart. But it is also a blessing, as there are always new connections waiting to be made. You are your synapses. They are who you are."[58] This is the double bind of living by virtue of the brain: its weakness is also its strength, and only through self-improvement can one stave off the inevitable breakdown.

Furthermore, these brain games orient responsible brain ˙health within media frameworks that reify particular cognitive values. Just as cognitive symptoms are modeled through media technology, its solutions are rehearsed through those same media practices and cognitive paradigms. In the case of a company like Lumosity, this relationship is built into its business model. It is similar to other digital products, where an individual's participatory data creates value for the company (say, Facebook), but it also shapes the parameters of individuality itself (your profile, networking abilities, social value, etc.). This is a by-product of increasing reliance on computers to facilitate, track, and model technoscientific identities—identities that are currently available and valuable not just to ourselves but to a range of other stakeholders.[59] In the case of companies like Lumosity, the exchange value is based on cognitive performance.

These media relationships can have a real impact on how we conceive of cognitive health and cognition's broader social values. Whether these brain games "work" to prevent Alzheimer's is almost beside the point. My argument about these media technologies is that they contribute to a cognitive meritocracy in the United States that overlaps with a broader ethics of media integration. That is a false model of agency that abstracts the reality of Alzheimer's. The idea that a brain game "can't hurt" or is simply good fun undermines the more pervasive influences that media's cognitive imperative might have on personhood. One of the big implications for the success of companies like Lumosity is that they will help shape the future of neuroscience and brain health—not only that, but they help shape the popular understanding of cognition itself.

Virtual Alzheimer's: From Risk to Empathy

One side effect of this kind of risk culture is that it can shape how the public understands people who already have Alzheimer's. While that kind of awareness can often be a positive development, all of this fear is also bound to lead to some stigma.[60] Alzheimer's stigma is in fact quite pervasive—especially in senior communities where prevalence continues to grow. Attempts to educate the public about the disease can help combat stigma. They might show the full spectrum of symptoms beyond memory loss, or they might reveal the potential that people with dementia maintain despite disease onset.

One educational tool that has caught on in the last decade is the use of virtual and augmented reality technologies to foster empathy for people with Alzheimer's. These interactive technologies replicate the symptoms of dementia through their media interfaces. The hope is

that, by actually putting someone in the shoes of a person with dementia, the user might better respect the reality of the disease. Given the
way media technology shapes cognitive empowerment, it is perhaps
not surprising that it also shapes its correlate in empathy.[61] Arguably,
these virtual reality empathy games are an extension of risk culture,
both in the way they normalize symptoms and in how they articulate
them through media technology.

A recent episode of the daytime television talk show *The Doctors* illustrates this relationship between risk and empathy.[62] The show addresses
various health topics in brief, easy-to-understand conversations between
a panel of doctors. Alzheimer's awareness and prevention is a common theme. In this episode, one of the four hosts, Dr. Sears, uses a
virtual reality kit to simulate the effects of the disease. He wears headphones designed to interfere with his hearing and to confuse him,
goggles to inhibit his sight, shoe inserts to alter his balance, and gloves
to interfere with his ability to handle and hold. The episode shows him
moving through a house trying to perform everyday tasks, such as getting a glass of water, buttoning a shirt, or finding a page in a book.
Sears narrates his difficulty with these tasks in a voice-over.

After the experiment, the episode cuts to the doctors' reactions.
Dr. Lisa begins to recount statistics: "One in ten men are affected by
this . . . one in six women are at risk, this can affect everyone you
know." Dr. Sears begins to cry, saying, "That was just a simulation,
but it really affects you to see what your loved ones can go through."
Dr. Travis contributes: "That was one of the most powerful pieces I've
ever seen on this show, because in an instant, you went from the Jim
we know to someone who couldn't do the tasks of daily living." The last
doctor, Dr. Ordon, then recounts the story of his own mother's death
from Alzheimer's. As he tells her story, he and two of the other doctors
begin to cry, and viewers are shown an old snapshot of Dr. Ordon with
his mother, smiling.

Dr. Travis then argues for the importance of media technology as
an empathetic bridge between illness and health: "I think what's so
powerful about your demonstration, Jim, is that I don't know that we
understand dementia unless we see it taking place in someone who

otherwise has their faculties." This statement shows that there is a clear relationship between respect for the challenge of the symptom in another person and understanding your own risk. Dr. Debra Cherry, introduced on the show as the executive vice president of the Alzheimer's Association, completes the argument with a description of early symptoms. She says that MCI can be so similar to normal brain behavior that it can be difficult to detect, and therefore we must all be vigilant. After all, despite a clear nod to the difficulties of care in this exercise, *The Doctors* is a show about health awareness and agency, not about caregiving.[63] This virtual reality experiment transforms empathetic witnessing into the inspiration for proactive self-care. In other words, this media experiment temporarily creates for Dr. Sears and the television audience the biopolitical formation that Alzheimer's mandates.

These Alzheimer's-oriented virtual experiences are becoming increasingly popular in health care training and public health outreach. For example, Second Wind Dreams offers a "Virtual Dementia Tour" that can be used to train families, caregivers, hospital staff, firefighters, or anyone, "anywhere that dementia is experienced."[64] While the program markets the tool as representative of "dementia," many of the experiences it models (problems with balance, hearing, pain, etc.) are in fact germane to aging more generally. In addition to prosthetics designed to simulate the physicality of aging, participants listen to something called a "confusion tape" that is designed to simulate cognitive deficit, "combining environmental noises, static fuzz, sporadic loud sirens and beeps."[65] Cynthia McFadden, a news reporter for ABC, took the tour on national television and found it eye opening: "I mean, I'm the queen of multi-tasking. I can do anything, I can do twenty things at once, I'm a mom, I'm a, it's very humbling."[66] The shock of the "reality" of Alzheimer's is the desired effect. The company says that "the Virtual Dementia Tour takes something intangible like empathy and makes it tangible by allowing participants to see themselves as impaired and behaving in ways that simulate their own clients, customers or loved ones living with dementia."[67]

Most virtual or augmented Alzheimer's experiences rely on digital media tools to generate this empathy. For example, British researchers

developed a smartphone app called *A Walk through Dementia* that sim-
ulates a trip to the grocery store, a family gathering, or a walk through
the street.[68] Anyone with a virtual reality (VR) headset (say, Google
Cardboard) can download the app to her smartphone and try the program for free in the comfort of her home. Empathy tools don't rely only
on VR headsets, however. A Dutch group created a social media campaign where Facebook users were tagged in old photos of events they
had never attended. The group digitally inserted the users' likenesses
into these photos, after which the users received a message saying "Confusing, right? You're now experiencing what it's like to have Alzheimer's
disease."[69] Alternatively, console or desktop computer games like *Ether
One* offer interactive environments meant to simulate the experience
of living with dementia.[70]

The purpose of all these media experiences is to create the conditions for empathy so people without symptoms can understand how
it feels to have dementia. The experience of Alzheimer's, however, is
more individual, both in the object of its "attack" and in the subjective
experience of the symptoms. How can a game or a costume represent
that individual experience? This is one reason why Michael Thomsen
argued in the *New Yorker* that empathy games are generally more conducive to self-interest: "If violent war games are driven by delusional
power fantasies, then empathy games are driven by a parallel delusion
about how caring we are in reality."[71] Thomsen's cynicism raises valid
questions: How much can VR experiences actually tell us about the
experience of dementia? How useful can they really be as instruments
of care? Might they in fact reinforce stigma rather than challenge it?

Another limitation of these kinds of empathy games is that they rely
on media technology as a means of translating symptoms. The designers of *A Walk through Dementia* said that they edited the video "in a way
that enhanced the feeling of confusion, blurring details and morphing
faces."[72] The simulation of symptoms is clearly constrained by these
basic media techniques. Of course, virtual media also offer tools like
story and character development, but the more direct tactic of these
experiences is to rely on the technological interface for the translation
of reality. Sometimes it is actually the dysfunction of that interface that

communicates the symptom. For example, Google Cardboard made me feel unsteady when I used it with *A Walk through Dementia* because of its rudimentary design. The fact that virtual and augmented reality technologies are still very much in development only adds to their effects. Aside from the impossible-to-verify, dubious claims on realism implicit in any virtual program (no matter how significant the contributions from people experiencing dementia), there is a clear claim made on behalf of media's cognitive imperative. Not only does the media technology shape our understanding of cognitive deficit but it prioritizes visual and cognitive symptoms in a hierarchy of embodied symptoms of Alzheimer's.

The very *idea* that virtual or augmented reality technology can allow access to the mind of the person with dementia indicates the limits of our understanding of the disease, from symptoms to solutions. Because these media technologies model, enhance, and perform cognitive abilities, they shape our understanding of what healthy cognition can be, ultimately contributing to a more broadly held ethic of mediated personhood. Even an optimistic approach to personhood is constrained through the software and media interface. What does it mean that empathy is defined as understanding through media engagement? What other kinds of empathy are lost in this model—empathetic perspectives or actions that might disregard the importance of media or even understanding itself?

What is the difference between an experience with a VR headset, a console video game, and a brain-training game like Lumosity? Aren't they all empathy games in that they allow users to compare their own everyday realities to another (future) reality? Don't they all translate cognitive abilities into functional goals and representational ideals? Even if they avoid narrative and simply allow for immersive experiences, they still provide a horizon of cognitive experience that translates symptoms into the logic of media technology. Media technologies that represent cognitive abilities may certainly provide an empathetic bridge between people with dementia and those without. But they also provide an ideological and technological armature for cognitive health that reinforces media's value.

4

PET Scans and Polaroids

Anachronizing Personhood

Historically, older bodies have not been represented in American popular culture in proportion to their demographics, while younger bodies remain abundant. This does not mean that aging is not open to representation. Quite the opposite: because human bodies are so susceptible to change, the physicality of the aging body "intrudes and insists on its attendant visibility."[1] It makes itself known *as* aged, and it cannot entirely escape its social judgment, no matter how healthy it might be. Another reason for this judgment is that aging is overwritten with various cultural narratives, and age-oriented stigmas thoroughly condition the aging body in the United States.[2]

Alzheimer's has changed the cultural response to the aging body, in part because of the presumed universality of disease risk but also because its effects are often assumed to be occurring in the brain in contrast to the body. While Alzheimer's does in fact often lead to bodily deterioration—and some of these changes can be quite radical—those external changes rarely feature in the dominant symptomatic codes. Instead, the body is seen as a kind of corporeal shell for the real travesty that occurs on the inside. This narrative rehearses a traditional mind–body dualism whereby the visibility of a basically healthy body is undermined by a mysteriously, invisibly sick brain. Rather than show people on life support, with bed sores or frozen joints, incontinent, propped up by pillows in bed, with feeding tubes or any of the other outward-facing signs that might signal later stages of the disease, most popular culture conceives of Alzheimer's as attacking the brain and the interior self.[3]

The invisibility of the symptoms can prove difficult for those wishing to use the image of Alzheimer's as a rhetorical tool. Psychiatrist Tom Kitwood describes how an agency seeking to promote dementia awareness asked a care facility for some publicity photographs of its patients. When the agency received the photographs, it sent them back "on the ground that the clients did not show the disturbed and agonistic characteristics that people with dementia 'ought' to show, and which would be expected to arouse public concern."[4] Public interest in a disease is often fundamentally tied to its visible codes, and the agency was frustrated by the difficulty in accessing those codes.

The fact is that the symptoms and experiences of Alzheimer's disease can be difficult to represent—especially through a static image. Because of this, an aging physicality is often supplemented by indications of a more profound interior crisis. Eyes are common tools in these efforts, and people with dementia are often reduced to images of wide eyes, alternatively vacant or frantic.[5] Representations of eyes are designed to give spectatorial access to the crisis occurring in the brain, as the figure of the eye is an important cultural link between interiority and agency.[6] Sometimes, if someone with the disease is agitated, then gesticulating or clutching hands indicate that inner turmoil. When we do see representations of behavior, aggression or emotional distress is far more common than more positive disinhibition like laughter, euphoria, or play. Usually, however, popular representations of people with Alzheimer's follow generic patterns of aging and a pathologized interiority.

Given these trends, however, it is important to note that the disease is still enormously open to imaginative description, and there is both space and demand for critical intervention at the level of representation. Tracing the many ways Alzheimer's commands both universal and epidemic status despite insecure etiological models is clearly important. Understanding how certain cultural patterns can actually disenfranchise people currently living with the disease is essential. This chapter addresses Alzheimer's in popular culture, paying particular attention to the ways representational media help shape Alzheimer's self and personhood. An important methodological point is that I do not simply wish to rehearse or contribute to the representational archive about Alzheimer's; others have written successfully to that end.[7] Instead, I will argue that links between certain forms of representation and cognition articulate collective concerns about the disease.

I focus in particular on the two most common aesthetics of Alzheimer's, the *snapshot aesthetic* and the *neuroscientific aesthetic*. Often engaged dialectically, the snapshot structures the self via memory and loss, whereas the neuroimage orients the self in the promise of the brain and neuroscience. Narratively speaking, the snapshot is analeptic, modeling the lossy self through nostalgia and degradation. And as I have argued in the first three chapters, the neuroimage inaugurates a proleptic tense, orienting solutions to Alzheimer's within technologies of innovation and an ideology of progress. In both cases, the pathologies of the present are "solved" through idealized and anachronistic models of interior value. What are the consequences of an anachronistic distribution of self through media technologies? More specifically, what are the consequences for Alzheimer's personhood? Given these aesthetics, how can media be a site of agency for people dealing with symptoms of dementia?

In addition to stigma or stereotypes about people with Alzheimer's, these dichotomous aesthetics indicate a social belief in the human capacity for mediation. We imagine the human brain as a kind of technology for representation. That technology offers a way of understanding cognitive deficit but also cognitive proficiency. The brain scan and the snapshot are temporal media artifacts, one indicating a collective relationship with the future, the other a haunted past. In a sense, *both* are neuroimages. What is being represented are investments in cognitive ability: memory, recognition, or other brain functions. The ways in which those figures of cognitive capacity relate to personhood and agency are precisely what need critical attention. The popular culture of Alzheimer's maintains a temporal logic of progress and loss that belies more pervasive and complex ideologies of cognitive value.

Making Progress: The Neuroscientific Aesthetic

Neuroimaging dominates the popular culture of Alzheimer's in the United States. It is difficult to find a television news report, a promising research profile, or advice for preventing the disease without encountering pictures of brains. These neuroimages reference the pathology of the cognitive symptom, but they also demonstrate strong belief in the industries of neuroscience. They haunt the background of media coverage of Alzheimer's in a kind of futuristic technoaesthetic, helping to articulate a progress narrative for the public. Not surprisingly, media coverage of neuroscience, like other biomedical sciences, focuses more on the speculative benefits of research than on the complexity of the media technology or research design. The neuroimage is often optimistic and anticipatory, even when discussing setbacks or failures.[8] It signifies sophisticated technology and innovation, but it also reminds the public that the struggle for a solution to Alzheimer's is an uphill battle.

In these progress narratives, Alzheimer's is not only an illness; it is also an enemy. It is mischievous, devious, and merciless.[9] It attacks, corrupts, and robs a person's self and identity. These words are often used to describe criminal behavior, and they lend Alzheimer's criminal status and an agency of its own. Alzheimer's steals a person's identity, her memories, and her connections to the world around her. Key in this discourse is the idea that Alzheimer's is a biological disease, but also more: it eviscerates the very thing that makes us human.

Narratives of Alzheimer's research, then, naturally portray the brain as desperately in need of a dramatic rescue. For example, an episode from the *The Dr. Oz Show* demonstrates this trend toward spectacle. Featuring Dr. Mehmet Oz's "disease detective," Dr. David Perlmutter, and his "revolutionary" hyperbaric oxygen treatment, the two doctors look at a brain scan projected onto a screen. Dr. Oz points out some brightly colored sections for the studio audience:

DR. OZ: Just to be clear, this image that we're showing is a real person's head, right, brain scan, and those bright little areas you see there,

they're not supposed to be there, all these little yellow little specks
there, that's the sign of raging fire that's going on in different parts
of the brain of someone who has Alzheimer's.

DR. PERLMUTTER: And this is what we call the Alzheimer's brain or the
brain on fire.[10]

The bright specks indicate the presence of difference within a simply
coded narrative of illness and health. While the discourse of "raging
fire" actually indirectly references a theory of Alzheimer's and inflammation, the doctors render neuroimaging a medical exercise akin to
heroic firefighting. Perlmutter's hyperbaric oxygen treatment is framed
as a promising new weapon in that fight.

Whether they show plaques, tangles, or inflammation, images of
the brains of people with Alzheimer's help naturalize a material bio-
genesis of the disease, despite that no specific biological etiology has
been secured.[11] That essential complication is rarely dealt with in scientific communication for the public. Instead, neuroimages communicate pathological processes like atrophy, the accumulation of excess
beta-amyloid, or, in this case, the brain "on fire." They illustrate the
highly magnified structure of the brain or the complicated interrela-
tionships of its parts. Alzheimer's in these neuroimages may still be
a mystery in terms of why or how, but not what. That is arguably not
just because the neuroimage can reduce a complex argument into a
clear effect but also because of its biological orientation.[12] The material
fact of the brain and its pathological changes are taken for granted.
The brain as image referent functions as an underlying truth claim
that reinforces the biological singularity of Alzheimer's. It helps sediment Alzheimer's as a material disease rather than, say, a more complicated intersection of environment, symptoms, and other actors.

After the Dr. Oz show aired, the Alzheimer's Association's NorCal
chapter publicly corrected Dr. Oz on its website, arguing that there is
no "substantive research evidence" to support the claims made on his
show on behalf of hyperbaric oxygen treatment.[13] That kind of correc-
tion did not seem to affect the show's reputation, however. This is no
doubt because of the medical authority that Dr. Oz maintained at the

time but also because what was being represented was medical progress and experimentation rather than proven results. In other words, realism in this kind of optimistic narrative is figured in the truth of the research objects ("a real person's head" or a "brain scan"), while the detective-doctor is merely searching for a better theory of Alzheimer's. This is research at its most optimistic and promising, and as such, it can be forgiven its factual problems. Public relationships with neuroscientific authority rely on a shared understanding of research as a work in progress.

The show, however, is a good example of how the research that accompanies neuroimages in the media is often simplified by both journalists and scientists for easier public consumption. Audiences for neuroimages are anything but secure, and those abstractions or simplifications are often an effort in rhetorical balance between persuasiveness and the communication of research results. The research is too complex to communicate the details of every new study. One common technique that helps researchers translate that complexity is the side-by-side comparison of healthy and sick brains. In his ethnography of PET, Joseph Dumit argues that this technique often uses "one word labels that emphasize differences between the subjects rather than qualify them."[14] In neuroimages of dementia, this often takes the form of a juxtaposition of a "normal brain" and an "Alzheimer's brain." The category of the Alzheimer's brain stands in for whatever is being tracked, traced, or studied. Neuroimages of these brains are often highly dramatic, with bright colors that simulate complex underlying processes at work. The fantastic complexity and illegibility of the brain maintain that image as spectacle, just as categorical opposition structures an easy logic of healthy and diseased.

The realism accorded to the practice of neuroimaging is simply not the same for imaging scientists as it is for the public. "What is really happening" in a brain scan for the nonexpert might be akin to cutting open the brain, putting it under a microscope, and seeing the truth of the thing. The illusion of transparency provided by the media technology can help shape public reception. A lay audience might assume the brain scan has the same kind of mimetic capacity as a photograph.[15]

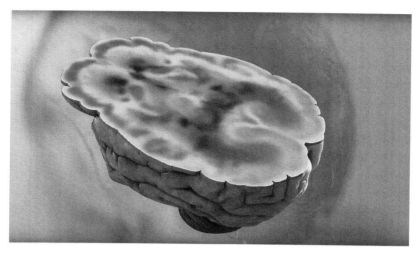

FIGURE 7. Interiority aesthetics: this image overlaps a neuroimage onto a cross section of the brain. Still from *How Alzheimer's Changes the Brain* (National Institute on Aging). https://youtu.be/oGXv3mHs9AU.

But for a research scientist, the value of an image is hermeneutic: it records specific, preselected signs and then translates them into a useful, meaningful representation.[16]

The transformation or translation of scientific information into an image can produce powerful rhetorical effects like realism and difference. This is not only because the public imagines a brain scan to be a device capable of photographic capture—although that kind of belief is common—but also because the public is invested in the neuroscientist's ability to successfully translate or read the image. Neuroimaging borrows on the cultural imprimatur of neuroscience more generally. A recent study found that the public finds neuroscience the most rigorous, difficult, and prestigious of the sciences, a belief that the authors correlate with neuroscience's "reductive allure."[17] In other words, the publicly available neuroimage is successful in its rhetoric not because of its presumed simplicity or transparency but because of trust in scientific ability to translate image complexity into something useful. Other studies show that viewers are more willing to trust scientific research if neuroscience is a part of its discursive presentation.[18] It is debatable whether it is neuroimages in particular that constitute the grounds for that trust or neuroscientific information more broadly. Regardless, it is clear that the science of brains offers a compelling aesthetic.

Unbalanced public faith in neuroimaging expertise has been well described and critiqued by social scientists, bioethicists, and medical practitioners, but that has done little to dispel the irresponsible use of these images in popular culture.[19] This "neurorealism" can be highly effective for helping to guide public policy and raise research funds, and it essentializes the brain as an object of inquiry.[20] That the images circulate as a part of popular culture certainly should not mean that the public is also held responsible for learning how to read those images. Despite mounting interest in the improvement of public scientific literacy, the average viewer of an image of Alzheimer's pathology cannot realistically be expected to understand its relationship to meaningful research. The broad circulation of neuroimages is simply an indication that their truth effects are valuable to that cultural sphere. In other words, it is precisely the *challenges* of legibility within the language of realism that make them so socially valuable. Some of the presumed superiority of the technology stems from its relatively restricted use and the professional expertise required for its operation.[21] The public is usually not exposed to debate or insecurity that diminishes the authority of the observer, not to mention the creative and productive faculties of neuroimaging technology itself.

The descriptive or diagnostic authority of the expert neuroscientific observer is not without its threats, however. For example, brain modeling is often reliant on digital tools, where machines, instead of human observers, are performing independent and figurative analysis. Anne Beaulieu and Sarah De Rijcke argue that rather than stand-alone images to be captured and analyzed, brain scans more commonly function within constitutive database logics, especially in the context of research. Those logics are comparative and exclusionary. "The iterative and relational aspects of neuroimaging," they argue, "are central to the specific kind of authoritativeness that comes into play when these images are used in making claims about the brain, the mind, and the self."[22] As regards Alzheimer's research, those "iterative and relational aspects" perform or redouble cognitive capacity, both in the modeling of presumably objective function but also in the remediation of cognitive authority through media's cognitive imperative.

There are of course a range of other challenges to neuroscientific authority, especially since the interiority that neuroscience describes can sometimes contrast with perspectives held by other social authorities on interiority, such as religion or self-help. Because of this ideological complexity, popular culture has not always framed neuroscience as heroic—especially in the battle with Alzheimer's. Some media frame research on Alzheimer's as a problem, often because it articulates the dangers of unchecked progress or the mysterious volatility of the brain. Even when cautionary, however, the neuroscientific aesthetic is still primarily oriented toward the future.

For example, in the 2011 sci-fi blockbuster *Rise of the Planet of the Apes*, the protagonist discovers a temporary cure for Alzheimer's by performing radical, dangerous research on chimpanzees. The consequences of this science are apocalyptic, as the research creates a population of intelligent super-apes that eventually take over the planet and enslave humans. This theme is similar to one that organizes the narrative of the 1999 action horror movie *Deep Blue Sea*. Sharks used to grow brain tissue that might one day cure Alzheimer's suddenly go out of control and kill a group of researchers on their floating research station. The film literalizes the cure to Alzheimer's within the overdeveloped brain of a giant shark. In an illuminating metaphor, the film's human protagonist eventually kills the shark by stabbing it in the eye with a cross that hangs from his neck. The battle between religious faith and faith in science is neatly summed up by a character responding to the sharks, "What in God's creation?" to which the scientist replies, "Oh, not His . . . ours." Like many other Hollywood narratives about scientific (often genetic) experiments, the film frames neuroscience as messing with sacred, biological, human boundaries. The fate of the people working with the apes and the shark represent the fearsome consequences of trying to find a cure.

Beyond the narrative of dangerous progress, Alzheimer's is also useful to these films for its generic traits as an incurable disease. Sentimental frames play a key role in these narratives, where personal relationships between scientists and loved ones dying of Alzheimer's motivate character behavior and allow the audience a certain measure of identification. The fact that Alzheimer's is incurable, however, raises the stakes of the plot to heroic levels. This kind of popular representation narrates neuroscientific research as inherently bent toward failure, maintaining the current status of Alzheimer's as an incurable epidemic for its audience.

Clearly it would be a mistake to say that the brain and its powers are secure in their popular imagination. Certainly this struggle over the legitimacy of neuroscience and Alzheimer's research is not new. As I pointed out earlier in this book, this battle for public support has been going on since its emergence as a public health crisis. Furthermore, public trust in the neuroimage derives in part from its historical relationship to medical truth making, but also from complex relationships to other media technologies.

As I have argued thus far in this book, the values of cognition are not merely set up by neuroscience. They are also oriented within a broader culture of computer and artificial intelligence. They are articulated through media technologies that reify cognitive abilities through their representational capacities. The neuroimage is a cultural icon and a discursive link between various registers of internal potential and promise: the brain, cognition, and self.[23] It is not alone in this work, however, and the remainder of this chapter explores other media artifacts that shape agency and cognitive capacity for people with Alzheimer's.

Imaging Loss: The Snapshot Aesthetic

The neuroscientific aesthetic is often used in tandem with a different media aesthetic: the snapshot. If the rhetoric of neuroimages enforces medical progress and cognitive empowerment, the snapshot negotiates lossy relationships with the past, regulating Alzheimer's personhood in the process. I use the term *snapshot* because the aesthetics of this kind of photographic object often signify its worn nature or its handled qualities. The almost tangible patina of an old photo communicates nostalgia for a simpler time but also a compromised relationship with memory. Because of its ephemeral nature, the snapshot reinforces the compromised nature of its subject, serving as a fragile memorial for the present.

By snapshot aesthetic, however, I am not referring only to references to old Polaroids or photos. Rather, the aesthetic embraces the way any form of media can articulate compromised relationships with time or durability. These formal tactics rely on the material characteristics of the media technology to communicate a philosophy of shared loss. Alzheimer's culture offers many examples: a black-and-white family photo juxtaposed with some other color component signifies its comparative age; a worn filmstrip references collective relationships with media progress and verisimilitude; the Post-it note is fleeting and ephemeral; the amateur qualities of a family film or photo album highlight threats to a shared past; blurry or degraded aesthetics in a point-of-view shot indicate a lack of lucidity or confusion.

Media objects and aesthetic tactics like these are common in the popular culture of Alzheimer's. They may depict the person with Alzheimer's, they may perform the perspective of symptom, or they may serve as a more incidental backdrop to stories about the disease. Regardless of approach, the aesthetic helps articulate social relationships with threats to self and memory. Just like the neuroscientific aesthetic, the snapshot aesthetic is an attempt to coordinate and control the symptoms of Alzheimer's. When Susan Sontag wrote that "photography is acquisition in many forms," she alluded to the photograph's ability to capture, possess, or consume something true.[24] Within the snapshot aesthetics of Alzheimer's, that truth can be understood as the threatened self of the person with the disease.

The snapshot aesthetic, then, is a social claim on Alzheimer's selfhood. It offers a retreat to a younger version of the person with the disease and an embrace of an authentic, uncomplicated self: one not ravaged by disease or symptom. At the same time, it references the cognitive symptom of the person with dementia, her fading capacities and representational loss. In both senses, it highlights a fraught individuality.

The "affiliative" nature of amateur, familial photos is important to understanding the social subject of Alzheimer's.[25] Perhaps more than any other form of media, the snapshot maintains intimate relationships with familial and collective memories. While the snapshot aesthetic orients its threatened subject as personal and elusive, that nostalgia for an uncomplicated memory is frequently shared.[26] A photograph might maintain an indexical relationship with the lived history of the person with dementia, but it does so also with her family, friends, and community. For this reason, a collective past, rather than the memories of just one person, is understood to be compromised.

In other words, selfhood is often figured as singular, but the self's intimacy is collectively shared through its reception and maintenance in media. These representational ethics disperse that self into a social network that also reinforces the importance of individuality. Of course, the context of reception is relevant to any media object's phenomenological relationship with time and self. But the cultural ubiquity of the snapshot in the last century affords us a measure of media hermeneutics, especially as it figures into contemporary economies of mobile photography.[27]

From the Brownie to the Polaroid to the digital selfie, a sense of self-agency has always been important to photographic practice. Especially after the advent of the digital camera and the popularization of smartphones, amateur images now permeate our highly mediated social landscapes, and the modern sense of self is caught up in that representational field. But the biographical content of the photo is increasingly less important than its curation in a social context. This is what selfie researchers have called the "sociotechnical phenomenon" of the self or a complex set of practices of the self.[28] In other words, agency lies in capture or performance but also in the curation and exchange of these photos. After all, social media platforms like Instagram and Snapchat are not so much photographic archives as network enablers and facilitators of social exchange. The self is not at all secure; rather, it is distributed in these media practices.

The snapshot aesthetic's affiliative, social nature helps to highlight the social nature of symptoms like memory loss. Take, for example, the

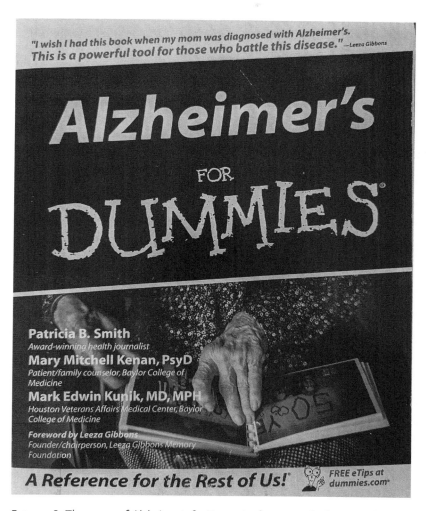

FIGURE 8. The cover of *Alzheimer's for Dummies* foregrounds the snapshot aesthetic.

cover of the book *Alzheimer's for Dummies,* part of the successful Dummies self-help book series.[29] Setting aside for the moment the way cognitive hierarchies are ironically naturalized by the Dummies brand name itself, one can see that the cover image employs the snapshot aesthetic quite effectively. In it, an older woman's wrinkled hands turn the pages of a small photo album sitting in her lap. The two visible pictures in the album show a group of happy, smiling people in front of a banner that says "50 YEARS," presumably indicating an anniversary of some sort. We don't see the woman's face, just aged hands flipping through memories in the album. Does this person have dementia, or is she a family member or caregiver? Does it matter? The use of the photo album on the cover reinforces the social values of memory just as it suggests what everyone knows: Alzheimer's is a threat to memory and social relationships for all. The reader only needs to understand that there exists a compromised relationship with the past to understand how Alzheimer's works.

The dominance of the snapshot aesthetic in Alzheimer's culture also contributes to the popular misconception that, despite the complex manifestations of its symptomatology, Alzheimer's is simply "a memory disease." Memory as a structure of knowledge is so overdetermined— as a media technology, human ability, or cultural construct—that it is no surprise that it informs this disease so fundamentally. Whether on a server or in cloud storage or on your personal device, memory capacities are increasingly taken for granted as a part of our media ecosystem. Those technologies often perform the requirements of remembering for us and, in so doing, help shape the shared values of memory.

Not surprisingly, Alzheimer's culture rehearses normative models of media memory such as a database or archive, and it is dismissive of the more complicated patterns of memory loss that can accompany the disease. For example, while most people with Alzheimer's lose the ability to make new memories, they may in fact enjoy talking about memories from earlier in life. A person might remember how to get to work but not how to drive the car. She might remember her wedding day but not the name of the person she married. How can the snapshot aesthetic perform these variabilities? If the person with Alzheimer's has any memories left, she is often stigmatized as "lost to the past" or "stuck in the past." In other words, the quality of these changes to memory is reduced to an aesthetic of media capacity. The snapshot aesthetic participates in broader conversations about what memory loss is but also about why that loss matters.

This correlates with another common cultural reference to the fragile memories of people with Alzheimer's: the Post-it note. Post-its are a common enough tool for people living with dementia that the brand even worked directly with the Alzheimer's Association in the promotion of its product and in the name of better care.[30] These brightly colored, sticky reminder notes litter the culture of Alzheimer's. For example, in Alice Munro's short story "The Bear Came over the Mountain," a husband begins to realize that something is wrong with his wife. It turns out that she is struggling with symptoms of dementia, a fact revealed by her use of Post-its:

> Over a year ago, Grant had started noticing so many little yellow notes stuck up all over the house. That was not entirely new. Fiona had always written things down—the title of a book she'd heard mentioned on the radio or the jobs she wanted to make sure she got done that day. Even her morning schedule was written down. He found it mystifying and touching in its precision: "7 a.m. yoga. 7:30–7:45 teeth face hair. 7:45–8:15 walk. 8:15 Grant and breakfast." The new notes were different. Stuck onto the kitchen drawers—Cutlery, Dishtowels, Knives. Couldn't she just open the drawers and see what was inside? Worse things were coming.[31]

This passage shows how the media artifact is not inherently pathological: the Post-it indicates a more typical desire to organize a busy life. As a common household object, it shows how important memory is, just as it shows how human memory often needs some help. The notes in Munro's story, however, also reveal a compromised memory. The pathology in the brain and the cognitive symptom are rehearsed in the material ephemerality of the small, disposable object.

The Post-it note, then, serves as an everyday memory aid, but it also reveals the social importance of memory in a productive society. In

Figure 9, a website for a pharmaceutical company uses that tension in an advertisement to enlist research participants for an Alzheimer's study. Handwritten script states "Please take note of our Alzheimer's clinical research study" under an image of several Post-its on a wall: "Milk, Eggs, Chips, Bananas," "I was in the Navy," "Call Bob Johnson," and so on. The ad codes memory as threatened but also as valuable and something worthy of saving.

Rather than a realistic rendition of a shared past, the snapshot aesthetic is generative of ever-shifting ways of thinking about the past. As Marita Sturken writes about photographs, they are "technologies of memory, not vessels of memory in which memory passively resides so much as objects through which memories are shared, produced, and given meaning."[32] This is also the work of the snapshot in the aesthetics of Alzheimer's—but rather than a particular shared memory, it is

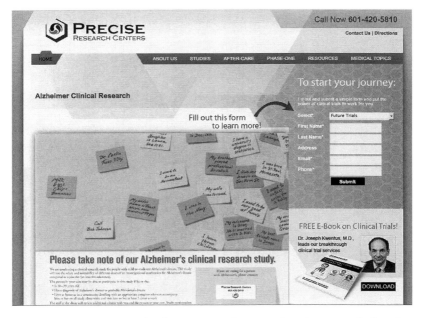

FIGURE 9. Precise research advertisement featuring Post-it notes, a hallmark of the snapshot aesthetic.

memory itself that is given meaning. This kind of aesthetic articulates collective fear of losing the past but also the fear of losing our selves. Geoffrey Batchen, writing of photography, death, and memory in his book *Forget Me Not,* argues that photographs do not so much capture a fleeting memory as they illustrate both the difficulty of depicting memory and the fear of its immanent loss (hence the imperative of his book title). Batchen writes, "Memorialization has little to do with recalling the past; it is always about looking ahead toward that terrible, imagined, vacant future in which we ourselves will have been forgotten."[33] It is at this level—the shared fear of loss of the past as the fear of the loss of self—that we can understand the deployment of the snapshot in the popular culture of Alzheimer's.

The snapshot aesthetic, then, is a kind of social negotiation with death, memory, and loss. Much has been written about haunting and possession in media technology that points to the uneasy relationship between a mediated presence and death.[34] While it may rely on some of those tropes, the snapshot aesthetic offers a different kind of spectral presence for Alzheimer's: nostalgia for a pure and sanctified self. It is aligned with what Roland Barthes claimed about the photograph's inclination toward death: "For Death must be somewhere in a society; if it is no longer (or less intensely) in religion, it must be elsewhere; perhaps in this image which produces Death while trying to preserve life."[35]

The televangelist Pat Robertson ignited national controversy in 2011 when he suggested that divorce is an acceptable choice for a spouse of a person with Alzheimer's disease because the symptoms are "a kind of death" and "'til death do us part."[36] Later in the book, I explore some of the ramifications of this perspective for Alzheimer's care, but for now it is worth noting Robertson's comparison of the symptoms of Alzheimer's to death. Despite widespread protests against his position, his comments are not an isolated incidence; rather, they contribute to a common stigma associated with the disease. People with Alzheimer's are often described as enduring a "living death" or a "social death."[37] According to this perspective, because the person with Alzheimer's cannot participate adequately in the world around her—to communicate, remember, or take care of herself—though the body is alive, the person is dead.

The overdetermined nature of the categories of life and death for Alzheimer's leads to all manner of confusion about best-care practice, living wills, and patient rights. Furthermore, if a person in late-stage Alzheimer's requires life-sustaining technologies, such as a feeding tube or drugs, caregivers face difficult ethical and economic choices over what constitutes death or a life worth living.[38] This confusion draws on other debates over the boundaries of death and life in twenty-first-century U.S. politics: assisted suicide, so-called death panels, fetal personhood, and abortion rights. These heavily politicized, often contradictory perspectives nearly always speak in the name of life: of protecting life, preserving it, or making it better. These moral perspectives penetrate the everyday experience of Alzheimer's in the United States, and they insert cognitive capacities into that moral economy.[39] They help shape complex familial and personal choices about how to care for people with dementia. Clearly the experience of Alzheimer's varies considerably as the disease progresses; MCI is judged very differently than the symptoms of someone experiencing late-stage Alzheimer's. But because the disease continues to shape the end-of-life experience for so many people, the public culture of Alzheimer's helps negotiate the terms and values of personhood around cognitive capacity.

Not surprisingly, then, the snapshot aesthetic often works in tandem with the neuroscientific aesthetic in popular representations of Alzheimer's. The combination of their codes demonstrates the way the disease is principally imagined through dichotomous temporalities of progress and loss. For example, an informational video about Alzheimer's available on WebMD dissolves images of a brain's neural circuitry with old photographs of unidentified people in a kind of interiority montage. In the background we hear the voice of the outspoken Harvard neuro-geneticist and author of *Decoding Darkness* Rudolph Tanzi:

> Who are you as a person? It is the sum collection of all your experiences your entire life, stored as memories, and then all your life as you experience new things you're associating that back on what you've already

learned. And that's memory. And based on how you're forming memories and learning, you're behaving a certain way and that's your personality. Alzheimer's disease robs every bit of that.[40]

While Tanzi speaks, we see a montage of old photos of people getting
married, couples laughing, children playing, each photo alternating
or overlapping with futuristic brain scans and illustrations. The aesthetics of the snapshot and the neuroimage are sutured within a montage of generalized interiority and articulated into a theory of mediated
personhood.

Key to the video's logic is the alternating degradation and sophistication of the images of interiority, ultimately answering the question "who
are you are as a person?" As the snapshot fades, so fade the memories,
brain, and person with Alzheimer's. But neuroscience provides a rhetorical balance to that lost personhood. The dichotomous opposition of
the personal, familial image with the neuroimage reinforces the truth
of each claim. The voice-over by the neuroscientist further establishes
a biomedical authority in the urgent effort to cure the disease. This is
a quintessentially modern representational tactic dependent on insecure but nostalgic relationships with older technologies as a way of
investing in the future.

This kind of media dichotomy grants personhood for people anach-
ronistically but denies it in the pathologized present. This harmonizes
with the way the category of personhood is often perceived as both a
rescue and an investment (debates over fetal personhood are a good
example of this). Indeed, much of the discourse in Alzheimer's care is
focused on salvaging selfhood as an agential move or as a kind of rescue. No matter how earnest the efforts, a culture that stares so longingly
away from the present stands a good chance of invalidating the lived
experiences of people with dementia now.

Claiming Selfhood: Media Agency

Given the ways cognitive empowerment is now shaped by engagement
with media technology, it should come as no surprise that media is
also used to treat people living with the symptoms of Alzheimer's. This

approach to media agency directly correlates to the snapshot aesthetic and its claims on personhood. For example, some argue that personal photographs can be used as a way to help people with Alzheimer's as a part of a popular form of treatment called reminiscence therapy.[41] Some research suggests that people with dementia can look at family photos, and it might spark increased focus, improved mood, and general well-being. The research does not go so far as to make recognition of photographic content a therapeutic goal, but it does situate the personal nature of the photo as necessary for successful intervention. And popular reception of these strategies is based on the media artifact's ties to memory. After all, it is called "reminiscence therapy" for a reason. Effectiveness aside, this kind of reminiscence therapy betrays more about social trust in the power of the photograph than the ability of someone with Alzheimer's to recognize the content of a photo. Despite the questionable nature of the research, many continue to use photographs and other forms of biographical media as a form of "memory aid."[42] This kind of care is not limited to photography, of course, as in theory, really any kind of media could be used in reminiscence therapy.

For example, the Minnesota Historical Society offers a free tablet or smartphone app called *My House of Memories* that allows users to "look through pictures of inspiring objects from a range of museums from across history to bring back great memories, brought to life with sound, music, and descriptions."[43] It was specifically developed as an activity to help people with dementia and their caregivers. Options include browsing photos, making memory trees, and participating in other "memory activities." In theory, users can also upload their own photographs to the app to inspire more personal memories. The app was created by a museum partner in Liverpool, England, and it emerged from a broader reminiscence program sponsored by the British government. The idea for the app came from a collection of memory suitcases: forty thematically curated suitcases, each containing objects that might appeal to different kinds of visitors with different kinds of memories.[44] According to the Minnesota Historical Society, that kind of culturally specific approach also applies to the U.S. version of the app; users have the choice to download "American" content when downloading it. That collection of objects was "curated by people living with dementia and their caregivers, including African-Americans who selected items that connect to the black community."[45]

Music in particular is quite popular as a form of care for people with Alzheimer's. One of the more well-known examples of this can be seen in the 2014 documentary film *Alive Inside*. The movie revolves around the idea that music has the power to tap into buried memories and ergo a buried identity. Early excerpts of the documentary went viral, garnering several million views on YouTube and extensive, celebratory media commentary.[46] In one sequence, a hunched, withdrawn man with dementia, Henry, is unable to recognize his daughter. We then hear her talking about positive memories of their family and the vibrancy of Henry's youth while the camera pans over a series of old black-and-white photos. A nurse then puts headphones over Henry's ears so he can listen to music he enjoyed when he was younger. The film's audience cannot hear the music, but they see the man dramatically respond. His eyes widen, he sits up, and he displays animated, excited behavior, singing along to the music.

The key to the video's popularity is perhaps the instantaneous and expressive transformation in the man's demeanor, a transformation made possible by the mysterious power of music. Precisely because of its seemingly magical effects, *Alive Inside* makes successful care look as easy as plugging someone into his headphones. Transformations like these ultimately reduce personhood to the mediation of lost memories; without that music, it's hard to see this man as anything but loss. Oliver Sacks, interviewed in the documentary, echoes this thesis, calling Henry "unresponsive and almost unalive" without the music. He argues that when people with dementia are "out of it," the music "will bring them back into it, into their own personhood, their own memories, their own autobiographies."

Another approach to reminiscence therapy is to create entire environments that reproduce some approximation of normal living from an earlier time of a person's life. One of the most publicized models of this kind of care is a residential facility in Amsterdam called Hogeway

(De Hogeweyk). Built in 2009, Hogeway was conceived of as a small "dementia village," complete with small homes, streets, a market, and a café. Because it is carefully managed, residents and the public have some freedom to use the facilities as they wish. The facility offers seven different lifestyle themes that might match up with the lived background of the residents, defined in their publicity materials as traditional, urban, arts and culture, etiquette, home, Christian, and Indian:

> It must be very similar to what the residents were used to at home. This means small-scale houses that look like "home." Life there must also be virtually identical to the resident's previous life. This may concern "big," important issues such as religion and culture but also the smaller things such as set-up, music, daily schedule and customs.[47]

The rationale for these different lifestyle areas is to re-create some sense of "normal" for people who live there, and not all of its residents will have similar interests and backgrounds.

That approach to care contrasts notably with one of its more publicized adaptations in the United States. Glenner Town Square, an adult day care facility in California for people with Alzheimer's, is designed to reproduce the experience of "main street USA" in the 1950s. Its facility also has a café, movie theater, pub, museum, newsstand, and other "stores," each featuring period-appropriate encounters for visitors. Visitors can "take a walk down memory lane with a loved one" or receive more structured clinical care through guided activities with staff, all a part of what Glenner calls "immersive reminiscence therapy."[48] The facility looks a little like a theme park—its miniature buildings were actually created by set designers from the San Diego Opera.[49] Glenner says it hopes its activities will lessen anxiety, encourage socialization, and help people get better rest at night, but its marketing seems perched on the promise to transport people with dementia back to another time. The company also claims that its approach to care is "revolutionary," a promise echoed or challenged by various media outlets. Robert Siegel on National Public Radio challenged the homogeneity of Glenner's version of the past as well as the potential confusion day visitors might have.[50] Maria Shriver adopted a more celebratory tone on the morning talk show *Today*: "there's a lot of creativity going on, trying to figure out different ways to activate the brain, music, you know, going back to a place like this, showing movies, looking at newsstands with the hope that that will bring the person somewhat back to you. . . . They feel like they remember and then they'll feel like they're themselves."[51]

Even if these kinds of activities do not help people with Alzheimer's the way some hope they might, many see reminiscence therapy as a valuable activity for families and friends of people with the disease. Really any kind of activity that brings some respite to caregivers can be seen as helpful, but a lot of focus is specifically placed on the preservation of threatened memories and identity. For example, a cottage industry that produces "memory books" offers to save valuable memories before they are lost to dementia.[52] The successful radio project "MemoryCorps" obeys the same media principle: record the stories before they are gone. The program is part of the public radio initiative StoryCorps, which circulates a mobile audio recording studio around the country. People with Alzheimer's and their families or friends can come to record their memories before they are lost. StoryCorps also encourages young people to record stories with their elders as a part of the "Great Thanksgiving Listen."[53] In 2015 the project sent more than 50,500 individual stories to the Library of Congress. StoryCorps reports that 96 percent of listeners say the program has increased their understanding of someone with a serious illness or disability.[54]

Certainly programs like these can have a meaningful impact on caregivers and people with dementia alike. An ironic side effect of interventions designed to restore or protect the identity of people with Alzheimer's is that they can overly emphasize their threatened individuality. For example, some people with Alzheimer's have taken an active stance in the maintenance of their own stories by writing autobiographies. The genre has helped clarify some of the difficulties involved with the disease, and their authorship could also be interpreted as a successful response to claims about the loss of agency or voice. But as Anne Basting points out, these autobiographies focus on the loss of the "I" in a way that leaves no room for other manifestations of the person. These authors often write their own stories to shore up the self in light of its impending loss. "Part of the reason," writes Basting, "is our strong focus on the individual. We think that this must be some *one's* story. Americans tend to think that people are either dependent or independent—we can't possibly be in between."[55] Indeed, one problem with any loss-of-self narrative is the excessive emphasis it places on the role of the self as a relational individual.

One interesting intervention into these representational dilemmas is an increasingly popular genre of patient-driven care that relies on collaborations around online social media and media gatherings on Zoom. Dementia Alliance International (DAI) is a membership program that offers forums for people with dementia to participate in live, online discussions and support groups. Ideally, this kind of care restores the agency of the person with dementia by providing opportunities for interpersonal exchange and socialization. The group doesn't give medical advice, claiming instead to combat stigma through educational webinars and advocacy. Echoing the disability activist slogan "Nothing about us, without us," DAI promotes the organization as "of, by, and for people with dementia." The alliance was founded in 2014 by a group of people from the United States, Canada, and Australia, but it now advertises itself as available to people with dementia from anywhere.[56]

Although DAI webinars are potentially open to outsiders, the online support groups have generally been restricted to people with dementia and their caregivers to preserve privacy. Participation in these groups is not necessarily about successful verbal exchange; one can participate simply by logging into a Zoom room. It is not even necessary to turn on the computer's camera, though that kind of participation is built into the design. The program is designed to emulate "an experience that is much like sitting around with a group of friends." Sessions are not only exclusive in membership; they are exclusive in time. According to DAI, nothing is recorded. The live encounter in these sessions transforms the temporal aesthetics of Alzheimer's into a different model of participatory agency. Selfhood shifts from an interior, identitarian condition to one of interpersonal activity. The DAI tagline "See the person, not the dementia" is enacted within the exclusive, live video chat between several people.

The critical question then becomes, does this example merely rehearse naive accounts of networked agency and techno-utopias so common in early accounts of new digital media? Or do the representational problems of Alzheimer's require that we reevaluate that critique in this instance? Given the way media so publicly shapes personhood, people experiencing symptoms of dementia are wise to consider how their own agential narratives are built into media environments. But the DAI sessions join a genre of dementia care that encourages both individual and group work around the creation of media representations not beholden to ideologies of salvation or capture. Instead, they open the door to a range of live social interactions. One of the crucial aspects of an intervention like this is that it is designed to create safe, social environments rather than preserve memories. The model of care seems little interested in rescuing a person's selfhood or identity within a media framework. That alone is an important victory in rethinking Alzheimer's personhood. Indeed, Alzheimer's networks like these might help us all reconceive of what personhood might already be.

5

Dementia in the Museum

Modern Art as Public Care

One recent afternoon, I sat with a small group in a well-lit, otherwise empty gallery of the New York Museum of Modern Art. The group was composed of six people diagnosed with Alzheimer's, several caregivers, and me. Before us, a MoMA educator stood next to *Sky Cathedral,* Louise Nevelson's large, flat, black wood sculpture.[1]

The educator briefly lectured us on the artist's background, discussing the sculptural style and how the piece was assembled. Some members of the group did not respond during this lecture, but other participants were quite visibly enthusiastic, smiling, nodding, and chatting softly (see the endnotes for clarification on the varied use of text and symbols in this chapter).[2]

EDUCATOR: Should I tell you the name of the piece now? It's called *Sky Cathedral.* Why do you think it's called that?

The group was hesitant. There was some murmuring, a cough or two, but no one spoke up. Todd, sitting beside his mother with a protective arm around her shoulder, raised his free hand.[3]

TODD: Mom has a different name. Yes, she calls it *puzzlement.*

Todd's mother, sitting more alertly in her wheelchair now, smiled and nodded.

MILLIE: Oh yeah, that's cool. I like that. That's good . . . *puzzlement.*

The woman who spoke, Millie, was apparently unrelated to this pair, but she sat next to them, and they seemed to share good rapport. Like Todd's mother, Millie had been diagnosed with Alzheimer's. She put her hand on Todd's mother's arm and squeezed it. Both smiled. The educator mentioned that there was a lot of black in the previous paintings we had looked at, and she asked how people felt about the black in this sculpture.

MILLIE: It's cool. Way cool. [*laughs*]

The group laughed with Millie, as she had already deemed many other artworks "cool" in this session. The educator read aloud a quotation from Nevelson that explained her perspective on black.

EDUCATOR: Maybe this will help: "It wasn't the negation of color, it was an acceptance. Because black encompasses all colors. Black is the most aristocratic color of all. The only aristocratic color. For me, this is the ultimate. You can be quiet, and it contains the whole thing." Now what do people think about that?
MILLIE: Veeeryyy coool. [*laughs*]
GROUP: [*laughing along with Millie*]
EDUCATOR: Cool huh? [*laughing too*] You like that? Why?
MILLIE: I don't know, it's just cool. Yeah . . . [*excited, nodding*] it's black . . .

Millie's voice trailed off into silence as she looked intently at the sculpture.

EDUCATOR: What do other people think?

Jill, another caregiver sitting on the other side of the group, spoke up. She leaned forward, facing the group but responding to the educator.

JILL: I don't know, I'm not sure I'm on board with the all black thing. It's not so comforting to me, it still has, I don't know, something dark about it. There's just too much black.

MILLIE, *nodding*: Yes, it's too black.

EDUCATOR: So it's not cool?

MILLIE: No, not cool. Definitely not cool.

This exchange details an encounter I had with MoMA's Alzheimer's education program, Meet Me at MoMA (also known as Meet Me).[4] The program invites people with early to mid-stage Alzheimer's disease and their caregivers to engage in monthly tours of MoMA exhibits in small groups. These tours, led by specially trained educators, usually last about an hour and a half, and they generally focus on just four or five works of art per visit. Meet Me is a good example of a popular psychosocial treatment model that figures art as potentially therapeutic or helpful to both people with dementia and their caregivers, each of whom might need help in the caring process. The psychosocial approach does not dismiss biomedical treatment outright; rather, it seeks to provide a more diverse set of nonpharmacological alternatives to Alzheimer's care and treatment.

Meet Me is a central component of the more expansive MoMA Alzheimer's Project, a special museum initiative that ran from 2007 to 2014. MoMA also coordinated educational conferences and participated in a support network for other institutions looking to develop their own dementia programs.[5] The museum even published a comprehensive book that illustrates how the program works, including interviews with program staff and commentary by professionals whose work deals with Alzheimer's.[6] MoMA also offered a DVD and book "module" for home or nonmuseum use that integrated potential education themes with artwork from the MoMA collection.[7] In 2007 the museum worked with the MetLife Foundation (the charitable wing of the MetLife insurance company) and New York University's Center for Excellence for Brain Aging and Dementia on a collaborative pilot project to "measure how programs such as Meet Me at MoMA positively impact people with early-stage Alzheimer's, as well as their caregivers."[8] This research led to more extended support for the project from MetLife.

MoMA runs Meet Me out of the Community and Access wing of its renowned Department of Education. In addition to offering both youth and adult education, the department provides programs for individuals who are deaf or hard of hearing, blind or partially sighted, or have learning disabilities. The MoMA Alzheimer's Project became a celebrated program for the Department of Education, garnering awards, press, and broad acclaim, which the museum promoted on its website.

Meet Me is a helpful case study for this book for two reasons: first, it illustrates still-developing perspectives about the value of art as a therapeutic tool for Alzheimer's care, and second, the program contributes to optimistic efforts to define and shape personhood through technologies of media. Because the program was designed for people with Alzheimer's *and* their caregivers, it allows for many different kinds of interactions while looking at art: the possibility for community and socialization, learning about art, positive feelings, and diminished anxiety. The diversity of modes of engagement leads to a productive confusion between the program as "art therapy" and as "art education." In an institution dedicated to the history of modern aesthetics and acclaimed artists, the program offers an unusual synthesis of the celebration of the individual mind and group-oriented affect.

Meet Me ultimately endorses the individual promise of *all* people, a utopian promise about interiority that people with and without dementia might share. This is a promise based at least in part on the media artifacts on which the program is based and the artistic genius required for their conception. While this kind of claim about access or capacity can certainly help challenge public perceptions around the loss of self, as a model of care, it does little to accommodate the structural differences that shape the lived experiences of Alzheimer's disease. Instead, it asserts the universal promise of modern art as an expansive tool in the service of care.

While Meet Me is a unique program at MoMA, I argue that it upholds two historical legacies of the museum's broader educational mission. The first of these legacies concerns the temporal alignment of the museum's modern art collection with the potential of progressive public education. The second regards an ideal of individual minds that unites artist and museum patron. Both of these legacies help shape Meet Me's model of care and its contributions toward mediated personhood.

Modern Times, Modern Selves—Some Historical Perspective

MoMA's approach to both educating and collecting has historically followed a progressive logic. While the past is acknowledged as vital—it is in fact a museum—MoMA has also prioritized the immediate future as part of its institutional mandate. For example, arguing for a mission of contemporary collection over gallery display, the museum's first director, Alfred H. Barr Jr., imagined the museum as a "torpedo moving through time, its nose the ever advancing present, its tail the ever receding past of fifty to a hundred years ago."[9] Later, in the 1960s, Barr said, "Looking back over the history of art is necessary and richly rewarding. But history begins with today. What will tomorrow bring? We look forward, impatiently."[10] Looking forward here helped a museum successfully to collect but also to negotiate the problem of an always transforming now: the elusive status of the "modern."

When temporality is part of an institutional logic—as it is with a modern art museum like this—it can be aligned with other social traditions that share similar relationships with time. For example, a 2012 advertisement for MetLife's Alzheimer's-related philanthropy neatly sutures MoMA's modernism and an Alzheimer's-based temporality into a kind of social fear (one ostensibly helpful for selling insurance). The Meet Me sponsor's advertisement depicts Snoopy in the third frame of a *Peanuts* comic strip. He looks back over the other two frames, which appear to be fading away. Beneath the strip is the tagline "Imagine forgetting your past."

Fear of losing the past is a common social attitude toward Alzheimer's, but the way that manifests into a museological ethic is significant. Lawrence Cohen's reminder that Alzheimer's helps society articulate broader relationships to time is relevant here: "The way senility marks a body as being irrevocably in time suggests a relationship between figures of the old body and temporal or political ruptures in the order of things. Senility becomes a critical idiom through which collectivities imagine and articulate a consciousness of such rupture and

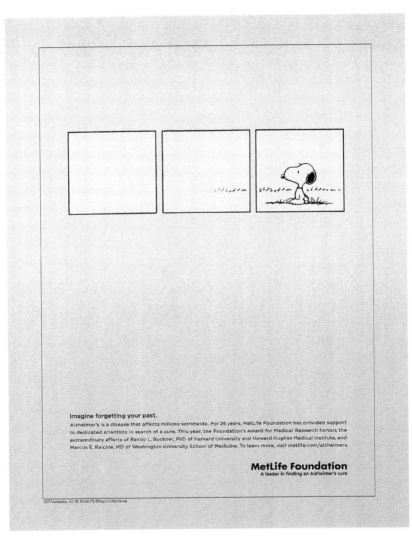

FIGURE 10. "Imagine forgetting your past." Alzheimer's temporality in an advertisement for the MetLife Foundation.

of the possibility of some sort of recuperation."[11] Meet Me clearly informs that "critical idiom." Cohen's description of rupture and recuperation is relevant to both MoMA's museological stakes and its educational mission. The rupture—and this is perhaps true of all museums—lies in the aesthetic claim: modern art. Modernity is always a temporal claim to collective progress, but as a museological, sense-making operation, it promotes a participatory aesthetics as the primary logic of that progress. Meet Me extends that logic into the universal promise of personhood itself. The program defends the history and value of modern art as a kind of universalizing rupture while also speaking to its recuperative promise for people dealing with dementia. Even though Meet Me encourages a presentist ethic of care, the reliance on these modern progress narratives anachronizes this universal promise.

For example, Meet Me's early slogan "Meet Me at MoMA . . . and Make Memories" is an institutional mandate toward the future that acknowledges the fragile state of its participants' pasts.[12] Here museological and biological memories collapse into a form of cultural memory, yoking fear to a kind of social responsibility to representation. This can be seen as a form of cultural memory precisely because of the slippery memorial values it promotes; as Marita Sturken argues, cultural memory reveals "the stakes held by individuals and institutions in attributing meaning to the past."[13] In this case, cultural memory is a form of individual and social empowerment. The slogan offers an uneasy mixture of the symptoms of dementia and the social promise of a museum.

It might be argued that these museological stakes seem more "postmodern" than modern, given these unstable relationships with temporality, but that perspective would miss the mark.[14] The way in which both the museum's education and curatorial programs claim a *particular* relationship to time reveals this ethic as deeply modern. Anxieties about loss, maintenance, rupture, and recuperation all support a moralizing claim about the status of the individual in and against time. This is not a metaphorical argument regarding symptoms of loss and dementia; it is, rather, a claim about the way certain social institutions organize collective relationships against the precariousness of the everyday.

That leads to the second of MoMA's educational traditions that organizes the status of the individual: in particular, the individual's autonomous capacity and, to a certain degree, her status as psychically unknowable. This model of interiority helps to frame both the individual artist and the individual viewer or museum-goer. In both cases, MoMA's practices might be understood as interdependent authorizations of a model of personhood that offers reciprocal social valuation of MoMA itself.

On one hand, MoMA promotes the artist as formidable creative talent to be respected: a unique and autonomous individual. But that artist also requires public study to ensure her status as a special individual. That happens in part through the museum's educational activities. Haidee Wasson argues that "formalizing an educational ethos [at MoMA] ensured sustained commitment to museum outreach, yet it also concretized the hierarchy between the serious and the popular, the properly artistic and the educational, within the museum's structure."[15] In other words, MoMA's educational practices consecrate the artist just as they structurally separate the artist from the public.

On the other hand, museological investment in individuality can also be interpreted as an investment in the museum patron as a self-made person. Aesthetic appreciation, creative intellect, and social potential: these are all capacities the museum might foster through educational outreach. Carol Morgan argues that midcentury progressive public education in the United States emphasized the potential of the individual citizen in much the same way that modern art fetishized the capabilities of the individual artist.[16] The progressive education that MoMA has historically valued fosters foremost an individual's capacity to grow. This tactic reinforces the developing status of the individual in question rather than her past.

According to these arguments, museological goals tether progressive temporality to both education and collection, and MoMA reinforces the essential power of the individual without compromising that important boundary between artistic genius and liberal populist potential. This explains how the museum can prioritize the products of unique creativity while still maintaining a foundation from which to organize popular education. The art allows access to interior, creative mystery and serves as the platform for collective education.

I argue that these educational traditions are still in play at MoMA today as lasting legacies of Western modernism, and they deeply inform Meet Me's promise as a psychosocial intervention. This is a temporality that in fact harmonizes with biomedical claims to the future and hope for a cure. The program helps the museum maintain an ethic of modern temporality alongside a philanthropic valuation of individual interiority. And it is precisely the art that helps forge this relationship. This is the universal promise of mediated personhood. Meet Me represents a social interest in modern art as a psychic, intellectual exercise, and it thus has the power to elevate, heal, and sustain a worthy population. If Meet Me's success is predicated on art's availability to a person with dementia *and* her caregiver, it is precisely art's ability to access an essential interiority that structures its value as a universal therapy.

The modern art object is authorized as a therapeutic tool in the service of public health, but it also participates in broader assumptions about the nature of psychic interiority. Take, for example, the following headline from the *AARP Bulletin* (a publication for Americans over fifty): "In Museums, Those with Alzheimer's Find Themselves Again: Art Revives Memories, and Sparks Flashes of Personality, Humor, and Perception."[17] This perspective validates the promise of art for a compromised mind. But it also comments ironically on the supposed capacity of the individual with dementia while reinforcing stigmas of lost selfhood, as the very viability of her personhood belongs to a younger version of herself. Celebrated in this discourse is art's power to "spark" or "revive" a buried, more valid past.

One cannot underestimate the importance of the art object and aesthetic mystery to the reputation of this program, as it offers a language for the public to reframe Alzheimer's personhood in optimistic terms. In this sense, it is not so much that the art object is, for example, abstract—and thus that it somehow harmonizes with the "abstract" mind of the person with dementia. Rather, I am arguing about collective relationships with time, mind, and value. As a creative encounter with the world, the art *matters* to this program. This aesthetic promise frames Alzheimer's personhood as viable in a future tense, abstracting the many differences that underwrite this disease under the vague banner of progress, potential, hope, and mystery. The next chapter further develops the biopolitics of creativity from the perspective of the individual artist, but for now it is important to grasp how art serves as a complex, discursive logic for progressive institutional and individual relationships to Alzheimer's.

From 2008 until 2012, I conducted ethnographic research on the Meet Me program. I performed interviews, observed sessions at the museum, and attended special educational events to learn how Meet Me works. I investigated both Meet Me's institutional discourse and the way people who work on the program understand their own roles as educators. In particular, I was concerned with the way public attitudes toward Alzheimer's and dementia encountered a tradition of modern art and progressive psychosocial treatment. How does Meet Me operate? How does it determine its own success? Why do other programs follow its lead? Is there a necessary relationship between Alzheimer's and modern art, aesthetic, ideological, or otherwise? What about Alzheimer's is understood to be modern? These are all questions I asked myself and the people who operate the program at MoMA.

As social nodes that enact a historically situated, developing subject of Alzheimer's, Meet Me sessions help to normalize and socialize the disease without necessarily fixing or curing. In this sense, they offer something akin to what Emily Martin describes in her analysis of bipolar disorder support groups: a "fabric of relatedness."[18] These fabrics help develop a sense of community and recognition of shared experience. They allow people dealing with the disease in different ways to come together in a loose community enacted by the disease without necessarily just being "about" that disease. Caregivers can discover, for example, that they share experiences similar to other caregivers'. Or people diagnosed with Alzheimer's might find comfort or perspective in sharing an activity with others with a similar diagnosis. My own participation in the Meet Me sessions wove me into this fabric of relatedness.[19]

Indeed, the material nature of my investigation is tricky precisely because of the social systems of description that historically give shape to this disease. My research needed to get beyond those traditions. Indeed, my fieldwork offers a useful kind of evidence that gets beyond the simple description of the construction of a disease category, instead helping to articulate the disease in context. Because of that, perhaps it can give voice to (and thus help respect) the variability of Alzheimer's as a lived process. I provide an extended account of a session here to convey something of the general tone and conversational style of a Meet Me session.[20] Given that finding "voice" can be a complicated challenge for people with dementia, I have tried to limit my interpretation here to the institutional tactics I discovered.

A Typical Session

MoMA sits along a few busy streets in the heart of Midtown Manhattan. One Tuesday, I arrived on the subway a block away and walked through the crowded streets toward the museum's side entrance. Walking into the museum provided immediate relief, as the filtered air and quiet, welcoming lobby contrasted notably with the cacophony outside. The museum is closed to the general public on Tuesdays, and so the few people who were there were either special visitors or museum staff.

I met with one of the many educational staff waiting at the desk to welcome Meet Me participants, and after giving me a name tag handwritten with my first name (bordered blue, to denote my group), she directed me to wait inside. Gradually the lobby began to fill up with arriving participants. Some used wheelchairs or walkers. One or two were quite active, shaking hands and greeting friends around the lobby. But for the most part, the visitors moved about in the caregiving groups of two or three. Not all of these caregivers appeared to be spouses—and of course it was impossible to tell based on their relative ages—but I presumed that some were paid aides and some were children, friends, or other (presumably unpaid) caregivers. One or two people appeared to be there alone. Outside of the relatively young educational staff (most appeared to be white, female professionals in their twenties or thirties), I felt I was the only "young" person waiting. I felt implicated, different. At the time, I was in my thirties.

It was always difficult for me to learn more about the program participants: where they came from, what their home care situations were like, their general backgrounds. While Meet Me visitors are encouraged to discuss their feelings or share stories during the sessions, they maintain a general anonymity. Aside from the requirement that one have dementia or be caring for someone with dementia, one's background is not central to the program experience. Indeed, as I will demonstrate, it is precisely their present potential that Meet Me values most.

At exactly two-thirty, our tour guide arrived with a blue name tag of his own, "Jean," dressed smartly in a blazer and blue jeans. He immediately took control of the waiting group, introducing himself in a clear, loud voice, even though it was evident that many in the group already knew him. Jean's introduction was concise, directed, and disarming. He maintained remarkable eye contact with the group throughout the visit.

> JEAN: OK, welcome, hello, let's get started. Lots of familiar faces here, some of you I have seen before, some maybe not on *my* tour. This is a different tour. I want to talk about what we're doing *today*. Sometimes when we come to a museum we look at lots of different works, today we're going to just look at four or five different works in depth and have a conversation about them. And let me emphasize that this is going to be a *conversation*. I want everyone to be involved. Our theme today is going to be *Spring Fever*.
>
> GROUP: [*many laugh along with Jean*]
>
> JEAN: Yes, I know, some laughter, but don't take it *lightly*. We're going to go into *depth*.

The manner in which Jean introduced the spring theme that day was not uncommon. Each Meet Me session generally has a theme (as do many education programs and nonmuseological art therapy exercises). While not all discussion necessarily follows that theme, it may help inspire contributions from reticent participants, and it also provides a useful tether for an educator in what often becomes a disparate conversation. Sometimes the educator will rely on the theme heavily; others dismiss it entirely. Occasionally, the show itself will provide the theme; for example, a show might cover a particular artist or a historical period, style, or movement.

We arrived that day at the galleries on the fifth floor, which were empty and quiet except for a faint echo of other Meet Me groups already under way in other parts of the museum. Sitting in a small group in front of *Starry Night,* or *Les Demoiselles d'Avignon,* or some such well-known artwork is a special occasion. But this is especially true when the museum is closed to the public, its galleries quiet, peaceful. It feels like that group is the only reason the museum is open at all, and thus the group is deemed vital as an audience. This is a relationship based on exclusivity. One of the institutional roles of the MoMA education programs, "providing access," acquires a multilayered valence because of this. It is no accident that anthropologists often use the word *access* themselves to describe their relationships with their informants and research sites. In both senses, access indicates exclusive relationships with the truth, and I think this is a powerful component of how the program does its work of recognition and validation.

We gathered in a loose group on fold-out stools around two paintings by Georges-Pierre Seurat. Everyone looked at the paintings for a moment before Jean began to lead the conversation. I watched and listened and found myself mimicking the crowd, nodding when they nodded, laughing when they laughed, almost anticipating their collective responses. I didn't do this intentionally. A woman with long gray hair kept turning to stare at me with a smile on her face, apparently more interested in me than the paintings. I smiled too, hunched forward in apparent interest, and tried to get her to look back at the paintings.

JEAN: What do you notice? What's similar about these two paintings?
SAM: Well, they're both nautical scenes.
JEAN: Yes, good, Sam, they're both—very advanced terminology—*nautical* . . . they both have boats and water. What else?

Readers will note that Jean, like all educators at Meet Me, was very conscious of each individual's ability to hear or process others' comments. This is of course not anomalous to this kind of tour. Devices to aid hearing were made available to participants, but they didn't necessarily solve all communication problems. A common tactic educators used to help was to identify each participant by name for the group and then repeat what the person had said in a loud and clear voice.

JEAN: What else?
PARTICIPANT: They're by the same painter.

Jean moved on to explain that yes, indeed, they were by the same painter, Georges-Pierre Seurat. Someone voiced the fact that the paintings have lots of dots, and—after agreeing—Jean spoke for a few minutes about the style of pointillism, optical theory, and the history of the artist. This was a relatively complicated account, and it was impossible to ascertain how much was learned. But many nodded throughout, and Jean worked through his lecture after a few minutes and quickly returned to the discussion.

FRANK: They're very serene.
JEAN: Yes, does everybody see this? These paintings are very *serene*. This goes with our theme of the day—spring—does everyone see that?
MABEL: I thought spring was supposed to be full of life, and energy, and new beginnings; how is that serene?
JEAN: OK, so Mabel says that maybe these *aren't* serene [*and then quickly moving on*], what are these round shapes here? What do we think that these might be? Someone who hasn't talked yet today?
NEW PARTICIPANT: Maybe they're shadows of the clouds on the water.
JEAN: *Yes* . . . shadows of the clouds on the water, did everybody hear that? See how he uses different color here to indicate the clouds' shadows?
HELEN: Maybe he's trying to show how the color of the water changes when it gets deeper or shallower.
JEAN: Well that's an idea I hadn't heard before. Did everyone hear that? Helen said she thinks that the color shapes on the water come from different depths of water.
HELEN: Yes, see how none of the boats are going in the darker patches, it . . . maybe it's because . . . maybe it's deeper there.

JEAN: You know, I know a lot about Seurat, and I've read everything there is to read about him, and I've never heard anyone make that comment before. You know you're right! There are no boats on the darker blue shapes. Maybe that's because it's a difference in water depth. OK, very good, so what else do you see? What's similar here?

DON: Well, these are both paintings about water and boats.

This was the first casual repetition of the day, something that happens frequently, and Jean took it in stride, reminding us all—as he often did as a matter of course—of what we had already talked about. He used a number of conversational tactics like this one, never negating, always encouraging. His style was one of affirmation or, if in a tight spot, deflection. This is standard practice for Meet Me educators. They rarely tell someone no or point out an error. In this case, he simply absorbed the repetition as normal.

Alzheimer's is never mentioned during Meet Me sessions, nor are its symptoms. The concept of memory, for example, rarely comes up. The only person I ever heard bring up Alzheimer's was an educator before or after a session in private conversation. The silence on the subject of dementia is intentional. According to educators, they are instructed not to allude to the disease. One educator thought of the program as a form of "escapism," or a chance to enjoy the art and the museum and not have to deal with dementia, hence the institutional suppression. Many educators find this to be Meet Me's primary benefit.

JEAN: Yes, right, very good, these are both water scenes, it's spring, it's colorful, we know there are these shapes on the water . . . what else?

PARTICIPANT: They're very colorful.

JEAN: Yes, they're colorful, let's talk about that. Mabel, you were here last month and we actually stopped at this painting and we talked about color. That was our theme last time, but now it's *spring awakening*.

GROUP: [*laughter*]

JEAN: What do we think about the color?

DON: There are boats here.

Remarkably, at this very moment of repetition, a number of young children in a school group walked through our gallery. They looked at us, and the participants looked at the kids the best they could—many couldn't turn their heads easily. There was an awareness of difference. They were there, perhaps, for different purposes. The kids moved on quietly, and Jean turned to a discussion of modern art.

> JEAN: This art is about the form—the artists are very conscious of form in their work. It's about what they're painting in the art, but it's also about the *practice* of art, the *materials* of art. Modern artists are very conscious of form, painting is about *painting,* sculpture about *sculpture,* film about *film.*
> MABEL: Well people were conscious about form before 1840.
> JEAN: Yes, you're right, very good, they were, but we're talking about Seurat now and the work in this gallery . . . so what else do you see?
> DON: They're all boating scenes.
> ALEXI: I see footsteps!

There were no footsteps in the paintings—at least none that I could see—and the comment diverted entirely from Jean's trajectory. Alexi was actually looking at a different part of the gallery entirely.

> JEAN: OK, good, footsteps, where?
> ALEXI: There.

Alexi looked pointedly across the gallery. Everyone looked at her for more information or guidance, expectant. Maybe she was looking at a different painting that we couldn't see, but she appeared confused. She began to get anxious, gesturing across the gallery.

> ALEXI: Down there! Over there!

Jean shifted the conversation, conscious of her anxiety.

> JEAN: OK, good, footsteps are another idea . . . so what do you think about these paintings? Do you like them?

PARTICIPANT: Yes!

JEAN: Why?

PARTICIPANT, *as if it's the most obvious thing in the world*: They're beautiful!

JEAN: Who else? [. . .]

MABEL: I like them. They're pretty. But he's an innovator. He's trying to do something here.

JEAN: Yes, he's an *innovator* [group laughter] . . . you're right. He's one of my favorite painters in *all* the museum. OK, shall we move on?

Everyone then slowly moved off into another gallery and a different piece of art.

This strategy of acceptance and affirmation dominated the sessions. Rather than correct, educators accept or ignore. And generally these educators are quite successful in eliciting responses. It really doesn't matter if someone makes an error. The rule is simply to repeat what someone says so everyone can hear it, affirm the validity of the person's

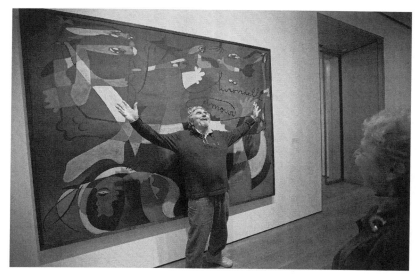

FIGURE 11. Participants in a session of Meet Me at MoMA. Courtesy of Marilynn K. Yee. Copyright *New York Times*.

statement, and move on to find someone else also to affirm or to make her own contribution. Repeat, affirm, and move on. You can always move on. This affirmation is designed to help participants dismiss their anxieties and develop positive feelings. And that positivity is a significant component of the public reputation of the program. As one *USA Today* headline quipped, "Alzheimer's Program Is One from the Art."[21]

In this sense the program functions through individual validation rather than purported education or learning. What matters is not so much what someone says in response to a painting but that the person responds at all, that she has a voice. One educator told me that it is vital participants get a "sense of understanding" via recognition as a part of the group. MoMA reinforces this—speaking, communicating, and being allowed to give your own input are central components. As another educator told me, for people with Alzheimer's, Meet Me "fulfills a basic human need to be heard." This approach is increasingly common in models of care, such as the popular dementia care tool developed by Anne Basting called TimeSlips. It encourages creative storytelling and validates all manner of contribution or engagement.

While error is tolerated as a matter of course by educators, it is perhaps important to point out that other participants did not always follow this logic. Sometimes participants would disagree or even argue, but these disagreements would never last long, as the logic of group harmony would often win out. The general mood at these sessions was happy, hopeful. Frequent laughter can be contagious, and it often overshadows performances of cognitive instability or conflict. The institutional avoidance of error in these sessions illustrates the unstable balance between the program's educational and therapeutic goals. While Meet Me educators want participants to learn something about modern art and their collection, the affective well-being of the participants is often more important.

The slippage between art education and art therapy in the Meet Me program is not incidental; in fact, under the rubric of "access," that slippage underwrites the logic of Meet Me's success. While the program is located thematically and institutionally in a department of art education and access, its primary goals are as much therapeutic or even palliative as they are educational. The program is presumably educational in that it attempts to teach both the person with Alzheimer's and the caregiver something about the art. The program is presumably therapeutic because of its power to access and heal an embattled interiority and to validate the person with Alzheimer's and her caregiver as sharing some essential human nature and present viability. The program makes no claims as to its status as an educational program or a therapy program; as an access program for people with Alzheimer's, it is special.

Part of the problem in determining program success in this regard lies in the different backgrounds of people who participate. Furthermore, Meet Me is geared toward people with Alzheimer's *and* their caregivers. It is designed to be helpful for people with cognitive disability and those without. As a psychosocial intervention into Alzheimer's care situations, the health of both sides of the caregiving contract is respected as potentially vulnerable. While educators often seem to focus their attention more on those people with Alzheimer's than on caregivers, the program allows for diverse modes of engagement and pleasure. The ambiguity of the role of education, access, therapy, and validation allows for that diverse engagement, inclusive of my own participation.

To be clear, art therapy often denotes *making* art rather than talking about it. In her book *When Words Have Lost Their Meaning*, Ruth Abraham argues that "the central feature of art therapy, which gives it such natural potential as a healing agent for the condition of Alzheimer's, is the fact that it bypasses the need for verbal communication."[22] Art therapy here is also called "expressive therapy." It allows for expression when, as Abraham argues, "words have lost their meaning."

According to this definition, Meet Me can hardly be called art therapy—at least not in the art-making sense. MoMA did also offer art-making sessions as a part of the broader Alzheimer's Project. They were often very quiet and peaceful, with only occasional instruction from the teacher breaking the silence. On the whole, they operated in the manner Abraham promotes—as a mode of expression that does not require much verbal communication for success. My understanding after watching these sessions is that participants very much enjoyed them.

But the Meet Me sessions upstairs in the galleries almost insist on validating each individual's contribution. Educators will often kneel down next to uncommunicative or nonverbal participants, asking them for their thoughts on a piece of art. This tactic does sometimes work to elicit some contribution from an otherwise laconic person, but the effort can seem herculean. Educators often seem pleased when they manage to include everyone with dementia in the conversation, even if the comments they elicit are not well received by other participants.

MoMA eventually introduced a new strategy to deal with those participants deemed to be at a later stage in the disease: those with more "apparent" symptoms were grouped together in a separate session. One educator called this the single most substantial change to the program since it began. According to Meet Me administrators, the idea behind this move was to provide these individuals with an experience in which the pace of conversation is slower and they can be included in the group dynamics. But the goal is still communication—at least in part—and looking and talking are still maintained as the central logic of therapy.

Locating Success: Aesthetics and Affect

Sometimes the therapeutic event has little to do with the artwork itself. For example, we ended that spring visit (led by Jean) in front of Claude Monet's triptych landscape painting *Water Lilies*. Jean asked the group if it reminded them of the theme of the day (spring). One of the participants, Bill, got very excited.

> BILL: I don't know about that, but when I was in grade school I was in chorus, and we had to sing a song called . . . the "Rustle". . . "*The Rustle of Spring*" . . . by *Christian Sinding*. I remember that because our teacher made us memorize it and it rhymed. [*singsongs it*] "The Rustle of Spring" by Christian *Sinding*. [*laughs*]
>
> HAZEL: You were in chorus? *I* was in chorus too [*laughing*]!

At this point the whole room broke out in voices, everyone talking about chorus or laughing or asking their partners what had been said.

Jean repeated the story for everyone in a loud and clear voice, and then Hazel told her own childhood chorus story about getting asked to be a "listener" because of her poor singing skills. Jean expressed disbelief that they had listeners and singers in chorus, and everyone roared with laughter because he did not understand. Jean was then somehow put on the spot as the person who did not grow up in New York City sixty or seventy years ago, when this practice was perhaps more commonplace.

This kind of incident is not uncommon. Educators are young, smart, and often creative artists themselves. They form a distinct body from the people looking at art: the people with Alzheimer's and their caregivers. But they also represent the museum. Along with the guards and the administrators, they serve as a kind of authoritative point of access, of giving, of teaching, of benevolence. But this is often refused (not necessarily intentionally) by the people with Alzheimer's and their caregivers. In this particular account, the memories were shaped by collective experiences of growing up in New York.

This form of shared memory was enacted by the social experience of Meet Me, but it was also dismissive of it. By dismissive, I mean to suggest that essential artistic components of the program—the works of art and the accompanying practices of looking—were not a required part of this interaction. This conversation could happen in any care group or community center, just so long as that space embraces the possibility of collective recognition. Certainly Meet Me encourages such "memory access," and it is framed as a positive side effect to the program.

I witnessed another incident during a different session in which the person with Alzheimer's did not exclude the institution but certainly changed the terms of the conversation and the relevance of the art. In this case, it was not ostensibly about memory access. A charismatic former artist with dementia named Sue was sitting in her wheelchair. She quite suddenly interrupted the teaching narrative of the educator.

SUE: *Hey!* [*shouting*] Look at me! . . . *Look at me.*

The educator stopped talking and looked over. And once she had looked at Sue, Sue blew her a kiss, narrowed her eyes, and grinned.

The educator looked a bit stunned, perhaps because this seemed to come from nowhere. She did not appear equipped to field the cue. After a long, silent pause, the educator cleared her throat and returned to her lecture.

This moment of the kiss fulfilled the institutional goals for participants: making memories, feeling good, positivity, smiling. But it also challenged those goals, literally in the command, *look at me*, and in the kiss: an invitation. To what? I have no idea. But it revealed an affective sociality that superseded the aesthetics or form of the art. People with Alzheimer's often "misrecognize" others, and perhaps she thought the educator was an old lover, friend, or partner. Perhaps this was simple social "disinhibition," common with Alzheimer's, and Sue just wanted some attention. What is clear about this situation is that Sue transformed the practice of looking at art into a vital, new social engagement.

This example returns us to the question of the importance of the art to the Meet Me experience. How important is the form of the artwork to the success of the session? Does representative art work better than nonrepresentative art? Is there a link between the abstraction of an artwork and some presumed abstraction in the brain of the person with Alzheimer's? MoMA is only one of many museums to now offer successful dementia access programs; even if it is a model, is there anything about MoMA's collection that makes it better suited to this kind of interaction?

In interviews, the educators disagreed over which art worked better. The debate over representational art versus nonrepresentational art, for example, did not play as central a role in participant engagement. In fact, the choice of artwork was often more reliant on the educator's familiarity with the piece or style and her corresponding ability to guide a conversation or to elicit contributions.[23]

In fact, the ambience of the looking environment plays a more significant role than the art under engagement. Because the museum is closed for Meet Me, sessions occur in a closed, controlled environment that is generally quiet and temperature stable. Outside distractions are not uncommon, however, and they are probably the single most difficult factor in a Meet Me session.

And of course, the participants might see artworks in radically different ways, even though they are looking together at the same art object. This is in part because Alzheimer's can affect visual perception; while some people with Alzheimer's actually report heightened visual acuity, many recent studies show that visual impairment can be understood as a symptom of Alzheimer's.[24] At Meet Me, the discordance in different visual perspectives often creates moments of humor, indecision, or conflict in the program.

For example, during one session, we were all seated in a ring in front of Henri Rousseau's 1910 painting *The Dream,* and the educator, Jonah, asked us what we saw.

> JONAH: Some things are kind of hidden, so look closely, be patient, I just want you to look at the whole painting and see what you see.

We started with perhaps a more obvious element in the painting, the elephant, and then moved on to other animals. Different participants called out different elements, usually caregivers speaking first. The conversation eventually moved to the woman in the painting, center left, lounging on the red divan.

> JONAH: Can she be Mother Nature? What do others think about that?

The figure had lighter skin than the other person in the painting, and this came up. Participants commented on her resemblance to Eve. This led to some debate over the sex of what was identified as the "dark-skinned" figure in the middle.

> AMY: Because of her skirt. She's shaped like a woman, she has hips.
> PARTICIPANT: Because she has no breasts!
> SPOUSE: She looks like a manimal.

The group appeared diverse with regard to gender and race, and these comments were potentially divisive. Jonah steered conversation away from any conversation about race, gender, or perceptions of difference.

People with Alzheimer's often say all sorts of things others might find inappropriate, and educators employ different strategies to circumvent conflict. Avoiding any social controversy like this is common practice, especially when anxiety can feel contagious.[25]

At this point, one of the participants in a wheelchair, Ellie, said that she could not see the figure in question. Jonah walked over to her chair and wheeled her closer to the painting, pointing at the figure when she got there.

> ELLIE: I don't see it. What are we looking at?
>
> JONAH: There's a figure right here. See her hair, and she's playing an instrument?
>
> ELLIE, *not seeing it and looking perplexed*: I don't see what you're looking at.
>
> JONAH: I can see exactly why you can't see it, there's a shadow here . . . I'm going to wheel you closer over here. [*she does, pushing her wheelchair*] Now can you see it?
>
> ELLIE, *with an exasperated laugh*: No!
>
> CAREGIVER: Wheel her back here.
>
> ELLIE: No, I can't see anything back there.

Jonah gave up at this point. Ellie simply did not see the figure in the painting, for whatever reason. What should be clear from these conversations is that not everyone in the session saw the same thing in the painting. The patterns of seeing were not necessarily bound to the experience of dementia. Ellie seemed to complete the lesson later that session when we were seated in front of another work painted in 1893 by Edvard Munch called *The Storm*.

One participant opened our conversation with a long narrative about what was happening in the painting. She offered that the house was on fire and everyone had run onto the street and "now they're freaking out." She knew the painting was by Munch, and she kept associating it with his more well-known work *The Scream*. Others continued to reference her interpretation as the best narrative, even though Jonah had attempted to communicate a different narrative. But Jonah seemed unwilling to correct any interpretation, and all agreed eventually that it was difficult to tell exactly what was going on in the painting.

> JONAH: It's hard to tell. That's something about modern art, modern art needs a viewer. . . . It needs you to complete it. . . . You look at it, there's something missing, and you can't quite put your finger on it. . . . Modern art keeps you looking at it. That's something these artists were doing, they were trying to get away from their formal training, and they were really championing the power of imagination.

Jonah's final comments reinforce my primary argument about MoMA's historical belief in each individual's ability to self-realize, regardless of disadvantage or disability. While the program certainly recognizes difference, Meet Me both homogenizes through recourse to the discourse of universal humanity and seeks to empower through an acceptance of each individual's capacity to contribute. While not intentional, this perspective can come across as vaguely utopian—at the very least optimistic—especially as many participants clearly are not contributing anything to the conversation. The Meet Me publication quotes the director of community and access programs, Francesca Rosenberg:

> The art acts as the spark for rich discussions and insights that we all hold dear. There's a buzz, a generosity of spirit, a connection that has been forged between the attendees and the staff. We're all thinking about the here and now. By the end of each program, everyone is uplifted.

Carrie McGee, the assistant educator, is also quoted:

> Most people in these individuals' lives "knew them when . . ." We didn't. We never met them before they were diagnosed. We accept them and value them as they are. We know them now. During the program, we're not thinking about Alzheimer's, we're just human beings, sharing an experience in the present.[26]

It is precisely modern art's aesthetic history that allows for that con-tribution, that spark, that "uplifting." Not only that, but according to Jonah's claim, modern art *requires* a viewer's contribution to succeed. This perspective orients potent individuality and personhood along-side one's capacity to participate in the modern puzzle. But it also places some responsibility on the person with Alzheimer's to be a successful viewer of the art as a function of successful personhood. I don't think anyone would suggest that MoMA expects people in this program to fulfill that mission unequivocally, but I do identify a ready acceptance of that promise in the person with Alzheimer's as part of a hopeful embrace of the program and its efficacy.

This emphasis on imagination and autonomy fulfills a broader assumption about personhood, one that insists on wholeness and inte-riority. The outside program that helped MoMA design Meet Me, ARTZ, echoes this language on its website: "ARTZ recognizes the wholeness that is inherent in each person, regardless of a diagnosis. We cele-brate each person's capacity to fully participate in the journey of life. We believe that access to creative expression is essential to our human experience."[27]

This perspective on its own would not, perhaps, be that striking, but in combination with a wholesale public interest in Meet Me's success, it becomes quite potent. MoMA is arguably one of the more well-known and admired museums in the world, and in a sense, it acts as a flagship institution of American high culture. As such, its reputation elevates its education and access programs in the public eye. Public and profes-sional interest in Meet Me was significant over the first decade of its existence, even though many other museums offer similar programs. This is evidenced by the program's strong press coverage, the success-ful conferences MoMA ran, and the awards the program won. This was one of the first of these access programs, and the museum's long history of public education and influence in the broader art education commu-nity has arguably helped it to succeed. Of course, the public visibility of the MoMA program also stems from the current visibility of Alzhei-mer's more broadly. The disease is still so misunderstood, so feared, that all sorts of potentially successful interventions receive press.

One of the educators told me that the constant attention from out-siders made the work difficult, even stressful: "It's always been a very special program with special attention. Anytime I'm giving a tour I'm being observed. I find that stressful. It's high stakes. I'm very aware of the stakes. I understand that it's experimental and we're allowed to make mistakes." The educator's anxiety is understandable. I witnessed many different visitors watching the sessions: a television crew, photog-raphers, and an almost constant stream of observers from other muse-ums, researchers like myself, and journalists. Carrie McGee, Francesca Rosenberg, project assistant Laurel Humble, and others engaged with running the program also circulated through the sessions, occasion-ally taking notes, shepherding visitors, and generally observing.

As a philanthropic institution, MoMA certainly benefits from the perception that both its collection and its access program can serve as a form of public health for all. And Meet Me can certainly be con-sidered successful as a psychosocial intervention that can potentially improve moods and quality of life, establish networks and communi-ties of care, and challenge some stigmas around Alzheimer's. But the way in which the museum's collections become depoliticized or uni-versalized participates in broader assumptions about what Alzheimer's is; conversely, it is precisely the disease's mystery that contributes to public interest in museological potential.

Ultimately, learning is not the most important logic of the pro-gram, even if it is a valued component. Psychiatry professor Margaret Sewell, commenting in an interview in the MoMA publication, said, "I think it's good that the outcomes are more quality-of-life or person oriented, rather than focusing on improving performance on mem-ory tests. . . . They're more meaningful, they're more practical, and they're more realistic for this group of people."[28] One concern for Meet Me, and indeed many psychosocial interventions into caregiving situ-ations, is that "this group of people" is a slippery category. If Meet Me is a program designed for both caregivers and people with dementia, it is perhaps easier to ascertain benefits and gains in categories such as quality of life and mood rather than in sustained cognitive improve-ment. This is one reason why the group's general mood is not only contagious but also a kind of barometer for educators in determining a session's success.

Unfortunately, Meet Me's successful track record in improving mood and quality of life for its attendees may in fact contribute to the divide between cognitive and affective health. As I have argued, this is a strong trend in approaches to Alzheimer's care: new biomedical interventions seemingly focus on cognitive success, while psychosocial interventions focus more on affective health and general well-being. While admittedly, many Alzheimer's patients are prescribed with all manner of psychotropic drugs designed to stabilize their mood, biomedical research of the magic pill variety is most actively focused on fixing cognitive deficits.

I have argued in this chapter that MoMA uses its modern art collection to foster or authorize personhood for all: a perceived individual interiority articulated via aesthetic community. But as Annette Leibing has argued, structural claims toward interiority and personhood in Alzheimer's research are culturally specific *moral* claims.[29] My goal with this chapter has been to integrate my own research within that moral claim to the future, not simply to render that discourse discrete but to argue that collective investments in the representational culture of Alzheimer's are never innocent. Indeed, it is precisely the representational culture presumed to be most universal and most progressive that reinforces individualized narratives of self. As we will see in the next chapter, this approach is dependent on more pervasive social ideologies that help frame the values of creativity and art.

6

Dementia on the Canvas

Art, Therapy, and Creativity's Values

The museum intervention described in the previous chapter belongs to a burgeoning research trend that explores how art can be used to address Alzheimer's. For scientists and a weary public increasingly desperate for ways to combat the disease, art represents a hopeful site of progress, despite only modest advances in understanding how art and dementia intersect. And for many, creative expression allows for the performance of the very individuality that Alzheimer's seems to threaten, and it does so in a progressive, optimistic manner antithetical to what is often stigmatized as loss.

A fundamental premise of this chapter is that Alzheimer's is useful for art, even though it is instead art that is often perceived as useful for understanding and treating Alzheimer's. Over the course of this book, I have argued that different forms of media help articulate and often reinforce social views on individual interiority. Art and the creativity that helps authorize it serve as the limit case of that representational ethic. Ideological ties between creativity and Alzheimer's personhood remain relatively undisturbed, in part due to broad social enthusiasm for creativity's values. I map some of that enthusiasm in this chapter, first in a brief review of the use of art as a means of understanding, treating, and living with dementia. Then, I explore the way creativity's unmarked positivity helps to structure personhood and its ties to representational culture.[1] Whereas the previous chapter focused on people with Alzheimer's looking at art, this chapter is about people with Alzheimer's making art. In particular, I employ two case studies of artists diagnosed with Alzheimer's to demonstrate social attitudes toward creativity and people with dementia.

The first examines the case of William Utermohlen, a painter who became famous for the art he made while living with symptoms of Alzheimer's. The reception of Utermohlen's work reveals pervasive assumptions about creativity's influence on individuality and interiority. I demonstrate how art can shape personhood based on a presumed connection between the material evidence of the artwork and pathological interiority.

The second case study focuses on Willem de Kooning, perhaps the most well-known artist with Alzheimer's. I describe a Meet Me session at MoMA's 2011 de Kooning career retrospective to demonstrate how creativity can enforce models of extraordinary selfhood, narratives of progress, and even forms of magical thinking. Referring to Willem de Kooning, Peter Gibson argued in *The Lancet* that "the act of painting may have had therapeutic value for him but no more so than basket making. The question of more general interest is whether a creative act, however overtly conscious, has any greater therapeutic value than basket making?"[2] I appreciate the way in which Gibson bracketed the intentional, creative act from therapeutic value. I would also add the supporting question, *for whom does the creative act have value?* Given the way in which representational culture dominates narratives of self and person, social enthusiasm for creativity's therapeutic values is entirely understandable. But the answer to this question also helps shape Alzheimer's personhood, as it reflects society's interest in particular, extraordinary forms of self.

I finish the chapter with some alternative ways to approach creativity and Alzheimer's—noting the need to recognize the value of art interventions while moving toward a more complex account of their place in a culture of self-production and a creative economy. What social investments do Americans maintain in creativity as a vehicle of self-expression and an indication of personhood? And what are the effects of those investments on the cognitively disabled? How does the act of making or creation enforce a temporal ethics of self and personhood? An ethics strongly complicated by the social orientation of Alzheimer's as foremost a crisis of memory? We need to take seriously the ideologies that authorize these creative practices, especially as they set up dependent relationships between art and agency and between personhood and representation more broadly.

Art, Creativity, and Personhood

Over the last twenty years, art has become an increasingly common tool in the efforts to understand Alzheimer's. One important research trend operates as a subgenre of the emergent field of neuroaesthetics, a field in part concerned with the neurological basis of the appreciation and production of art.[3] Much of the related Alzheimer's research focuses on the correlation between compromised brain function and creative practice. While not labeled as such, cognitive tests that involve art (drawing clocks, for example) have long been a standard component of diagnostic practice. It is an easy leap to translate that approach into more complex forms of representation. People with dementia often experience changes in those artistic abilities linked to perception, cognition, and expressive inhibition. Looking at these changes can help researchers understand the relationship between dementia and art but also the neurology of art more broadly.[4] Researchers have focused their inquiry on both professional artists and nonprofessionals with different kinds of dementia diagnoses to compare and map neurobiological artistic function.[5]

Art therapy is also now a popular component of Alzheimer's care.[6] Art therapy can include a range of different creative activities, such as painting, sculpture, music, dance, and storytelling. While art therapy is used both for people with Alzheimer's and for their caregivers, most related research has focused on those diagnosed with dementia. By investigating the relationship between symptoms and the skills presumed to be useful in art practice, investigators have begun to learn how art therapy can respond to particular neurological dysfunction.[7] While conclusions are difficult to generalize, studies have shown that art therapy can impact participants in a range of different ways, including quality of life, mood or affect, self-esteem, alertness, and social and physical engagement. These interventions can directly target symptoms or provide meaningful social activity.[8]

Despite the use of control groups in some of these studies, it is still difficult to discern how and even if the artistic practice itself is responsible for these impacts. While many researchers now agree that "artistic engagement may improve behavioral symptoms and the quality of life in patients with dementia," it can be difficult to separate the influence of socialization, environment, or other forms of validation that might accompany the creative act.[9] Indeed, part of the problem with evaluating the success of these programs is in the lack of rigor or clarity in research design, as well as the lack of systematic descriptions of the art, who is affected by it, and the mode of delivery.[10] It is also important to take seriously the different actors involved in the broad array of arts interventions and their expectations and definitions of health outcomes, all of which might impact the understanding of how art works.[11]

Beyond research and care, art therapy can also be helpful for the public as a means to better understand the persistent abilities of people with Alzheimer's. This is the perspective of the 2009 documentary film *I Can Remember Better When I Paint,* which, according to the film's website, seeks to demonstrate to the public "the positive impact of art and other creative therapies on people with Alzheimer's and how these approaches can change the way we look at the disease." This kind of audience is not limited to the general public; rather, it can help medical professionals as well. The creative storytelling activity TimeSlips was the focus of a study that looked at how art therapy can help medical students develop "positive attitudes" toward people with dementia.[12] Another study showed that staff in a long-term care facility who participated in TimeSlips reported positive interactions and developed "positive views" of people with dementia.[13] Studies like these illustrate how the visibility of creative therapies can help combat some of the stigma that often accompanies Alzheimer's.

While making art and appreciating art are clearly different practices, they tend to fold together in the event of their social reception. Art therapists will likely voice the objection that these practices are foremost dismissive of the tangible artifact that is produced—that it is the making that matters rather than the work of art itself; however, this is not always the way it is received. Art created by people with dementia is often scrutinized by the public and science alike for evidence of pathological interiority or the spectacle of the disordered mind. Furthermore, as I described in the last chapter, art making is also tied to narratives of art conservation, display, museology, and other forms of value ultimately antithetical to the proposed aims of a pure creative therapy, aims that are ostensibly dismissive of the final product.

Despite uncertainty about *how* art works for people with dementia, there is an insistent, often public claim *that* it works; broader social interest in art maintains these interventions as universally positive. Groups like the National Center for Creative Aging have coordinated and funded large-scale efforts to integrate art into healthy aging. Memory care frequently relies on art as part of its daily activities. The cottage industry of Alzheimer's prevention promotes art practice as a valuable activity for cognitive health. This celebratory culture is echoed by a news media anxious to provide some hope, even if there is a lack of good evidence to show how art works. PBS, for example, produced a two-part series called *Art and the Mind* that promotes art's positive powers. Creativity's optimistic ambiguity is of course linked to the social ambiguity of "art" more broadly and its vague ties to exceptional selfhood.[14]

Indeed, one benefit that is often accepted unequivocally by both practitioners and the public is art's power to communicate or express interiority. In other words, art can restore a sense of self to the person with Alzheimer's. Art therapy is also known as "expressive therapy" precisely because of its ability to bypass verbal communication while still allowing for personal or social expression.[15] How much of this is based on art's social values? Is creativity's purest ideological promise individual interiority? If personhood for people with Alzheimer's is often granted some representational presence, then creativity might be understood as a kind of hopeful authorization of that representation, an indication of interiority and mediated personhood.

In other words, creativity is a way of making the self. It is a pure expression of individuality, an almost magical form of self-agency.[16]

And it is often understood to be universally available. Opposing "culture as standardization" in youth education, "creativity expert" Ken Robinson claimed in a 2013 TED talk that creativity is "the common currency of being a human being."[17] The logic of Robinson's truism echoes in the dementia intervention literature. For example, art therapist Cathy Malchiodi argues that "creativity has come to be defined as a human potential, a capacity we can develop in ourselves if we want to."[18] This is the perspective adopted by the National Center for Creative Aging, an organization "dedicated to the vital relationship between creative expression and healthy aging . . . for older people of all cultures and ethnic backgrounds, regardless of economic status, age, or level of physical, emotional, or cognitive functioning."[19]

This discourse reveals creativity to be both universal and agential. It is a deeply human form of productivity or progress. That creativity implies a movement forward in time not insistent on a compromised past is the root of its promise as a psychosocial or psychotherapeutic intervention for people with dementia. But if creativity is a language of human progress and becoming, it is also enormously available to magical thinking and ideological slippage.

Given its influence on self and personhood, *creativity* is a term that needs to be more carefully explored within the context of art-based interventions for Alzheimer's. This is especially true given the difficulty in assessing creativity's role in these models of care. With that said, I am less concerned with what creativity *is* than with the ways in which it achieves historical, institutional, and formal logic in the context of Alzheimer's care. This includes both public perceptions of art and dementia and increasingly professionalized art interventions. What is it exactly about creative art that harnesses such public interest and optimism, specifically as an intervention for Alzheimer's? Does it have something to do with the social space of art as something mystical or mysterious or as an embattled expression of individuality? As neurologists, gerontologists, and therapists continue to research the potential benefits of art interventions of all kinds, it is critical to acknowledge the kinds of myth making that accompany the social reception of these practices.[20]

William Utermohlen:
Social Attitudes toward Art and Alzheimer's

William Utermohlen was an American artist who lived most of his life in London. After he was diagnosed with Alzheimer's in 1995, he painted a series of self-portraits. This was not unusual, as he had also created self-portraits in earlier stages of his career. But these new self-portraits were more abstract than many of his older ones. In fact, one could argue that they became progressively more abstract as he aged and the disease progressed. Not surprisingly, it was only after his diagnosis that his work developed a popular, international appeal, precisely because of the way his art appeared to reveal some essential truth about the subjective experience of the disease.

The popular reception of these self-portraits often specifically addresses the way the aesthetics reflect his fading selfhood. For example, commenters on an art blog focused on the sadness of the transformation and his evident loss of identity.[21] An article in the *Huffington Post* garnered similar public response, but respondents commented most actively on the aesthetics of the paintings. One called them "cruelly representational," while another said his work "takes us into the mind of an Alzheimer's victim like no other written word has ever accomplished." Commenters also oriented those aesthetics within a modern tradition, citing figurative resonance with the work of painters such as Van Gogh, Picasso, and Munch.[22] Importantly, in this discourse, the creative nature of the representation allows for a kind of communicative tether between healthy and diseased people. This is purportedly something that only art can achieve. As commenters pointed out, the artistic representation does what words and science cannot.

Key to the reception of Utermohlen's work is the way the successive orientation of paintings provides a kind of time-lapse montage of mental decline. The juxtaposition of Utermohlen's healthy work with those paintings produced during different stages of his illness provides both popular appeal and a narrative structure. This also tends to make the narrative of loss more dramatic. Frédéric Compain's 2010 documentary *Glassy-Eyed* followed this popular trend, narrating Utermohlen's decline through a montage of the artist's paintings set to music. This technique adds some narrative drama to the process, even as it authorizes the decline narrative of Alzheimer's more broadly.

Journalists covered Utermohlen's story rather extensively, and the thread that unites those stories is this idea that the art is reflective of an internal pathology. In turn, most presume that the art gives a viewer access to the normally hidden workings of the mind of the Alzheimer's patient. For example, Andrew Purcell writes in the *New Scientist*, "Despite this suffering, Utermohlen's dedication to his art provides viewers today with a unique glimpse into the effects of a declining brain."[23] Denise Grady wrote in the *New York Times* that "the paintings starkly reveal the artist's descent into dementia, as his world began to tilt, perspectives flattened and details melted away."[24] An Associated Press article offers even more dramatic language: "The works shortly after his diagnosis convey terror and isolation. Those feelings later give way to defiance and anger. Then shame, confusion and anguish. Then, in the shadowy final pair of portraits, little more than afterimages of a creative and talented spirit whose identity appears to have vanished."[25]

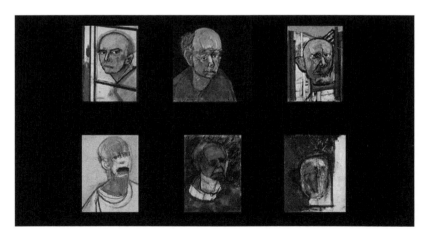

FIGURE 12. Utermohlen's self-portraits, progressively arranged in the film *Glassy-Eyed*.

Aside from the popular appeal, another important reason for the dissemination of his late work is that Utermohlen wanted to put his art into dialogue with medical research on Alzheimer's.[26] At least, he willingly engaged in research that examined the relationship between his symptoms and his art. A group of researchers working with Utermohlen published a case study in *The Lancet* in 2001, citing numerous interpretations of the changes to his artistic style, including professional colleagues, family, the artist's own comments, and measures of his cognitive function. The researchers concluded in part that "the abstract style may provide an outlet for expression unhindered by the restrictions imposed by realism and the unattainable accurate replication of colours, forms, angles, proportion, and perspective."[27] This analysis seems to orient agency more on the style than on artistic intent, even if the symptoms still maintain distinctive relationships with aesthetics. In a later publication, however, two of the study's original authors foreground the problem of artistic intention as the threatened aspect of creative practice.[28]

The researchers' focus on intentionality is not surprising, given how public celebration of artistic legitimacy is largely predicated on that trait. Tobin Siebers, who wrote about art and disability, points out that according to this kind of perspective, any loss of intention would denigrate the quality of the art in the public eye:

> Genius is really at a minimum only the name for an intelligence large enough to plan and execute works of art—an intelligence that usually goes by the name of "intention." Defective or impaired intelligence cannot make art according to this rule. Mental disability represents an absolute rupture with the work of art. It marks the constitutive moment of abolition, according to Michel Foucault, that dissolves the essence of what art is.[29]

It is helpful to see how intentionality as a component of artistic creativity is what is both valued and pathologized in social judgment of mental illness. Much of the reception of Utermohlen's work is predicated on a temporal orientation of both healthy and pathological production, where agency is still attributed to the remnants of a healthy self. In other words, sometimes it is the original, embattled selfhood that is valorized for its productive capacity; it is no accident that one of the most common words public commenters use to describe Utermohlen's late work is "heroic."[30]

Intentionality aside, it is interesting to note the assumptions that bind popular and scientific treatment of Alzheimer's in relationship to artistic production. While a neurological researcher might attribute changes in the formal properties of a painting done by a person with Alzheimer's to changes in her visuoperceptual and visuospatial function, a nonspecialist might interpret this as some evacuation of selfhood. But both support the idea of creativity and the artistic individual as *both* resilient to and fundamentally affected by this disease. And they find that a source of hope or inspiration, despite its sadness. For example, referencing Utermohlen's paintings, gerontologist Desmond O'Neill said that "even with the most feared illnesses of later life, art can afford insights into the preservation of our humanity and continuing need for self-expression."[31] Here is the central paradox of the relationship between art, creativity, and Alzheimer's: on one hand, social attitudes toward the disease frame people with Alzheimer's as disabled in a way that allows their minds to paint the world in special or unusual, albeit broken, ways; on the other hand, the art also shows them as somehow reductively human—at core they are perversely *more* normal as they reveal something universal that unites all humans.

The reception of Utermohlen's work therefore reveals three primary assumptions about art and Alzheimer's personhood. First is the presumed connection between an artist's selfhood and the aesthetics of the art. This might simply be a result of the indexical relationship between the labor of production and the art artifact, but it draws on a more pervasive ideology that links creativity and self-production.[32] As researchers Maurer and Prvulovic conclude in their study of another artist with Alzheimer's, "observing his artistic changes with the progression of the disease may help to better comprehend the inner world of patients with Alzheimer's disease."[33]

The second assumption is based on the idea that Alzheimer's attacks the substance of that interior self, thus compromising personhood.

This is now a standard perspective in public attitudes toward the disease and well described in this book, but what is novel in this instance is the assumption that the self has a kind of representational presence, much like the pigment on a painting. Any change to that presence reflects this new claim on personhood. This is further evidenced by the fact that the artist with Alzheimer's often only has public value *as* an artist. Utermohlen died in 2007, but he stopped painting many years before then; public reception of his work orients the timeline of his personhood squarely within a narrative of his creative production.

Third is the assumption that Alzheimer's irrevocably alters our appropriate progression through life. Margaret Gullette argues that Americans often live out their lives through particular narrative structures, progress being one of the mostly deeply felt. They often understand their own aging process through notions of progress like improvement, accumulation, fulfillment, and success.[34] Gullette calls this the "American dream as a life-course narrative," or a "life-course imaginary" of the way it should go, the way it has gone, internalized through recourse to narratives of progress and decline.[35] The myth of Alzheimer's is that it disrupts the life-course narrative. It disrupts narrative itself, stripping the future and destabilizing individual and collective relationships with past and self. Narratives of economic productivity, national progress, and technological transformation, for example, imply a cognitive demand perhaps counter to the compromised abilities of aging citizens.[36] Athena McLean destabilizes this myth, asking whether it is all "narrative" that is threatened by Alzheimer's or a particular notion of narrative: "persons with dementia may employ creative strategies to adjust to their cognitive impairments and preserve their selves. Social identity can only be guaranteed when others acknowledge their stories."[37] How does art fit into this kind of practice? Is creativity not a reassertion of the progress narrative as individual self-realization?

I would argue that "preservation" should not be a key objective for Alzheimer's care, because it overly values an identity predicated on the past. The language of preservation, in other words, hinges on an ethic of self based on memories or other cognitive abilities ultimately threatened by dementia. However, McLean's argument is useful here because it offers a language and politics of creativity that are not necessarily bound to aesthetic production. Opportunities for creative encounters with self exist in countless social activities. All this begs the question, what is it about art making that is so appealing as a tool for dementia care? Is it the material evidence of that activity that demonstrates a kind of successful intervention? Or is it something perhaps more insidious, tapping into a long-standing social narrative that unites mental pathology and artistic ability? The next case study should help answer these questions.

Exhibiting Loss: The de Kooning Problem

The artist Willem de Kooning famously had Alzheimer's or some related form of dementia, although his exact diagnosis was controversial. Unlike Utermohlen, de Kooning never participated in any published research on the relationship between his symptoms and his art. Consequently, art historians, therapists, and neurologists debate how his later paintings reflect or were affected by that dementia.[38] Many of the assumptions that undergird Utermohlen's self-portraits also reverberate in the debates about de Kooning's later work. Central are the notions of authenticity, intentionality, and value that link selfhood and artistic creativity. Is his later work the true act of creative genius, is it the result of latent or embodied memory, or something else? How did projection or repetition change the work? Was he helped by his studio assistants? I take the substance of these debates to be further evidence of the importance of creativity as an indication of personhood.[39]

In late 2011, the New York Museum of Modern Art celebrated the life of de Kooning with a full career retrospective, a massive exhibit spanning a full floor of the museum. In addition to being the most famous artist with Alzheimer's, de Kooning is arguably one of the most well-known modern artists in general; the admirable size and scope of the show echoed that fact. The exhibit was designed with a trajectory that began with his earliest works and moved progressively through different hallmark periods of his career, concluding with his final decade. This retrospective format is a traditional way to think about a person's life after he has died, and it reflects the life-course narrative so often tied to healthy aging. But it also reveals MoMA's perspective on artistic practice as shaped through a narrative of progress.

I observed a Meet Me session of the de Kooning show, and my experience bears heavily on this argument around creativity and Alzheimer's. Our group was composed of about fifteen people, as usual made up of people with dementia and their caregivers. We looked at several artworks, slowly moving through de Kooning's life and talking about the paintings. The educator never talked about Alzheimer's or the dementia de Kooning encountered at the end of his life. This was in line with the general practice of never mentioning Alzheimer's during a Meet Me session. But beyond that, the exhibit did not reference the disease or symptoms in the final decade galleries either. MoMA seemed generally unwilling to foreground the subject of his illness, perhaps because the subject has received so much previous attention in the international art world.

For example, the San Francisco Museum of Modern Art produced a de Kooning show in 1995, and Alzheimer's was highlighted as a key aspect of de Kooning's later work. Corresponding with that show, two physicians working on Alzheimer's participated in a panel discussion with art historian T. J. Clark. Each addressed possible correlations between de Kooning's later work and his physical and mental condition, but they all urged care in making formal connections between aesthetics, creative ability, and his symptoms. Still, the primary focus of that panel was Alzheimer's and de Kooning's late art.[40]

In 1997, MoMA staged its own show of the late work of de Kooning, including forty paintings from 1981 to 1987. Acknowledging the popular reception of this work as perhaps pathologized, curator Robert Storr argued instead that this was a productive, creative, and inventive time period for de Kooning, the paintings a product of a "superior aesthetic intelligence exploring the furthest limits of consciousness itself."[41] While Storr did not make definitive connections between Alzheimer's and de Kooning's aesthetic style in this commentary, he did use the language of mind to make his point. However, like the 2011 show, this show did not include any of de Kooning's very last works—those painted after 1987, ostensibly when his Alzheimer's too seriously affected his artistic abilities.[42] MoMA's chief curator emeritus of painting and sculpture, John Elderfield, said that this was a difficult curatorial decision, but one clearly based on aesthetic evidence. Elderfield said, "The pictures after '87 are a different species of painting. They are transitional to something else that never happened. I didn't want to end on a lesser note."[43] Elderfield's comments demonstrate a broader commitment to the artist's career trajectory so evident in the retrospective.

These three de Kooning exhibitions reveal clear tensions about the relationship between Alzheimer's and creativity. I will not argue that the 2011 MoMA show covered up his dementia, but it certainly did not foreground it. Rather than reduce his career to a diagnosis or a symptom, the museum chose to focus on other aspects of his life. His declining "abilities" were mentioned, but the show refrained from citing this as Alzheimer's or dementia. If symptomatology appeared at all, the exhibit installed those symptoms within the logic of the aesthetic production. Words used in the wall text in the final two rooms, such as "diminish," "lessening," and "atrophy," ostensibly described the aesthetics of de Kooning's painting, not his cognitive abilities. Here cognitive disability is translated into the spatial or figural description in the paintings.

What is fascinating is the manner in which MoMA incorporated the subjectivity of Alzheimer's without even mentioning the disease. This became even more clear in my Meet Me tour. As we walked into the final room of later paintings, the educator asked us all just to look for a moment at the art. We stood in the middle of the final gallery in the exhibit, surrounded by approximately ten to fifteen of de Kooning's paintings from the 1980s. The wall text (and audio tour, more extensively) described this as "reminiscent" of work done in earlier periods. As an observer, I found the moment somewhat fraught because I anticipated some sort of declaration of solidarity, perhaps offered by the Meet Me program. But my anticipation of a frank conversation about dementia and art never manifested. Many of the participants enjoyed the work, just as they had enjoyed the earlier paintings. Perhaps the paintings of the final decade elicited a more effusive response. It is difficult to say. Murmurs of "oh, I like these," "these ones are good," or "beautiful" made no necessary claims to psychological affinity. It was simply a room of paintings with certain appeal. People were tired after the hour and a half tour of the exhibit, and it was time to leave. But in an ironic moment, the large doors at the end of the exhibit were locked, and we could not exit. The educator leaned heavily on the doors, grimace on her face, to no avail. Instead, we had to retrace our steps all the way back through de Kooning's life, revisiting the paintings we had already seen, shuffling along as a group, finishing the way we began.

The museum made two primary comments on de Kooning and creative value through the structure of the exhibit. First, the museum reinforced the idea of de Kooning as a master artist and an individual whose illness (however unmentionable) had a necessary relationship with his aesthetic output. Individuality was validated through recourse to extraordinary modern selfhood—a selfhood that waned or failed as did, eventually, his art. Second, the retrospective organization of the show asserted a life-course narrative as one of progress and creative realization. Each of these strategies coincides with more traditional museological practice.

Despite the exclusion of Alzheimer's from the show, I would argue that MoMA benefited from a much older tradition of associating modern art with mental illness. This is of course a pattern beyond the museum's control, but it arguably fed the publicity. According to this perspective, the unusual or creative aspects of the art originate in the unusual aspects of the mentally or socially ill mind. Be it Jackson Pollock's excessive alcoholism or Vincent van Gogh cutting off his own ear, popular histories of modern art frequently associate exceptional talent with apocryphal tales of "mad behavior." This kind of discourse also illustrates an uneasy slippage between the reception of genius and the mentally ill as concerns creative practice. The art historian T. J. Clark commented on this problem in the panel talk associated with the San Francisco Museum of Modern Art's de Kooning show:

> I should hate the painting of de Kooning's last ten years to be canopied by the glamor of pathology. There is a danger of that happening, I think. Maybe many of us would like to be shown that modern art at key moments

was (literally) pathological, because that would allow us to forget that for much of the time it was metaphorically, or deliberately, so.[44]

Clark clearly references a broader social myth of the artist as mentally ill or deranged. However, he also shows how this mythology transfers "pathology" from a dispersed, modern condition to an identifiable and individually held illness. Is it out of the question to wonder if the public fascination with Meet Me or the 2011 de Kooning show follows similar assumptions about mental illness and modern art? Not at all. The aforementioned public responses to Utermohlen's paintings almost assure that it is so.

Creative Value

Alzheimer's and art are each so overdetermined as social concepts that it seems natural that social attitudes toward their relationship would remain open to a range of interpretations. Aging and creativity pioneer Gene Cohen commented on the relationship thus: "the energy coming from the visual art itself engages in ways that are so unexpected, and actually they're quite mystical, so I don't think anyone knows why this happens."[45] By this logic, it doesn't really matter how people with Alzheimer's can benefit from interactions with art; this perspective is not isolated. Creativity is a kind of magnet for magical thinking. As Frans Meulenberg opined in *The Lancet*, "does dementia undermine creativity or does it change its energy? It is impossible to give an answer."[46]

To return to my earlier challenge, then, the better question might be, for whom does creativity have value? Certainly not just the people doing the creative work. Creativity is enormously influential to modern life, but in the last few decades, creativity has become a particularly important force in the emergence of an online, digital economy. Creativity is one of the central capacities that help authorize a cognitive meritocracy in the United States. In fact, creativity is often discursively linked to cognitive ability as a mode of production, especially within these digital networks.[47] It is through that kind of discourse that creativity becomes open to exploitation and commodification. As critics of the creative economy have noted, "art seems to reveal not only the sublime essence of humanity, but also the very treacherous and nega-tive character of contemporary capitalism, namely its parasitic nature."[48] Creativity is vulnerable to those processes in part because it appears to be so universal, so autonomous, and so liberatory.

Of course, not all modes of creativity are commodifiable or exploit-ative. Recognizing that creativity is symptomatic of broader patterns of contemporary labor and economic innovation is not an argument against creativity and Alzheimer's, nor certainly a suggestion that people with dementia should opt out. The value of creativity depends on the degree to which it "conforms" to the expectations of the social context of which it is a part. This is especially true in the ways that creativity shapes social expectations of mental illness or mental behavior.[49] Cre-ativity, however, cannot be allowed the status of magic, and it should not be relished for its individuating effects. Those ideological effects are precisely the mode by which creativity articulates a false vision of emancipation.

After all, the concept of creativity only entered popular discourse in the United States in the middle of the last century. In her history of the concept, Camilla Nelson argues that part of its power arises from the idea that it is very old or very human.[50] That it appears universal is central to its appeal. Showing how the discourse of creativity is in fact useful in the contemporary moment should help dispel some of its less helpful effects. I offer the following suggestions that might help researchers collectively destabilize creativity and its attendant social attachments in the current moment.

First, without dismissing the significant progress in the fight against social stigmas of aging and cognitive disability, we ought to question the essential *positivity* of art: the social insistence on the value of positive outcomes both in their productive, creative sense and as they seemingly always oppose the negative aspects of Alzheimer's. The next chapter of this book explores this unmarked positivity in greater depth.

Next, we need to take seriously the way creativity's positivity sets up dichotomous relationships with biomedical interventions that offer different forms of evidence. Clearly those dedicated to psychosocial interventions for Alzheimer's are frustrated with the overwhelming dominance of biomedical treatments for the disease. As I have shown, psychosocial interventions are often framed as an alternative to biomedicine, as they promise a fresh perspective into a frustrating medical situation without known cause, cure, or satisfying treatment. As just such an intervention, art steps in as both hopeful and progressive, a perspective that harmonizes with broader public appreciation for art's values. Given that creativity is often linked discursively to human nature, it is no surprise that it should be claimed by the arts (and humanities) in contradistinction to biomedicine. However, dichotomizing biomedicine's failures with art's success does not allow for complex, sustainable models of personhood for people with Alzheimer's.

Perhaps one way forward is to diversify creativity's logic, not simply by recognizing that biomedicine is itself consistently engaged in creativity, but also by radically reconfiguring what gets to "count" as an artistic intervention. Here we might articulate a new ethics of creativity in dementia care that embraces all manner of embodied acts under the rubric of art therapy. Or we might look for ways art and biomedicine are—while distinct—also complementary, sharing in components conducive to desirable health or social outcomes. Despite the potential variability of these engagements, this should harmonize with de Medeiros and Basting's call for a "stronger understanding of the mechanisms at work in cultural arts interventions."[51] This diversification implies a different kind of relationship with progress and the future that involves confronting both representational and institutional hierarchies as well as a radical openness to what creativity might be. Furthermore, this kind of practice will naturally help combat the ideology of human universalisms so prevalent in creativity discourse and consequently respect the differences that impact the lived experiences of Alzheimer's.

Of course, art therapy is already good at diversifying creativity's modes and values, but as I have argued in this chapter, this perspective is often not reflected in its institutional or public reception.[52] The two brief case studies on Utermohlen and de Kooning demonstrate the many ways dementia is useful for art when it is precisely the reverse ethic that frames the wellspring of the creative industry in Alzheimer's care. More research is necessary to investigate the ideological slippage between art and Alzheimer's, research that can map the way creativity has historically structured claims of personhood, interiority, authenticity, and value. That information should help not only in the arena of public health education but in the delivery and exercise of art interventions themselves.

Given the rise in public, philanthropic, and governmental interest in creative therapies, it would behoove those invested in art's value as a psychosocial intervention to take seriously the representational ethics that provide its context. This involves understanding how art fits into the more diverse regime of mediated personhood described in this book rather than hailing it as special or magical. By honoring creativity as a banal process of the everyday rather than as heroic or genius, we might lessen the social insistence on creativity's value while still honoring minor, humble performances of social relevance. This locates value within—and not dismissive of—the ambiguity of loss. Perhaps here individuality will lose some of its social relevance, and creativity might be reborn as a mode of social collaboration and play.

7

Loved Ones

The Capacity for Representation, Recognition, and Care

Lisa Genova's 2007 novel *Still Alice* ends on a high note. The best-selling book tells the story of a fifty-year-old Harvard University professor of cognitive psychology, Alice Howland, who is battling early-onset Alzheimer's disease. Genova narrates primarily from Alice's perspective, giving the reader a detailed, personal account of her symptoms and the frustrations and suffering they entail. She experiences progressive problems with memory loss, disorientation, and changes in mood, judgment, and emotion. Much of the novel focuses on Alice's increasingly strained professional and familial relationships and her inability to perform everyday tasks at home and work.

By the end of the book, Alice is experiencing serious cognitive disability, but her daughter is doing her best to still communicate and maintain some sort of optimism. Her daughter, an actress, performs a scene from a play, but she does not want Alice to try to understand the narrative. Rather, she asks that Alice simply say how the scene makes her *feel*. Alice watches her speak and gesture, but Alzheimer's renders her unable to follow along except at an emotional level. Her daughter finishes playing out the scene to Alice's muted tears:

> The actress stopped and came back into herself. She looked at Alice and waited.

"Okay, what do you feel?"

"I feel love. It's about love."

The actress squealed, rushed over to Alice, kissed her on the cheek, and smiled, every crease of her face delighted.

"Did I get it right?" asked Alice.

"You did, Mom. You got it exactly right."[1]

This is how the novel ends. Alice has lost her ability to communicate in the ways she values most, her family is fighting over where to put her and how to manage best-care options, and the entire novel has detailed all the ways her life, career, and relationships have fallen apart because of this disease.

But in this moment, all of those problems are set aside. While the book shows how Alzheimer's makes it easy to get everything wrong, finally Alice gets something exactly right. Love is experienced as a kind of temporary solution to the loss of memory and all of the other symptoms of the disease. Furthermore, Alice's entire person, her entire self, is reduced in this moment to love. It is a momentary perfection, narrated through interpersonal possibility. Love here signifies not an end to the story but a beginning, as if the sequel is just around the corner. Genova offers this implied sequel to readers as a collectively oriented future.[2]

So often the stories we tell about disease in America involve love. Lost loves. Love defeated. Love regained, renewed, redefined. Alzheimer's disease is no exception; in fact, love is the dominant language used to understand this disease in popular and public culture.

One reason for this trend is that the narrative of Alzheimer's generally involves more than just one person with a disease; symptoms permeate a broader social network of friends, family, and caregivers. Because the disease affects one's ability to remember shared experiences and even other people, and because many care situations take place inside the home with the help of family and friends, Alzheimer's can be a profoundly interpersonal disease.

The overflow of symptoms across bodies and social fields leaves open the question of who exactly is responsible for managing those symptoms. Currently in the United States, the majority of that responsibility falls on informal caregivers, intimates responsible for in-home, direct care practice. Because Alzheimer's has no known cause or cure, long-term, informal care cannot be understood simply as a solution to a medical problem; rather, its labors are woven into the fabric of everyday living. The way in which interpersonal, familial affects like love are tethered to neoliberal health care as forms of obligation, agency, and endurance complicates assumed boundaries between public and private feeling. Thus the public life of Alzheimer's is most clearly articulated through a historical turn toward love as a kind of sentimental logic.

This chapter examines the loving logic of Alzheimer's, showing how that affective promise is oriented within aggressive utopias of health practice. It traces the discourse of love through a diversity of popular representations of Alzheimer's, and it explores how caregiving is comprehended, narrated, and legislated as and through love. I frame this as a kind of socially comfortable slippage between love and care. This slippage is a form of covert myth making that renders certain social, mainly familial structures essential components of long-term public viability.

The historical framework for my argument roughly overlaps with the rise of popular media in the United States that explicitly deal with Alzheimer's: from the mid-1990s until the mid-2010s. Those two decades have also seen growth in the attention to the experiences and well-being of caregivers.[3] This is for good reason: until the turn of the century, caregivers had gone largely unrecognized in their labors. While caregiving can be rewarding, it can also be enormously taxing, often injurious to caregiver health, wealth, and social life. Increasing attention has been directed to care as a viable site of scientific research, social policy, and philanthropy. Some training is also available to help facilitate and improve care in the home, even as financial support is quite limited.[4]

Much of the new attention to caregivers, however, has led to the unintended consequence of leaving the person with Alzheimer's untended, her voice unrecognized. While the battle to recuperate the value of the person with Alzheimer's is now long entrenched, the rise of love-care might ironically strip personhood from those it seeks to enfranchise, introducing an interpersonal politics of representation and recognition structurally unavailable to the cognitively disabled.

At its core, the crisis of love is framed as a problem of recognition, in other words, "does my loved one still recognize me or not?" We are understandably often more concerned with someone's ability to recognize us than with the person's ability to understand how to operate a microwave. But the idea that Alzheimer's threatens recognition while elevating that ability as essential to personhood is crucial for understanding the imbrication of love within the representational culture of dementia. This makes for a compelling failure. As Sara Ahmed argues, "the impossibility that love can reach its object may also be what makes love powerful as a narrative."[5] I don't have the space in this chapter to do more than gesture toward this collective addiction to the ethic of recognition—perhaps as a defining crisis of modernity itself—but it is worth acknowledging here, as it conditions our focus on love and care in Alzheimer's media.

This ethic of recognition is profoundly operative in the public discourse around the disease, as anthropologist Janelle Taylor has described in her own experiences of caring for her mother.[6] She argues that the problem of recognition needs to be made secondary to other ways of thinking about care. Lawrence Cohen responded to Taylor's essay by pointing out that its "power lies in establishing that the object for the anthropologist and any other observer is a relation between these bodies [meaning both a caregiver and a person diagnosed with Alzheimer's], a relation that Taylor shows us remains subject to extraordinary pressure to name itself as failure."[7] I would argue that it is also a relationship that is under dichotomous pressure to regulate itself under the sentiments of love. In other words, even if recognition is admitted as a failure, it is love's viability in collective judgment that is the true benchmark for human life and personhood. And love as a primary act of recognition validates recognition foremost as a site of agency.

If love's ultimate promise is recognition of the other, and if Alzheimer's most devilish symptom is the way it befuddles that recognition, where does that leave the person with dementia in the love-care contract? The popular country musician Glen Campbell released a compelling song that reflects aptly on the subject called "Not Gonna Miss You." Campbell became a public face of Alzheimer's in 2011, when he embarked on a final Goodbye Tour and released two albums, a music video, and a documentary film after he was diagnosed with the disease.[8] The song's lyrics describe the position of the person with Alzheimer's succinctly: "You're the last person I will love. You're the last face I will recall. And best of all, I'm not gonna miss you." Julian Raymond, who cowrote "Not Gonna Miss You," says that the original sentiment came from Campbell.[9] The song describes the unsustainability of love from the position of someone with dementia, if not because of the loss of memory, then more certainly because of the eventual loss of life.

Arguably, the discourse of love recognizes all parties of the caregiving contract, but it does so by rehearsing the practices of care via representations of sentiment. My position is not, of course, that love has no place in care. But the more that love is seen as an essential logic of successful caregiving, the more it becomes a kind of mandate that restructures the policies of health care itself. With this, love is articulated into neoliberal models of health, aging, and labor, and the autonomy of the family unit is made instrumental to later-life health care. That is a presumed autonomy that "masks" the way that certain families are systematically disenfranchised in America.[10] This essential positivity is made to make up for the deficiencies of everyday health care, a relationship often experienced as lack: from symptom to insurance to cure. Alzheimer's care in the United States thus fits into a longer biopolitical tradition that frames affective agency as essential to both personhood and national welfare.

The evidence in this chapter ranges quite broadly from entertainment to advertising and from movies to television to the internet. Despite the apparent disparity of these media forms, the representational culture of Alzheimer's that focuses on care maintains surprising consistencies across a range of forms and audiences in the United States. It is through popular representations that love-care aspires toward universality and normativity.[11] Of course, it is not love itself but precisely love's normative aspirations that must be questioned.

A related concern, then, is exactly how one defines *love,* as the ambiguity of the term contributes to love's viability as a mode of governmentality.[12] Love can be defined infinitely according to its purpose, and it is not my task to do that work here. More valuable is to describe the way it relates to purpose itself or the ways love acquires a logic of capacity and agency. This logic of love describes the capacity for care when other resources fall short, but it also describes the capacity for recognition within relationships of dependency.

The love-care slippage is oriented around the pure possibility of representation. As Lawrence Cohen argues about dementia, "forms of care are not merely cultural patterns or individual or collective strategies, they are critically public and mediated phenomena."[13] As an aspirational affect, love preys on representational ideals. That is, love in these narratives crystalizes around the ideal of who the person with Alzheimer's was before, memories for the most part, and advocacy for the ideal of that person now. Alzheimer's, however, forecloses on those memories, and it certainly hinders the practice of making new ones unadulterated by the disease. As I have argued thus far in this book, Alzheimer's is often conceived as the failure of representation. I would argue that it might also sometimes be about the failure of love. It should perhaps be allowed to be so.

Love and Nation

On November 5, 1994, President Ronald Reagan released a statement to the press disclosing that he had been diagnosed with Alzheimer's disease.[14] The letter was personal and handwritten with laborious penmanship and crossed-out words, a fact not lost on the press. Reagan addressed the letter to "My Fellow Americans," followed with this curiously phrased opening statement: "I have recently been told that I am one of the Americans who will be afflicted with Alzheimer's Disease." This statement is remarkable because it connects his own individual diagnosis to a kind of national diagnosis: he will be afflicted, just as many Americans will be afflicted; this is our collective fate. The intimacy of the address coupled with the magnitude of the disclosure and his audience (the American people) confuses notions of public and private in the service of a very abstract notion of health.

Reagan was clear, however, that his intention in going public with his diagnosis was an interest of national security, awareness of the disease being a key component of public health. "In opening our hearts," he wrote, "we hope this might promote greater awareness of this condition." Reagan promotes public awareness as coming from the heart— his and his wife's in particular. The public informatics of the disease are here *born* of love; love allows the disease to be seen and known:

Nov. 5, 1994

My Fellow Americans,

I have recently been told that I am one of the millions of Americans who will be afflicted with Alzheimer's Disease.

Upon learning this news, Nancy and I had to decide whether as private citizens we would keep this a private matter or whether we would make this news known in a public way.

In the past Nancy suffered from breast cancer and I had my cancer surgeries. We found through our open disclosures we were able to raise public awareness. We were happy that as a result many more people underwent testing. They were treated in early stages and able to return to normal, healthy lives.

So now, we feel it is important to share it with you. In opening our hearts, we hope this might promote greater awareness of this condition. Perhaps it will encourage a clearer understanding of the individuals and families who are affected by it.

At the moment I feel just fine. I intend to live the remainder of the years God gives me on this earth doing the things I have always done. I will continue to share life's journey with my beloved Nancy and my family. I plan to enjoy the great outdoors and stay in touch with my friends and supporters.

Unfortunately, as Alzheimer's Disease progresses, the family often bears a heavy burden. I only wish there was some way I could spare Nancy from this painful experience. When the time comes I am confident that with your help she will face it with faith and courage.

In closing let me thank you, the American people for giving me the great honor of allowing me to serve as your President. When the Lord calls me home [text crossed out] whenever that may be, I will leave with the greatest love for this country of ours and eternal optimism for its future.

I now begin the journey that will lead me into the sunset of my life. I know that for America there will always be a bright dawn ahead.

Thank you, my friends. May God always bless you.

Sincerely,

Ronald Reagan

As a part of his public visibility, Reagan was also careful to acknowledge the effects of the disease on caregivers and families, writing how he wished he could "spare Nancy from this painful experience." He wrote of his confidence that the nation would provide support for his wife. The press was quick to pick up on this aspect of his statement, and much of the public dialogue in ensuing weeks dealt with the effects of the disease on caregivers and families.

In fact, the majority of the public attention in the next ten years before his death was focused on his wife's role as caregiver and the couple's great love.[15] Four years before he died, Nancy Reagan even published a volume of their personal love letters in *I Love You, Ronnie: The Letters of Ronald Reagan to Nancy Reagan.* His death was eventually commemorated in article after article by virtue of the couple's love. Tempered to a certain degree in these public eulogies were stories of family strife—something that was certainly known in the public during his presidency—or many of the difficult details of his final ten years of life. In fact, Reagan was largely absent from the public in this time, as Nancy Reagan prohibited photographs in the interest of protecting his public image.[16]

The irony of this new invisibility, however, is that with this letter to the American people, Reagan became the new national face of Alzheimer's, catapulting the disease into the public eye. The letter's closing stanza evokes his movie star cowboy image. "I now begin the journey that will lead me into the sunset of my life," he wrote. "I know that for America there will always be a bright dawn ahead." His journey aligned with America's journey, but through love, through this new public visibility, there was hope. America finally realized that it had to account for Alzheimer's.

In 2008, four years after Reagan's death and fourteen years after he helped suture caregiving to national biopolitics, the U.S. Postal Service (USPS) released sixty-four thousand limited-edition Alzheimer's stamps to spread awareness of the disease and the problem of care. The *New York Times* describes the image succinctly: "A pensive, muted stamp, it features the unsmiling profile of an elderly woman with the hand of an otherwise unseen caregiver resting gently on her left shoulder. One upper corner is sunlit; one lower corner fades away into purplish shadow. Hope and sadness juxtaposed as subtext."[17] The dominant tropes are all present: the slip from light into darkness; affective polarities of sadness and hope; and the blank, unsmiling visage of the person with Alzheimer's guided by the angelic, disembodied hand of the caregiver. The stamp was successful enough that the USPS renewed it for another fundraising run in 2017 (it simply reversed the image so the woman faced the other direction). Money raised by the stamp was earmarked for the NIH.[18]

The concept for the image was developed by the prolific stamp designer Ethel Kessler, who was quite vocal about her own connection to the disease: "It's one of the most emotional projects I've ever worked on," she said. "I'm not even sure my mother remembers my name now. She hasn't said it in a long time."[19] Kessler designed the stamp with the help of advocacy organizations, friends, and the NIH, but her own role as the daughter of someone with Alzheimer's indicates a kind of emotional subjectivity that is concomitant with other kinds of caregiving media. "The whole notion of caregivers is critical," Kessler told the *Washington Post*. "They provide the care that Alzheimer's patients need to live, and they suffer a terrible loss of their own. It took us 10 or 15 false starts before we finally figured that out."[20] It is worth noting here that the solution to the stamp's design problem only arrived through the inclusion of the caregiver in the aesthetics of the disease.

Caregiving is represented as angelic, as pure, and it comes from the light—not the dark to which the diseased is faced. Caregiving is the answer to an otherwise haunting and depressing subject matter.

Much like Reagan's letter before, the intimate, innocuous nature of the delivery and the absorption of the disease within the theme of love-care help shape the message. The size of the stamp and the banality of its purpose offer closure to the difficulty of its content by making it small and manageable. But aside from the form of the media, the emphasis on caregiving also offers some containment of the disease. The comforting hand on the shoulder of the woman with Alzheimer's is designed to highlight the vital importance of care in any conversation on Alzheimer's. Just as a letter is sent from one person to another by virtue of a small investment in a national service, caregiving is a simple but vital interpersonal service that reverberates in the national effort to defeat Alzheimer's. Buying the stamp is a small choice that each citizen can make in the nationally oriented battle against Alzheimer's. Like Reagan's letter, it conflates scales of public and private in the service of U.S. public health.

Love for Now, Science for Later

According to a recent report from the Alzheimer's Association, in 2020, more than eleven million Americans provided more than fifteen billion hours of unpaid Alzheimer's care. The association estimates that labor as worth more than $256 billion.[21] Eighty percent of Alzheimer's home care comes from family members. Caregivers are more prone to stress, emotional duress, chronic disease like hypertension and heart disease, and early death.[22] They are also susceptible to economic duress, often giving up on careers and jobs to provide care. Two-thirds of these caregivers are women. Nearly one-quarter of caregivers have children under age eighteen; they are called the "sandwich" caregivers, so called because they are caught between two charges: their children and their parents with Alzheimer's.[23]

These are the statistics championed by the primary advocacy and philanthropic organization in the United States, the Alzheimer's Association. They accompany a major surge in attention to the issue of care across the board, including academic research, labor organizations, pharmaceutical companies, professional caregiving, new industries to aid informal home care, and federal and state initiatives and policy. Another major Alzheimer's philanthropic and advocacy group, the Alzheimer's Foundation, long rallied behind the slogan "Caring for the nation, one person at a time," ultimately echoing Reagan's epistolary charge. In fact, this organization has promoted the idea of caregiving at the expense of all else. Its recent "Together for Care" telethon and fundraising campaign was resolute: "For now, there is no cure for Alzheimer's disease. Care makes all the difference. It's that black & white." There were care-oriented consumables available in the online store; from fleece blankets and jackets to T-shirts and coffee mugs, a range of products (in black-and-white colors) allowed you to express your dedication to care as the most important issue for Alzheimer's.

The emphasis on care above all other priorities could be considered contentious and perhaps even reactionary to the overwhelming

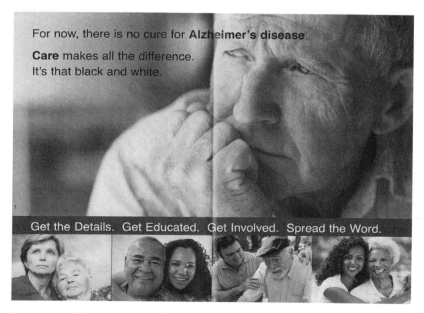

For now, there is no cure for **Alzheimer's disease**.

Care makes all the difference. It's that black and white.

Get the Details. Get Educated. Get Involved. Spread the Word.

FIGURE 13. Alzheimer's Foundation "Together for Care" mailer.

predominance of biomedical research oriented around diagnostics, cause, and cure. These Alzheimer's advocacy groups simply do not see eye to eye when it comes to investment and philanthropic priorities. The Alzheimer's Association has argued that it is for care and science but also that it is highly invested in discovering a cure, whereas the Alzheimer's Foundation has historically prioritized care. Limited resources make this debate occasionally acrimonious. The Alzheimer's Foundation has even been engaged in litigation with the Alzheimer's Association over, among other things, fraudulent handling of money donated through wills.[24]

The dualism articulated by these two advocacy organizations echoes through the social, institutional, and governmental structures of Alzheimer's. Science and care are the fundamental targets of advocacy and education, and they are generally maintained as separate categories. I should be very clear that these categories are not necessarily oppositional; rather, they articulate distinct logics in the public health of Alzheimer's. Love-care mandates responsibility now on behalf of a compromised past, while science orients proleptic or anticipatory research on behalf of that increasingly compromised present.

Perhaps the most comprehensive public health media campaign on the subject of Alzheimer's in the United States—and a good example of this trend—is HBO's *The Alzheimer's Project*. Having premiered on Mother's Day in May 2009, the project offers a multitiered, comprehensive examination of a range of Alzheimer's issues. It was produced in coordination with the Alzheimer's Association and the NIA. The content of the project is vast, including four feature-length documentaries, fifteen smaller web-based documentaries, a book and related DVD, and extensive integration with advocacy and support networks. It not only provides a broad introduction to the disease, but it attempts to show the latest developments in scientific research.

The project alternates between two dominant rhetorical modes, science and care, framed as fundamentally separate. According to critics, this largely matched HBO's intentions: alternating feelings of hope and realism, emotion and science, sending "viewers on an emotional roller coaster as they confront the anguish of a current diagnosis and the potential better news for future generations."[25] Interestingly, the NIA was in charge of regulating the scientific content of the films, but oversight on the subject of care was left more to HBO and the Alzheimer's Association. This rendered the caregiving component emotional and personal rather than scientific—a vital distinction.

One of the four feature documentaries, *The Caregivers,* details a range of individual caregiving narratives as a way to demonstrate the complexity of the problem of care. It explores themes like financial burden, employment issues, community outreach and access, strategies for successful care, and, most centrally, the emotional and mental health of caregivers. One segment recounts two love stories in one. Titled "Pat and Terry . . . and Suzanne," it details Terry McKenna's care for his wife, Pat, while she had Alzheimer's. After she dies, he is able to find love and happiness again when he marries a different woman, Suzanne. Critically, agential love is the tool he values most while taking care of his partner with Alzheimer's, but it is also still available after she dies. McKenna explains the challenges of caregiving at home:

> You're one on one, that's the toughest kind of caregiving. For the most part it was a lonely difficult existence. I have always said a caregiver can't be a caregiver if he doesn't love the person he's caring for with this disease. No way. It's very demeaning. When I put her in that home, I used to do the private duty all day Saturday and all day Sunday because I didn't think the home was qualified enough to take care of my wife. But once she got to that point where she couldn't speak anymore but that girl is going and going and going and is eventually gone.

As the audience hears McKenna's words, HBO provides a visual montage of several snapshots of Pat with the song "As Time Goes By" playing in the background. Each shot in the montage shows her appearing older, less capable, and less focused, until a final snapshot shows her in a wheelchair, wearing a neck brace to keep her head up, mouth open, looking away from the camera. "Pat McKenna 1936–2006" is written beneath it. So HBO has taken a seemingly innocent comment about love as a kind of commitment and transformed it into a reprise of *Casablanca* in exorable decline, a classic romantic love story with only one possible ending.

This segment makes visible many of the sad narratives of Alzheimer's, but most importantly, it foregrounds the assumption that when someone's ability to communicate is gone, when her cognitive abilities are compromised, all that's left is love, and that this is what keeps one going. The memory of their love is what a caregiver needs to endure the illness. Even if it fails to save the life of the person with the disease, love offers an enduring narrative structure for a situation in which narrative itself is threatened. Love is your responsibility as a caregiver, and the rest (according to HBO) can be left to science.[26]

A strange twist in this socially inscribed dualism between science for the future and love-care for now is in the shifting structure of medical inquiry itself. Researchers are actively integrating categories of emotion and affect (and quality of life) into the study of Alzheimer's on a broad scale. This mode of research, however, is largely invisible in the public conversation on scientific progress. Of course, the centrality of emotional connection as a substitute or alternative to cognitively oriented exchange is a major focus of Alzheimer's caregiving in the United States today. Dementia ethicist Stephen Post, for example, is a strong proponent of the viability of love in caregiving relationships. He argues that "even when cognitive capacities wane, the emotional and relation power of love can still remain powerful."[27] Person-centered care has long emphasized that people with dementia offer the capacity for noncognitive connection, along with the possibility of emotional honesty and spiritual awareness.[28] On the basis of these traditions in care, other Alzheimer's arenas are increasingly integrating affect and emotion into their research.

In 2006, the NIH, the NIA, the National Institute of Mental Health, and the National Institute of Neurological Disorders and Stroke sponsored a major push for the recognition of the affective dimensions of aging and dementia called the Cognitive and Emotional Health Project (CEHP). Its goal was to assess the state of "research on demographic, social, and biological determinants of cognitive and emotional health among adults, [and] to determine how these pathways reciprocally influence each other."[29] Recognizing the historical separation of these two categories in dementia research as a problem to be corrected, CEHP strongly recommended the active articulation of categories of emotion into the sciences of cognition and aging. These categories of emotion included depressive symptoms, anxiety symptoms, and positive and negative affect.

This new national focus on emotional health was arguably an important step in the development of a more complex model of personhood for people with Alzheimer's, in addition to theories of cause, cure, and prevention of the disease. Certainly the emphasis on emotion—especially at the level of something as abstract as "positive and negative affect"—asserts the viability of love as integral to successful aging. While CEHP does not in fact raise the concept of love per se, it is difficult to imagine its exclusion in *any* contemporary discussion of care whereby the emotional health of interpersonal familial relationships is a subject of concern.

Given the significant structural transitions in dementia research in the United States over the last decade, one might argue that Cartesian dualisms are on their way out. Important trends include the national emphasis on emotional health as a vital and integral part of cognitive health for both caregivers and people with Alzheimer's, the enfolding of caregivers into the way that health is monitored and integrated into scientific research practice, and the increasing standardization of categories of emotional health. But the structural accommodations of categories of affect within scientific research still leave these two categories as distinct, despite their apparent integration.

Loved Ones: The Subject of Alzheimer's

The national orchestration of love-care for now and science for later puts enormous pressure on the sustainability of love within caregiving situations. In an interview featured on the Oprah Winfrey Network (OWN), celebrity "lifestyle icon" B. Smith and her husband, Dan Gasby, described their relationship as a model of how to live with Alzheimer's. During the segment, the couple is seen walking on the beach, enjoying a drink on the deck looking over the water, a fruitful garden, their dog, and a nice house. Even when B. shows fear or insecurity, Dan is there to provide support. In the interview, there is a discussion of how "time is elastic" in the experience of Alzheimer's. Here they are reflecting on the problem of memory loss. Viewers hear Oprah's voice in the background, explaining how to combat that elasticity: "Dan says the disease has taught them to live in the present, the way a person with Alzheimer's only can." However, Dan continues the narrative with a comment that reveals his obligations to the future: "this is a marriage, this is love, but this is a friendship built to last."[30] Beyond the obvious way in which the OWN video masks financial and social caregiving resources through the discourse of love, it begs the question as to limits of sustainability: what happens when that love is no longer adequate?

In 2012, prominent businessman Charles Snelling killed his wife, Adrienne, and then shot and killed himself in their upstate Pennsylvania home. Adrienne had Alzheimer's disease, and Charles had helped care for her in their home since her diagnosis six years earlier. In a public statement, Adrienne's family said, "After apparently reaching the point where he could no longer bear to see the love of his life deteriorate further, our father ended our mother's life and then took his own life as well. . . . We know he acted out of deep devotion and profound love." When covering the story, many news organizations referenced a short essay Charles Snelling had written for the *New York Times* the previous December describing his love for his sick wife and their life together. Alongside the coverage of the murder-suicide, an article titled "Tale of Love and Illness Ends in Deaths," the *Times* republished Snelling's essay with an Associated Press photo of the smiling couple taken in 2007.[31]

The news coverage was especially challenging because of the way it turned the story of a homicide into a nostalgic romance and a tale of "unconditional love," when it is clear that his love had very clear conditions. The Snelling case is no anomaly. It is in fact part of a small pattern of murder-suicides in Alzheimer's care, but the *Times* coverage focused more on the Snellings' love story than on the murder and suicide.[32] This had the effect of almost excusing or explaining the acts through the logic of love. More broadly, this trick turned the realities of caregiving into a romantic aesthetic, a sad, nostalgic gloss that subsumed any discourse that might help solve this pervasive crisis in care. The logic of love is channeled through the defensibility of the choice to end Adrienne Snelling's life, a decision that elevates the importance of the caregiver's perspective over that of the person being cared for, even as it imagines a more relational morality.

A good example of this subjective position—and one category of affect that remains widely used but undertheorized—is *loved one*. *Loved one* in Alzheimer's parlance is often code for a person diagnosed with Alzheimer's. This phrase is common throughout the broad range of Alzheimer's representations—not just in popular discourse but in scientific journals, care literature, and public health. President Obama's use of the phrase in 2009 is a good example: "The physical and emotional demands of caring for a loved one with Alzheimer's can be overwhelming, but no one should face this disease alone."[33]

In a banal sense, the phrase reveals a kind of semantic slippage between love and care. Used in this way, it articulates the person with the disease into a social relationship that can ironically erode personhood. In other words, the caregiver maintains agency, while the person with Alzheimer's is simply "loved." Contemporary caregiving is fundamentally structured around the recognition of the enduring person in Alzheimer's. However, that personhood is still understood primarily through social systems of meaning and a bioethics of belonging.[34] Personhood, therefore, is made *conditional* to love.

This problem of "ones" and "twos" and "I" and "we" bears special mention because of this complex subjectivity of Alzheimer's. Richard Taylor, whom the reader may remember from chapter 3, is worth quoting at length on the matter, in part because he had dementia but also because he represents a movement to recognize the perspective of the person with Alzheimer's as unique and worthwhile in its own right. He wrote,

Caregivers remain members of their "we" grouping, whereas the person for whom they are caring slowly become a group of one. Some—dare I say many—healthcare professionals and experts who pontificate about what I should do, what "we" should do, are not (from my perspective of course) sensitive to the fact that I am less and less part of a "we." Caregivers are offered advice about how to handle us "we's," what to say to us "we's," what "we" are thinking, and what "we" want and need. Unfortunately, awareness of the changes in how we communicate with each other is more and more in my caregivers' minds, not in mine.[35]

What is in the caregiver's mind is obviously of great importance to the person being cared for, and Taylor is at pains to make that clear. But too often what is in his mind is made secondary, and his perspective is too often ignored.[36] Popular representations of Alzheimer's mimic this model of care subjectivity in easily recognizable patterns. One pattern well described in this book is the general focus on memory loss above all other kinds of symptomatology, a symptom especially troubling for notions of "we."

One way that popular media fetishizes memory and love is through recourse to the flashback—a relatively simple narrative tool to demonstrate the evolution of love over time and the way Alzheimer's affects that relationship. Generally speaking, the viewer can identify with the memory of the love of the couple in their youth via the flashback and then experience the heartache of love threatened by disease in a more present day. This strategy harmonizes with the more general use of cinematic, biographical devices that authorize the decline narrative for Alzheimer's.[37] Because the viewer is encouraged to identify with the agency of memory, the flashback foregrounds that subjective space even as it demonstrates the limitations of the person with Alzheimer's. Several popular movies rely on this narrative structure to recount dramatic love stories of Alzheimer's, including *Iris, The Iron Lady,* and one of the more iconic Hollywood love stories of the twenty-first century, *The Notebook.*[38]

Iris was one of the first movies to focus overtly on the experience of Alzheimer's and gain both critical and box-office acclaim. It details the story of the British writer Iris Murdoch, who died of complications due to Alzheimer's, and it is largely based on the recollections of Murdoch's husband, John Bayley, in his memoir *Elegy for Iris*. The film utilizes flashbacks to show the healthy, intellectually fervent love affair of their youth alternating with present-day dementia and a love threatened. The film's younger star, Kate Winslet, told *USA Today* that the narrative structure was required to understand their love: "you wouldn't feel the impact of the tragedy if you didn't have the love story that comes before."[39] What this statement implies is that their love is situated on a foundation of memory. Indeed, suturing memories of past experiences of love to care today is a dominant theme in caregiving. Many caregivers claim that the reason they care is because of what came before, and caregiving is only possible because of their earlier love.[40]

In a review of *Iris* directed toward medical ethicists, Solomon Liao argues that this subjective position is about human relationships: "Ultimately, when all else is stripped away, the ability to love and receive love is what makes us human. . . . What this movie and dementia itself teach us is that personhood is about relationships and the ability to love."[41] But if Liao is correct, and personhood is about the ability to love, then what do these representations say about the person who has Alzheimer's? What does the "ability to love" even mean? Ultimately, their personhood is encapsulated by a "we" rather than an "I," and their care is perched on the possibility of that love's sustainability.

One of the more popular movies to orient the experience of Alzheimer's around love is *Away from Her*, directed by Sarah Polley and based on a short story by Alice Munro. The film was understood to show something about the realities of caregiving—a love story stripped of all melodrama. This is largely because the love-threatened narrative comes true—if only for a while. The film recounts the story of a man who checks his wife with Alzheimer's into a long-term care facility. While there, she loses her ability to recognize him and gradually falls in love with another resident. Like the HBO narrative, the film celebrates the possibility for new love even as the old love fails. *Away from Her* demonstrates that if popular narratives of Alzheimer's don't resort to love as a solution, it is still the litmus test we use to decide whether the person is valuable. The person with Alzheimer's is still worth thinking about precisely because they can still love or be loved—in some fashion.[42]

Christopher Filley, a professor of neurology and psychiatry, wrote a review of the film in *Neurology* celebrating the film precisely for its affective coherence: "Neurologists accustomed to intellectualizing the clinical phenomena of dementia will find themselves immersed in the personal tragedy of cognitive decline through Polley's powerful cinematic vision." This statement poses a problem in the way it distances intellectual or professional labor from the amateur affairs of culture and the heart. The film is first rendered a populist token—despite the skill with which it is delivered—then it is praised for its sophisticated rendering of love and care: "the film does succeed . . . at reaching a measure of gentle resolution to alleviate the suffering, confirming an unusual but genuine love story."[43] The review therefore rehearses the now standard theme: science will take care of the future of Alzheimer's so long as love can serve as a public, personal answer to the problem of the disease right now.[44]

Away from Her raises another critical issue for love-care, and that is the way in which love impinges on nonfamilial caregiving situations—ultimately eradicating the easy boundary between "formal" and "informal" caregiving. Not all structures of care take place in the home between familial intimates. A significant and growing trend in Alzheimer's care is the use of paid workers inside the home. This will lead to expansive growth in the care industry; the Committee on the Future Health Care Workforce for Older Americans at the National Institute of Medicine estimated that the United States will need an additional 3.5 million paid caregivers by 2030 just to maintain the current ratio of caregivers to the population.[45] The resources provided to facilitate home care for people with Alzheimer's are meager and intermittent. Respite care (temporary care used to provide relief for caregivers) has increased over the past few decades, but it is still only used by one-quarter of dementia caregivers.[46] While Medicare pays for some acute care situations and hospice care, it does not cover the long-term, sustained home care necessary for many people with the disease.

The increase in paid home health care is an interesting lacuna in the national imagination of dementia care, and it directly correlates to the uneasy relationship between love and care in these situations. Home care workers have always held a complicated relationship with state recognition of their conditions of labor due to the "hidden" nature of their work inside the home. Since the 1960s, paid home care workers in the United States were never really granted the status of employee, despite receiving federal assistance through state institutions like welfare and Medicaid.[47] Eileen Boris and Jennifer Klein argue that the national discomfort with the status of home health care is a direct result of the intimate nature of the labor: "neither public employment nor private service, combining aspects of health care and household labor, home care existed in the shadows of the welfare state."[48] The history of federal home care policy belongs to the "realms of welfare, poverty, health, and aging," but not labor standards. This has led to a systematic economic devaluing of home care inclusive of low wages, no protection, and little representation.

This blind spot also applies to representations of paid home care in stories about Alzheimer's. There aren't many. Despite the interpersonal requirements of this kind of labor, affect rarely figures into the labor situations of Alzheimer's health care workers, and their stories often go untold. Part of this is because love is the dominant discourse, and care workers are supposed to be dispassionate medical professionals. Boris and Klein point out the contradiction at the heart of paid care: "we seek respect and dignity for aging and disabled people but not for those who make it possible for them to live in the community."[49] If paid home care workers *do* play a role in developing an ethic of Alzheimer's care, they simply function in the popular imagination as a fulcrum for the real characters in the story: generally spouses and children of people with the disease.[50] Our image of Alzheimer's renders caregiving the provenance of either the family at home or some sort of bewildering bureaucracy if outside of the home, and variability in this dichotomy is difficult to accommodate.

Adaptations: Normativity, Closure, and Care

The 2014 Oscar-winning film adaptation of *Still Alice* ends in almost the same way as the novel on which it is based. Just like the book, Alice's daughter is performing a scene from a play. But this time, the play itself is a significant part of the scene. Instead of an unnamed play, the daughter performs dialogue from *Angels in America, Part Two: Perestroika,* Tony Kushner's tribute to the multivalent experiences of HIV/AIDS in America. By introducing this discourse, the film makes a clear claim on the centrality of Alzheimer's to national identity, just as it articulates Alzheimer's into a longer history of disenfranchisement and disease. This time, the last line the daughter performs is "Nothing's lost forever. In this world, there's a kind of painful progress. Longing for what we've left behind, and dreaming ahead. At least I think that's so." After a pause, the daughter again asks her mother, did she like it? What did she think it was about? And again, Alice answers: love. The film fades into the snapshot aesthetic. Its last shot is a grainy, 16 mm family video of mother and daughter walking toward the beach, an easy arm around her daughter's waist, dreaming ahead.

I have argued in this chapter that the problem with love is that it has become the primary logic of care across popular, scientific, and civic arenas in the United States: a way forward in the absence of a cure. It maintains Alzheimer's as a public crisis while it pretends to ameliorate stigma. It is a mode of collective endurance through which we both recognize and authorize Alzheimer's personhood and imagine a national solution to care. As the Kushner tribute points out, this situation is not specific to Alzheimer's. Other diseases certainly harness affect under narratives of care, but Alzheimer's in particular maintains a public face in the United States as love and love threatened. Perhaps this is because Alzheimer's is unique in how it is most often understood through problems of lack or absence: the absence of memory, the loss of cognitive skills, the loss of recognition, the absence of cure or definitive cause, or the oft-maligned absence of self. These kinds of narratives can be devastating to public narratives of hope and dreams of a cure. But they also have the tendency to isolate a kind of "all that's left" feeling in any discourse that is twisted around hope for a better future. That is, if good care is articulated as the capacity to love the person who is already or almost "gone," all that's left for all parties involved is love. The representational media I have analyzed in this chapter salvages "all that's left" and then recuperates it as essential labor in a politics of care. Perhaps, as critics, we might reorient that process.

Needed is a model of Alzheimer's care that respects the love potentially implicit in familial care situations but does not rely on it as a narrative for good care. Fortunately, there is a range of well-considered practical and theoretical models (beyond the obvious need for financial assistance).[51] For example, Alzheimer's care could be improved by forms of social reciprocity Eve Feder Kittay calls "doulia," in which "nested dependencies link those who need help to those who help, and link the helpers to a set of supports."[52] This model of care and protection acknowledges that dependency and care are always socially situated rather than a contract between individuals. But it also acknowledges the social fact that we have all been in positions of dependency at youth, and we are all destined to a position of dependency in old age. It reorganizes the futurity of Alzheimer's (as fear, as progress, as cure) into a temporal ethic that respects a mantra of disability studies: that we will all be disabled someday.

This chapter contributes to an ongoing critical conversation about the entanglement of private and public sentiment in public, popular culture, and it participates in a genealogy of pathology, care, and personhood already deeply familiar to feminists and queer theorists.[53] Ann Cvetkovich points out that one of the primary goals of the affective turn in cultural studies and critical theory has been to "depathologize negative affects."[54] This makes sense when critics address marginalized or minoritarian social groups for whom negative affects contribute to the networks of political orientation and shared histories, but what about the relationship between positive affect and pathology? Neville Hoad, writing elegies and aesthetics of poetry in the South African AIDS pandemic, acknowledges the critical viability of the pathological, arguing that "reading . . . critically, reparatively, mournfully, works to reanimate the words of the dead and to keep the spectacle of the dying painfully, shamefully and politically in us and with us."[55] Might critics reorient the goal and pathologize positive affects in the mediatics of Alzheimer's care? There is a politics to that kind of description simply because it disrupts neoliberal dependencies on love. More simply, it helps disarticulate love from care. There is no cure; this much is true, so perhaps we need to lessen our affective demands.

This is a kind of articulation—not necessarily of the ideological vein—but a disambiguation of the ambiguities created by U.S. health care policy and by insecure, still nascent cultures of Alzheimer's care. Close attention should be paid to the way love is utilized across public and private structures of health care and functions to close down biopolitical belonging in particular ways. Charting such affective closure as a problem of representation reorients Alzheimer's care in a way respectful of an alternate agential politics. This is important because of the ways in which health care often structures individual agency.

While not beholden to them, love certainly fits into neoliberal formations of health care in the United States in the natural overlap of biopolitics and liberalism. Mitchell Dean describes how this works through technologies of agency, those technologies of government that depend on the capacities and agencies of individuals. What is vital about this framework is that it is through an exercise of our own freedoms that we help to achieve the interests of the state and its integrated economic interests. But it is disguised through recourse to free will, powerful feelings, and a range of apparent rights and self-empowerment discourse—inclusive of our efforts in the academy to locate agency.[56] Dean makes clear in this analysis that technologies of agency employ social agreements (such as love-care) as way to "contract out" biopolitical obligation, risk, and responsibility.

Those who enact these technologies of agency do not do so out of public service. Their disguise as love is part of their operative logic: individuals in a love-care situation act through immediate relationships of dependency and obligation. Though they may not directly act out of national support, they do certainly act with an awareness of others in like situations. Their individual, agential feeling often contributes to a greater structure of feeling, a situation compatible with what Lauren Berlant describes as an "intimate public." The representational culture of Alzheimer's is an operative component of these intimate publics because of the way in which it helps enact a sense of the commonly held feeling and a "fantasy" solution to the problems that bind the public in the first place. Berlant argues, "The culture of true feeling has no inevitable political ideology. . . . Its core pedagogy has been to develop a notion of social obligation based on the citizen's capacity for suffering and trauma."[57] This particular intimate public is only made possible through collective recognition of forms of care as obligations of love.

I am specifically arguing here against the fixing of love and the ways love's normativity actually gets in the way of good care. One of the ways love becomes normative is through the dichotomization of love and cognition: apparently love is all that remains after the mind is gone.[58] We should challenge this dichotomy. Love is often disguised as cognition's other, but given the primacy of recognition as a social optic, love might be better understood *as* cognition in our current conjuncture. Furthermore, given the immense volume of decisions, tactics, and intentions that go into everyday Alzheimer's care, it should be evident that cognitive capacity is integral to care. Love is cognitive engagement disguised as noncognitive affect. As I have argued throughout this book, that cognitive engagement is profoundly orchestrated through media technology and representational culture. What other ways might we reconsider the affective agencies of Alzheimer's and their relationships with representational culture?

One difficulty of the slippage between love and care for Alzheimer's is the way in which it eclipses other kinds of interpersonal affects, such as humor, confusion, boredom, and anger. When news leaked that Will Ferrell would play Ronald Reagan in an upcoming satirical film about the president called *Reagan*, the public backlash was swift and uncompromising. The Alzheimer's Association publicly condemned the film, a stance that reverberated in the media. Reagan's son Michael also tweeted his displeasure: "#Alzheimers is not a comedy to the 5 million people who are suffering with the disease, it first robs you of your mind and then it kills you."[59] Within a few days, Ferrell dropped out of the film, and *Reagan* appeared to be on the chopping block itself.[60] Michael Reagan's perspective is understandable as a defense of his father's public image, but his position on the value of humor and comedy for people living with dementia is wrong. However, it also clearly demonstrates the sacred status of Alzheimer's in the United States and the difficulty of introducing alternative affect into stories about the disease.

Future work might pay heed to the way in which any affective clarity can be naturalized and utilized by economic and political interests as an effect of governmentality. This is, after all, how modern governmentality works—through the free affectual capacities of citizens. Love (and its companion fear) just seems to be most available to our approach to aging and dementia. With that said, perhaps an important further step would be to explore affective contradictions in order to intervene in the hegemony of love. These technologies of agency can certainly overflow their apparent, legislated, commoditized capacities. In fact, they already are. As scholars, critics, and activists, we just need to draw attention to that practice as a part of our own representational politics.

Love will always haunt care. But perhaps if one insists that representations of Alzheimer's care not be beholden to love, other affects might intrude. This kind of critique restores some of the person with Alzheimer's to its embattled subject; at the very least, it is more honest. I'm not aiming for answers, and closure is an unacceptable response to a system without a cure.

"How to Not Forget"

In a recent television commercial, someone types "how to not forget" into a Google search bar.[1] The results of his search reveal that this is a common concern, but Google provides a range of solutions to the problem, solutions the ad will go on to demonstrate. We hear an old man's voice, "Hey Google, show me photos of me and Loretta." Old snapshots appear of a couple smiling for the camera. The man chuckles, "Remember: Loretta hated my mustache," to which Google replies, "OK, I'll remember that." He searches Google for "that little town off the coast of Juneau," and he finds information about Sitka. "Remember: Loretta loved going to Alaska and scallops." Google replies, "OK, I'll remember that." Google then provides a montage of different mediated memories, each answering a different nostalgic prompt: "Show me photos from our anniversary" reveals an aged, cracked snapshot of the couple; "Remember: she always snorted when she laughed" is answered with a home movie of Loretta laughing and looking at the camera; "Play our favorite movie" inspires a brief sequence from the film *Casablanca*. Google then summarizes his memories, ending with "Loretta always said, don't miss me too much, get out of the dang house." The man laughs in response, "Remember: I'm the luckiest man in the world," and we hear a screen door creaking open as he takes his dog out for a walk, following Loretta's advice. The commercial ends with the tagline "a little help with the little things."

The commercial, titled *Loretta,* was very popular when it first aired in 2020; in addition to sizable audiences of both the Super Bowl and the Oscars, the ad garnered more than fifty million views on YouTube in just the first two weeks after it was broadcast on television. It also attracted considerable attention in the news and social media.[2] The commercial's conceit is also its purported wisdom—that we ought to have a life outside of media—and yet, it is evident that it is increasingly difficult to live without these cognitive media prosthetics. Although users of all ages and abilities rely on media technologies for assistance, aging people like the man in the ad often articulate the threat to memory, identity, and relationships.

And this is indeed a threat, as the man searches, not for ways to remember, but for ways not to forget. Forgetting is the problem that Google helps solve. The ad shows how media technology often articulates common fears around memory loss but also how that media provides a practical solution. Memory may only be "a little thing," but it is something we need help with, especially as we age. The ad reinforces the value of memory by showing all the different ways Google remembers. Not only is Google an effective search engine but Google Assistant is a tool to help manage personal information, valued memories, and intimate relationships.

The commercial reflects many of the themes of this book: the collective fear of memory loss, the way media technology both models and supports cognitive disability, and the media aesthetics that often describe Alzheimer's disease. There is in fact no direct mention of Alzheimer's in the commercial, but the man's fears of memory loss and his apparent age certainly raise the specter of dementia. The commercial also borrows the snapshot aesthetic, contrasting the proficiency of a digital assistant with more personal, analog media: fading snapshot photos, old home movies, and a black-and-white Hollywood film. It is clear from the ad that memory is instrumental to our sense of self but also to our relationships with others. Loretta serves as a figure for the nostalgic memories of love lost and the person who came before the disease. Not surprisingly, the majority of the video's comments on YouTube focus on sadness and crying, and a great deal of them also mention family members with dementia or Alzheimer's.

As I have argued in this book, it is difficult to understand Alzheimer's without acknowledging the way the past and future so overwhelmingly structure the disease—ultimately anachronizing the present. The dominant temporal narratives of Alzheimer's are progress and loss, simultaneously described through the unifying logic of cognitive capacity. Popular investments in media technologies both reveal and reinforce these temporal logics. The correlates to the snapshot aesthetics of *Loretta* are the anticipatory, proleptic work of the neurosciences, the promises of artificial intelligence, and the broad spectrum of media technologies that shape everyday digital experience.

In this book, I have explored a range of precarious media, such as ephemeral Post-it notes, fading Polaroids, and various forms of art and music that serve as the dominant technologies for understanding lossy Alzheimer's personhood. Their aesthetics ostensibly pay respect to the ways people with dementia seem lost to the past, but an unfortunate consequence is the disavowal of these people's viability in the present. In contrast, I have documented the way the anticipatory structure of the neurosciences echoes in media practices of self-improvement, creativity, and aspiration. These perspectives are seen as hopeful because they offer a kind of media agency, but they put great pressure on all of us to integrate and adapt to media's cognitive imperative. Whether lost to the past or looking to the future, Alzheimer's is abstracted out of the present as a part of the broader play of these media temporalities.

These anachronistic values, however, are easily challenged. One tactic, for example, that can destabilize the culture of threat is to absorb disability studies' orientation with time: the familiar mantra that "we will all some day be disabled."[3] That perspective does not ignore the difficulties of living with Alzheimer's, but it might help lessen the impact of cognitive deficit—both the pathology and the threat. Old age is too commonly understood in this country as a problem that needs to be *solved,* and Alzheimer's sutures mental performance in particular to this dilemma of successful aging. If old age is indeed a universal promise rather than a guarantee, perhaps it is better to embrace the variability of how it might unfold.[4]

At the same time, it is also important not to embrace a false presentism, the increasingly common rebuttal to the hectic mandate of modern advance. Take something like mindfulness, the path to enlightened neuroliberal success—especially prominent in corporate media environments like Google. The doctrine of mindfulness purports to save us from technology burnout through clarity and pause, but it is still intentional neuropractice. Mindfulness is present practice for future success and health, an instrumental tactic that improves one's capacity for other kinds of cognitive labor and cognitive belonging.[5] It speaks the same language as the quantified self or social networking: the daily maintenance of an online profile and the vigilant exercise of self as the skills of communicative capitalism. It simply pretends otherwise. This is a sad paradox: the "selfless" pursuit of a better self. All of this adds up to a better cognitive you, and it ultimately augments that model of self that Alzheimer's disease in its incurability so powerfully threatens.

This book began by calling for the separation of the categories of self and person because their conflation can disenfranchise people with dementia. What, then, in the end, is the difference between self and person? I have argued that personhood is the public, social claim on selfhood and that it is primarily in its mediation that selfhood acquires value as personhood. That form of representation is so pervasive that it seems impossible to challenge on a comprehensive scale, especially because the business of self and identity drives entire media industries and forms of social belonging. But for Alzheimer's in the United States, the mandate on selfhood has a clear history that opens up a space for activism. There is already a movement dedicated to redefining the terms of personhood—a battle fought both by people with dementia and on their behalf. This book has joined that movement by specifically addressing the role of media in the articulation of cognitive health and the construction of personhood.

In many ways, this book has been a plea for the reconsideration of representation's value. At the same time, it also allows that representation is not always in our control. Lessening our demand on representational mastery is not to lose sight of its value or of the critical importance of its truths. Given the attacks on science, evidence, and truth from the Right in America, and the concordant threats to minoritarian agencies, we should continue to defend the many values of representation.

Ultimately, however, it is important to destabilize the representational ground of Alzheimer's and aging. To do so is not to work against a cure. As I have argued in this book, diversifying our research paradigms holds promise, and biomedicine's monopoly on resources is not likely to topple any time soon. But destabilizing homogenous narratives of personhood, cognition, and representation is likely to enable a more pragmatic approach to a future.

Even if one is not diagnosed, Americans live out their lives in a relationship with Alzheimer's because of their shared interest in the brain and its agencies. The declaration that Americans live in the "century of the brain" finds its sibling in the oft-bandied claim that Alzheimer's is the "disease of the century." To accept both is to accept our collective fate under the logic of our brains, diseased or not. As Georges Canguilhem noted, "in the case of disease the normal man is he who lives the assurance of being able to arrest within himself what in another would run its course."[6] This is not to say that Alzheimer's helps to define a norm by virtue of its radical alterity. On the contrary, this is not a rare condition. It is increasingly something universal in its visage, helping to describe the future of an aging nation. The economic, affective, and technological stakes that drive and adhere to these processes of normalization are diverse precisely because of the everydayness and perceived inevitability of the symptoms. Conversely, they cohere in the media coordination of cognitive symptom and solution and in the technological imagination of our threatened selves.

In this conjuncture, the biomedicalization of cognitive ability crystalizes in the social and diagnostic category of Alzheimer's, but it is broadly reinforced through media technologies that model cognitive abilities. My critique of Alzheimer's reflects the insertion of cognitive capacity into the very coherence of a life well lived. Understanding Alzheimer's in the U.S., then, means coming to terms with the way media technologies already shape agency, self, and person. For those working to improve life for people with dementia, this does not mean dismissing the many uses of media; rather, it means we must address the way media can shape cognition's values.

Acknowledgments

This book would not have been possible without the advice, expertise, and support of a great many people. While it has grown considerably since, much of the early thinking for this project took shape with the help of the faculty and doctoral students at New York University and Columbia University. Foremost among them is Marita Sturken, my doctoral advisor at NYU's Department of Media, Culture, and Communication. I am grateful for the interest she showed in my ideas from a very early stage, and she remains a trusted mentor. This book would not exist without her. The rest of my committee, including Nicholas Mirzoeff, Emily Martin, Mara Mills, and Brett Gary, each contributed his or her own helpful perspectives, and I am grateful for the ways they pushed me to think differently.

At NYU, I received funding and institutional support from the Institute of Fine Arts; the Graduate School of Arts and Science; the Steinhardt School for Culture, Education, and Human Development; the Hemispheric Institute; the Council on Media and Culture; and several different scholarly working groups. The Humanities Initiative Graduate Research Fellowship offered not only funding support but also an enjoyable, collaborative work environment and smart feedback.

I was fortunate to spend three years as a postdoctoral fellow in the Michigan Society of Fellows at the University of Michigan, certainly one of the most valuable intellectual experiences a young scholar might dream of. My fellow fellows were generous in thought, quite brilliant, and remarkably committed to the difficulty of interdisciplinary work. They include my cohort of Beckett Sterner, Michael Garratt, Yasmin Moll, Leslie Rogers, and Chelsea Wood, but also Damon Young, Mac Cathles, Tarek Dika, Lauren Gutterman, Sarah Loebman, Jennifer Nelson, Martha Sprigge, Eric Plemons, Sarah Besky, S. E. Kile, Erik Linstrum, Seth Marvel, Lucas Kirkpatrick, Adedamola Osinulu, Beth Pringle, Carrie Brezine, Rebecca Wollenberg, Amanda Alexander, Amanda Armstrong, Lydia Beaudrot, Jana Cephas, Alice Goff, Ying-Hsuan Lin, Allan Lumba, Ben Winger, Tierra Bills, Kevin Ko, Zhiying Ma, Ana Vinea, Kelly Wood, Aniket Aga, and Clare Croft. A number of senior fellows whose contributions shaped my project also helped round out a wonderful academic community. In particular, I acknowledge the professionalism and guidance of Don Lopez, truly peerless in that institution, and the support of the indefatigable Linda Turner.

At Michigan, I was also made to feel welcome by the staff, students, and faculty of the Department of Communication Studies. This manuscript benefited from the perspectives of Susan Douglas, Christian Sandvig, Paddy Scannell, Derek Vaillant, Julia Sonnevend, and Aswin Punathambekar. Each of these people also provided significant mentorship and helped shape my perspective as a media scholar. I learned a great deal through the community provided by Gabrielle Hecht, Paul Edwards, and the various faculty affiliates of the Science, Technology, and Society Program.

Thank you to my colleagues at the University of Arizona, to my many students in the minor in health and human values, and to my fearless colleagues Victor Braitberg and Laura Berry, whose passion for teaching was contagious and an inspiration. I was lucky to have Eric Plemons as a colleague at both Michigan and Arizona. Eric's encouragement and wisdom enriched my project considerably.

I also appreciate the collegiality of the faculty and staff of the Department of Communication at Portland State University. Our chair, Jeff Robinson, helped provide institutional support that was extremely helpful during the final stages of this book's publication.

Many others read portions of this manuscript as it developed into the text you now have in front of you. This includes a diversity of faculty from the institutions already listed. I owe particular thanks to my good friends Hatim El-Hibri, David Raskin, Wazhmah Osman, and Kate Brideau for their thoughtful comments on drafts of this work. This book would most certainly not have made it to press without the help of my family, and in particular my wife, Amber Hansen. In addition to her relentless support and encouragement, her professional experience and knowledge consistently grounded my research in more valuable questions.

Research for this book took place at a number of archives and libraries, including the New York Public Library and the Schomburg Center for Research in Black Culture; the Center for the History of Medicine at Harvard University's Francis A. Countway Library of Medicine, Boston University Medical Center; and the History of Medicine Division of the National Library of Medicine in Bethesda, Maryland. In addition to financial support, many of the archivists at these institutions made significant efforts to help me find my footing in their collections. This is a book that draws on many different fields, and the librarians at my home institutions were helpful with my varied research questions, especially at NYU and Michigan. Chapters 6 and 7 of this book would not be possible without the help of Laurel Humble, Carrie McGee, and Francesca Rosenberg and the entire Department of Education at the New York Museum of Modern Art. They provided remarkable access to a program still in process, and I am grateful for their contributions to this book.

And last, I would be remiss not to acknowledge the many people living with symptoms of dementia and the people who help care for them. Over the years that I worked on this book, I met many of you, each with your own stories to share. I have tried to honor your experiences here. We all still have a great deal to learn about Alzheimer's, and no one is a better guide on that journey than those who are dealing with the disease each and every day.

Notes

Introduction

1. Kontos, "Embodied Selfhood," 196.

2. A popular example of this kind can be seen in the film *Alive Inside*. For more on art and music therapy, see chapter 6 of this book.

3. Vidal, "Brainhood," 7.

4. Rose and Abi-Rached, *Neuro*, 3, 22.

5. It would be easy to argue that these increasingly ubiquitous media technologies make the body irrelevant, allowing for more immaterial identity play. While the affordances of media prosthetics are expansive, I would argue that the human body and its limitations are not so easily cast aside. The brain continues to matter deeply. The natural response to the posthuman promise is the reauthorization of the requirements of the human, and this is most evident in the contemporary fascination with the brain and its mysteries.

6. As Amit Pinchevski and John Durham Peters wrote about autism, "media sit at the switch between disability and ability, a spot of fierce contestation." See Pinchevski and Durham Peters, "Autism and New Media," 2509.

7. Chess, "For Early Signs of Dementia."

8. Lyketsos et al., "Prevalence of Neuropsychiatric Symptoms in Dementia and Mild Cognitive Impairment"; Zhao et al., "Prevalence of Neuropsychiatric Symptoms in Alzheimer's Disease."

9. Albert et al., "Diagnosis of Mild Cognitive Impairment Due to Alzheimer's Disease."

10. Covid-19 temporarily complicated this hierarchy. See polls from Marist (https://maristpoll.marist.edu/1114-alzheimers-most-feared-disease/) and Harris

Interactive   (https://www.metlife.com/content/dam/microsites/about/corpo
rate-profile/alzheimers-2011.pdf).

11. There is some debate over whether the prevalence and incidence of Alzheimer's are in fact rising. Inclusion in either category is of course dependent
on how you define the disease, a practice that is itself constantly under revision
and debate. Two studies that argue for a lowered incidence are Satizabal et al.,
"Incidence of Dementia over Three Decades," and Langa et al., "A Comparison
of the Prevalence of Dementia."

12. National Institute on Aging, "About Alzheimer's Disease," https://www
.nia.nih.gov/alzheimers/topics/alzheimers-basics; Alzheimer's Association,
"2021 Alzheimer's Disease Facts and Figures," 19; Prince et al., "World Alzheimer Report 2015," 4; Weuve at al., "Prevalence of Alzheimer Disease in US
States."

13. Researchers define CTE as a "progressive neurodegenerative syndrome
caused by single, episodic, or repetitive blunt force impacts to the head and
transfer of acceleration-deceleration forces to the brain." See Omalu et al.,
"Emerging Histomorphologic Phenotypes." Much of the current attention to
CTE stems from 2007, when a retired National Football League player committed suicide because of cognitive problems that led to withdrawal and depression.
The neuropathologist who performed his autopsy said his brain looked like
"that of an 85-year-old with Alzheimer's disease." The story was widely discussed in the media, and the journalist who broke the story, Alan Schwarz, was
nominated for a Public Service Pulitzer Prize for his reporting. See Schwarz,
"Dark Days Follow Hard-Hitting Career in NFL" and "A Suicide, a Last Request,
a Family's Questions." As a disease associated with aging, the threat of Alzheimer's can be seen as directly oppositional to the athletic prowess of these
athletes in their prime. Discourse that frames CTE as a kind of Alzheimer's-
oriented symptomatology gives fans a narrative structure to comprehend the
gravity of the condition. For example, researcher Bob Stern told the *Boston Globe*
that CTE is kind of like Alzheimer's but that it affects *young* athletes, and this
is the primary cause for public concern: "We've seen this disease in people
who've just played college ball, just played high school ball, we've seen it in
people who've died way prematurely at age seventeen, eighteen, twenty-one.
What we need to do is think about the youth. We need to protect these games
for our youth so they can enjoy them and not grow up to have these devastating problems with their brain." In other words, what makes CTE special
is not so much its symptomatology as its distinct connection to specific activities and injuries and the way it affects young people "prematurely." See Smith,
"Be Well."

14. Butler, "Is the National Institute on Aging Mission out of Balance?"

15. Adelman, "Alzheimerization of Aging."

16. Whitehouse and George, *Myth of Alzheimer's*, 4.

17. Lomangino, "How the 'Optimism' Narrative in Alzheimer's Helps the Drug Industry and Harms Patients," https://www.healthnewsreview.org/2018/08/how-the-optimism-narrative-in-alzheimers-helps-the-drug-industry-and-harms-patients/.

18. Lock, *Alzheimer Conundrum*, 229.

19. Wu et al., "Latinos and Alzheimer's Disease," 5; Mayeda et al., "Inequalities in Dementia Incidence"; Alzheimer's Association, "2016 Alzheimer's Disease Facts and Figures," 18–19, http://www.alz.org/facts/overview.asp; Alzheimer's Association, "2021 Facts and Figures," 24–26.

20. Alzheimer's ethicist Steven Sabat tells a story of an Alzheimer's physician who complained that "treating an Alzheimer's patient is like doing veterinary medicine." The story is revealing of the stigma the personhood movement had to confront, common even within medical culture. Sabat, *Experience of Alzheimer's Disease*, 114.

21. Leibing, "Divided Gazes," 250.

22. Kitwood, *Dementia Reconsidered*.

23. Fazio, *Enduring Self in People with Alzheimer's*, 7.

24. Kitwood, *Dementia Reconsidered*. See also Sabat, *Experience of Alzheimer's Disease*; Basting, *Forget Memory*; Fazio, *Enduring Self in People with Alzheimer's*.

25. Leibing, "Divided Gazes," 242.

26. Leibing, "Entangled Matters," 190.

27. Comprehensively, see Cohen and Leibing, *Thinking about Dementia*. More directly within that account, see Kontos, "Embodied Selfhood"; Kaufman "Dementia-Near-Death." See also Ballenger, *Self, Senility, and Alzheimer's Disease*, 152–87.

28. Respectively, see Taylor, "On Recognition"; Lock et al., "Susceptibility Genes and the Question of Embodied Identity"; Moser, "Making Alzheimer's Disease Matter"; McLean, *Person in Dementia*.

29. Those efforts are a part of a long-standing tradition that addresses the subject: critics like Marx, Freud, and Foucault, for example, theorized subjectivity to argue how the self is dispersed through or structured by relationships, social institutions, and forms of knowledge. In contemporary critical theory, the concept of the subject is often a way of describing disenfranchised people and—in some cases—affording agency. As such, it has been integral to political projects that seek to understand the uneven experience of race, sexuality, gender, and other areas of identity and difference. Theorizing subjectivity is as old as theorizing knowledge, and critique of the autonomous agent will likely always be important.

30. Perrin and Anderson, "Share of U.S. Adults Using Social Media."

31. Banet-Weiser, *Authentic TM*.

32. As Hélène Mialet argues in *Hawking Incorporated*, this is not a contradiction but a defining aspect of modern identity. She calls this the "distributed-centered subject," as the more distributed a self is, the more "singular" or recognizant that self is. Mialet is writing specifically about Stephen Hawking but more broadly theorizing subjectivity and individuality. Her understanding of subjectivity is worth quoting at length here: "Though one might conclude that because Hawking is a cyborg, a totally distributed postmodern subject, an actor-network composed of humans and nonhumans that constitute his mind, his identity, and his body, we necessarily lost sight of the subject, I argue on the contrary, that it is precisely because of this material-collective process that we can grasp his singularity. This is not a contradiction. Rather, by showing the (re)distribution of competencies to nonhumans and humans as an antidote to the image of the ethereal, rational, subject, I have tried to reframe questions of singularity and individuality. Indeed, they are central to this project. Thus, it is not because Hawking is outside the social and material world (i.e., the brain-in-the-vat) that he is the most singular; rather it is because he is the most materialized, the most collectivized, the most distributed, and the most connected that he is the most singular. He is what I call a distributed-centered subject" (192).

33. In a democratic society, this is exacerbated by the idealized cognitive capacity of its citizens. See Simplican, *Capacity Contract*.

34. There is a sizable body of literature on this topic. See Gilman, *Picturing Health and Illness*; Gilman, *Seeing the Insane*; Gilman, *Disease and Representation*; Hacking, *Representing and Intervening*; Lynch and Woolgar, *Representation in Scientific Practice*; Daston and Galison, *Objectivity*; Hentschel, *Visual Cultures in Science and Technology*; Van Dijck, *Transparent Body*; Cartwright, *Screening the Body*; Treichler, *Visible Woman*; Jones and Galison, *Picturing Science, Producing Art*; Pauwels; *Visual Cultures of Science*.

35. Coopmans et al., introduction to *Representation in Scientific Practice Revisited*, 3–4.

36. For his description of scientific visualization as argument, see Wise, "Making Visible." Alternatively, see the Latourian "inscription device" in *Laboratory Life*, 51, 88.

37. Dumit is largely concerned with the ways neuroimages come to signify or the way people understand them: their meanings. Therefore personhood is based on the neuroimage's facticity or "how facts come to play a role in our everyday category of the person." While indeed an important part of neuroculture, this model of personhood reduces agency to a hermeneutic question. See Dumit, *Picturing Personhood*, 157.

38. Taylor, *Public Life of the Fetal Sonogram*, 28.

39. Serlin, *Imagining Illness*, xxvi.

40. In *Biomedicalization*, Adele Clark posits a helpful way of thinking about this kind of historiography through what she calls "healthscapes." Clark et al., *Biomedicalization*, 105.

41. Reckwitz, "Status of the 'Material'"; Coole and Frost, *New Materialisms*; Bennett, *Vibrant Matter*; Lemke, "New Materialisms"; Parikka, *What Is Media Archaeology*; Durham Peters, *Marvelous Clouds*; Kittler, *Gramophone, Film, Typewriter*. See also a longer tradition of media ecology, notably Marshall McLuhan, *Understanding Media*.

42. Mayer-Schönberger, *Delete*, 50–91; Jones, *Ctrl + Z*.

43. For example, Clay Shirky says the overlap of the social human and the computer contributes to a "cognitive surplus," a social potential based on the aggregate of free time among "educated populations" and the ability of digital technologies to mediate that time. See Shirky, *Cognitive Surplus*, 27.

44. Vradenburg, "Alzheimer's."

45. The representational presence is a part of what N. Katherine Hayles calls the "cognitive nonconscious." See Hayles, "Cognition Everywhere," 201.

46. In a limited sense, processes of visualization make the hidden operations of media legible for a human audience. As Orit Halpern argues specifically about data interactivity, "visualizations are about making the inhuman, that which is beyond or outside sensory recognition, relatable to the human being." See Halpern, *Beautiful Data*, 22. My argument is that humans are not always an audience to the operations of media technologies, and they are disproportionately disenfranchised within the operations of "relatability."

47. Post, *Moral Challenge of Alzheimer Disease*.

48. Within the projects of visual culture or media studies, the concept of "visuality" often refers to the diversity of regimes of the visual: seer, seen, representation, technology, practice, meaning, etc. It is an encompassing term, even if it has a more particular genealogy. In *The Right to Look*, Nicholas Mirzoeff argues that although "visuality" is commonly used as a "trendy theory word meaning the totality of all visual images and devices," it has a specific and powerful meaning in relation to colonial power and history (2). Mirzoeff reorients this perspective by offering a genealogy of the term. Visuality, I would argue, also demands that we take into account the ways cognitive ability underwrites practices of representation and mediation. It describes not just the thing being looked at or the activity of the viewer but the power of recognition and identification. It adds the *how* to the who and what of representational critique. That question of how is increasingly answered by media technology, algorithmic activity, and software processes rather than purely by human agents of sight. This use of visuality invigorates the term as a critical, political tool, more a function of bioethics or disability critique than simple reception or perspective. It also allows critics to consider the embodied experience of use,

spectatorship, and interactivity, and thus it requires a critical interrogation of the media armatures of that experience.

49. See Chen, "Brain Fog"; Johnson and McRuer, "Cripistemologies"; Carlson, *Faces of Intellectual Disability*; Burke, "Introduction"; Kittay and Carlson, *Cognitive Disability*. Much of the work on cognitive disability and representation has focused on autism. See Osteen, *Autism and Representation*; Pinchevski and Peters, "Autism and New Media"; Savarese and Savarese, "Superior Half of Speaking." For other disability scholarship on media and communication, see Ellis and Kent, *Disability and New Media*; Ellis and Goggin, *Disability and the Media*; Mills, "Deaf Jam"; Mills, "On Disability and Cybernetics"; Sourbati, "Disabling Communications?"; St. Pierre, "Cripping Communication"; and Ellcessor, *Restricted Access*.

50. Moulier-Boutang, *Cognitive Capitalism*.

51. This is an ideal. Jennifer Simplican argues in *The Capacity Contract* that "no human can emulate the disciplined and idealized cognitive demands of the fictive democratic subject, and yet we maintain it as a model of democratic politics" (4).

52. As detailed in chapter 2, this gap in historical medical consciousness is first described by Jesse Ballenger in *Self, Senility, and Alzheimer's Disease*.

53. Jennifer Wolff, "Re-created 1950s City Helps to Ease Dementia's Grasp," December 7, 2018, http://www.aarp.org/health/dementia/info-2018/glenner -town-square.html.

1. Origin Myths

1. Alzheimer, "Concerning a Unique Disease of the Cerebral Cortex," 3.

2. Maurer and Maurer, *Alzheimer*, 164–69.

3. A central paradigm in Alzheimer's historiography is rooted in geriatric and gerontological perspectives on healthy or successful aging. These historians attempt to locate Alzheimer's discovery on a continuum with the historical study of aging and dementia more broadly, thus illustrating the ongoing debate over the diagnostic categories of normal and pathological aging. See, e.g., Torack, "Early History of Senile Dementia"; Gubrium, *Oldtimers and Alzheimer's*; Beach, "History of Alzheimer's"; Berchtold and Cotman, "Evolution in the Conceptualization of Dementia"; Ballenger, *Self, Senility, and Alzheimer's Disease*.

4. Zaven Khachaturian even calls Alzheimer's study approach "the template for the NIA's." Khachaturian, "Diagnosis of Alzheimer's Disease," 410.

5. There is a strong social constructivist perspective that questions how and why Alzheimer's as a disease entity embraces such an ambiguous, diverse, and misunderstood symptomatology. See, e.g., Torack, "Adult Dementia"; Berrios, "Alzheimer's Disease"; Gaines and Whitehouse, "Building a Mystery."

These critics often question its place in nosology or its history within broader classificatory schemes that developed during key moments in the history of scientific professionalization. Because the disease is so overdetermined, its etiology so open, its social life so diffuse, a single eponym strains under the descriptive and referential weight. Therefore historians have struggled to provide some cultural and social context for the discovery narrative that helps make that clear. See, e.g., Holstein, "Alzheimer's Disease"; George et al., "Evolving Classification of Dementia."

6. Perhaps most broadly, historians of science and medicine seek a detailed account of the actors who have informed the disease throughout the past century. These historians generally frame the origin of the disease from a realist standpoint, arguing that better research can provide a better account of the actors' labor. This strategy is often about clarifying and organizing truth. The disease's material nature as something "discoverable" contributes to that realist narrative. See Berrios and Freeman, "Alzheimer and His Time"; Katzman and Bick, *Alzheimer Disease*; Maurer and Maurer, *Alzheimer*; Dahm, "Alois Alzheimer"; Cipriani et al., "Alzheimer and His Disease."

7. Berrios, "Alzheimer's Disease"; Bick et al., *Early Story of Alzheimer's Disease*; Rocca and Amaducci, "Letter to the Editors"; Goedert, "Oskar Fischer and the Study of Dementia."

8. Maurer et al., "Auguste D and Alzheimer's Disease," 1546.

9. Numerous popular writers and journalists also reflect on the Alzheimer's origin myth, often to provide historical context for readers, to question the "truth" of the disease, or to add narratological complexity. See, e.g., Franzen, "My Father's Brain," or Shenk, *The Forgetting*. The origin narrative helps ground Shenk's hypothesis about the unstable status of the Alzheimer's epidemic "as old as humanity that, like nothing else, acquaints us with life's richness by ever so gradually drawing down the curtains. Only through modern science has this poignancy been reduced to a plain horror, an utterly unhuman circumstance" (252). In other words, Shenk argues that Alzheimer's is nothing new; science, technology, and conditions of modernity have simply given new visibility to the disease.

10. Foucault, *Birth of the Clinic*, 146.

11. Among the many historical narratives of Alzheimer's, Martha Holstein and Jesse Ballenger have provided an excellent foundation for the social history of Alzheimer's in the United States. See Holstein, "Aging, Culture, and the Framing of Alzheimer Disease"; Holstein, "Alzheimer's Disease and Senile Dementia"; Ballenger, "Biomedical Deconstruction of Senility."

12. Hagner and Borck, "Mindful Practices," 508.

13. Ellard, "Struggle for Identity," 4.

14. Cartwright, *Screening the Body*, 52.

15. Ellard, "Struggle for Identity," 19.

16. Lanska, "Role of Technology in Neurologic Specialization," 1722.

17. Bonner, *Becoming a Physician*, 251–55. In particular, there was some concern about the replacement of personal patient experience in medical training with large lecture classes.

18. Bonner, 272–73.

19. German proficiency in histology in this time period was driven largely by bacteriology. See Bracegirdle, "History of Histology," 91–92.

20. Roelcke, "Biologizing Social Facts," 387.

21. According to Allen Thiher, Kraepelin believed that good psychiatry recognizes foremost "the 'mental condition' of the patient, by which Kraepelin meant inner experience. Inner experience became the object of medical classification—though with perhaps insufficient reflection on the epistemological conditions that permit definitions of mental conditions." Thiher, *Revels in Madness*, 213. Thiher's latter comment about the limitations of diagnostic categories as an epistemological issue is helpful for this study because it demonstrates the tenuous status of nosological practice in early German psychiatry. This problem becomes even more evident when confronting the fact that the nosological categories largely predated the empirical research that described those categories. Roelcke, "Biologizing," 386–88. Kraepelin was a realist in that he wanted to detect natural disease categories rather than constructing them. This philosophy left him entirely open to critique, given the lack of empirical proof in his research.

22. Star, *Regions of the Mind*, 73–76.

23. Rosen, *Madness in Society*, 282; Jablensky, "Living in a Kraepelinian World."

24. Pickstone, *Ways of Knowing*, 211.

25. Berchtold and Cotman point out, "The tendency to emphasize Kraepelin's involvement in the 'politics of science' undermines his involvement as a basic scientist." Berchtold and Cotman, "Evolution in the Conceptualization of Dementia," 181. That separation is untenable.

26. Maurer and Maurer, *Alzheimer*, 107, 109, 129, 133.

27. Maurer and Maurer, 111–12.

28. Ann La Berge has argued that journalists helped legitimate microscopy not only as a tool for scientific inquiry but also in its very relationship to truth making. In La Berge, "Debate as Scientific Practice."

29. Kraepelin and his colleagues practiced a theatrical pedagogy in a teaching amphitheater, resulting in a somewhat dramatic, visually oriented description of mental illness. See Thiher, *Revels in Madness*, 231.

30. Richter, "Brain Commission of the International Association of Academies," 446.

31. Germany's involvement in this cooperative effort was complex, especially because of the overlap of neurology and psychiatry in the German approach to mind. Even within Germany, competing scientific approaches to the brain, neuronal theory, and localization severely affected the manner and scope of that cooperation. See Hagner, "Cultivating," 2001.

32. Maurer and Maurer, *Alzheimer*, 130–32.

33. Maurer and Maurer, 130.

34. Kaplan and Henderson, *Solomon Carter Fuller*, 37.

35. Engstrom, "Researching Dementia in Imperial Germany."

36. Dahm, "Alois Alzheimer," 14.

37. Richter, "Brain Commission of the International Association of Academies"; Hagner, "Cultivating."

38. Kraepelin, "Loss of Three German Investigators," 93.

39. Maurer and Maurer, *Alzheimer*, 60.

40. Indeed, in his 1904 review of Alzheimer's Habiltationsschrift, Kraepelin commended, "His attempt to place diverse anatomic images beside the finer clinical differences of individual disease processes distinguished by him, practically for the first time, makes it possible for psychiatry to appear to be equal to other fields of medicine in its mode of research and its results." Reproduced and translated in Maurer and Maurer, 116.

41. Hammond, *Camera Lucida*, 81.

42. Maurer and Maurer, *Alzheimer*, 85.

43. Hammond, *Camera Lucida*, 155.

44. Berrios and Freeman, "Alzheimer and His Time," 7.

45. The integration of Abbe's theoretical microscopy with Zeiss's manufacturing prowess led to widespread international popularity and the translation of the microscopic technique from "artisanal craft to scientific practice." Feffer, "Ernst Abbe," 23.

46. Not all histological training required dead humans; most histological training relied on dead animals. See Anderson, "Facing Animals in the Laboratory."

47. Clark et al., *History of Staining*, 142–45.

48. Castellani et al., "Microscopic Investigations," 172.

49. Daston and Galison, *Objectivity*, 121.

50. Daston and Galison, 324–29.

51. Castellani et al., "Microscopic Investigations," 172.

52. De Juan and Pérez-Cañaveras, "How We Teach," 788.

53. Engstrom, "Researching Dementia in Imperial Germany," 410–11.

54. Maurer and Maurer, *Alzheimer*, 18, photo 21.

55. This same argument could be made for a successive case study by Alzheimer on "Johann F." See Graeber and Mehraein, "Reanalysis of the First Case of Alzheimer's Disease," III/11.

56. Stengers, *Invention of Modern Science*, 24–25.

57. Alzheimer, "Concerning a Unique Disease of the Cerebral Cortex," 3.

58. An antagonist to Kraepelin's method, Alfred Hoche, would use these words to describe his techniques. Quoted in Berrios et al., "Schizophrenia," 132.

59. Foucault, *Birth of the Clinic*, 14.

60. Jelliffe, "Obituaries: Alois Alzheimer," 475–77.

61. Kaplan and Henderson, *Solomon Carter Fuller*, 56.

62. Westborough Massachusetts State Hospital, *Annual Report of the Trustees of the Westborough State Hospital* (1911), 21, https://archive.org/stream/annual reportoftr2027mass.

63. Fuller, "Photomicrographs for Illustrating Histological Objects."

64. For more on the history of photomicrography, see Wayne, "Photomicrography"; Normand Overney and Gregor Overney, "The History of Photomicrography," 2011, http://www.microscopy-uk.org.uk/mag/artmar10/go-no -history-photomicro.html. Many authors erroneously claim that Fuller invented the photomicrograph; see, e.g., a 2010 NIH consensus paper on Alzheimer's disease: Daviglus et al., "National Institutes of Health State-of-the-Science Conference Statement."

65. Like Alzheimer, Fuller believed the camera lucida and the photomicrograph were each valuable in its own right but that the former was an excellent pedagogical tool. Fuller, "Photomicrographs," 81, 84.

66. Fuller, "A Study of the Miliary Plaques Found in Brains of the Aged," 156.

67. Fuller and Klopp, "Further Observations on Alzheimer's Disease," 26.

68. Multiple American authors contributed to the debate at the time via recourse to microscopic and macroscopic evaluation—with or without acknowledgment of Alzheimer's contribution. See, e.g., Russell, "Senility and Senile Dementia"; Pickett, "Senile Dementia"; Southard, "Anatomical Findings in Senile Dementia"; Southard and Mitchell, "Clinical and Anatomical Analysis of 23 Cases of Insanity"; McGaffin, "An Anatomical Analysis of Seventy Cases of Senile Dementia"; Barrett, "A Case of Alzheimer's Disease with Unusual Neurological Disturbances"; Hoch, "Dementia of Cerebral Aterio-Sclerosis"; Alford, "An Analysis of Fourteen Cases of Senile Dementia."

69. In particular, Alzheimer provided more details on Auguste D. and a further case study of Johann F. in 1911. See Graeber et al., "Rediscovery of the Case Described by Alois Alzheimer in 1911."

70. Southard and Mitchell, "Clinical and Anatomical Analysis of 23 Cases of Insanity"; Alford, "An Analysis of Fourteen Cases of Senile Dementia."

71. McGaffin, "An Anatomical Analysis of Seventy Cases of Senile Dementia," 649.

72. Bracegirdle, *A History of Microscopical Technique*, 76.

73. New England Society of Psychiatry, "Proceedings."

74. Meyer, "Henry A. Cotton."

75. In particular, Cotton translated Alzheimer's "The Present Status of Our Knowledge of the Pathological Histology of the Cortex in the Psychoses."

76. Bracegirdle, *A History of Microscopical Technique*, 333–35.

77. Schickore, *The Microscope and the Eye*, 250.

78. Fuller, "Study of the Neurofibrils in Dementia Paralytica," 425.

79. Fuller, 461.

80. Langdon, "Biological Aspects of Dementia Praecox," 681. Daston and Galison have argued that an appreciation for the "doctrine of science as endless work" and the attribution of genius to that doctrine are in fact germane to narratives of scientific labor in the second half of the nineteenth century. This is, perhaps, a part of that legacy. See Daston and Galison, *Objectivity*, 228–30.

81. Burnham, *How the Idea of Profession Changed the Writing of Medical History*, 22, 41–43.

82. As Alder Blumer argued in his 1906 lecture to the American Medico-Society, "the history of the term 'dementia' epitomizes that of psychiatry itself." See Blumer, "History of Use of the Term 'Dementia,'" 337.

83. Ludmerer, *Time to Heal*.

84. Flexner, *Medical Education in the United States and Canada*, 53.

85. Critics of this science-oriented medicine saw it as a revival of a dangerous rationalism with no clear benefit. These opponents saw in the laboratory the "potential for the remystification of medical knowledge," the kinds of mysticism that positivist science had fought so hard to overcome. See Warner, "Fall and Rise of a Professional Mystery," 131.

86. Warner, 140–41.

87. Holtzmann-Kevles, *Naked to the Bone*, 22.

88. Cartwright, *Screening the Body*.

89. Fox and Lawrence, *Photographing Medicine*, 41–54.

90. David Serlin argues, "The visual culture of public health . . . arguably represents the confluence of two mutually dependent innovations: the emergence of modern medicine's reliance on sophisticated media to represent diagnosis and treatment, and the emergence of modern communication's reliance on sophisticated media to fulfill particular institutional or ideological goals." Serlin, *Imagining Illness*, xxii.

91. Brown, *Health and Medicine on Display*, 4, 9.

92. Brown, 175–77.

93. Lears, "From Salvation to Self-Realization."

94. Tomes, "Merchants of Health."

95. The historically precise scientific profession, then, that these histological practices help shape is a way of thinking about Alzheimer's without recourse to the description of a definitive subjugation of people with mental illness. Social

scientific hermeneutics of disease might unwittingly participate in that sub-jugation by showing how doctors "map" themselves, their fears, and their gen-eral dominance onto the patients, in a sense "creating" their illnesses through history. I have tried to resist describing large groups of medicalized peoples historically by virtue of reductive models. This chapter's approach does not definitively separate scientific practice from social practice because it only con-ceives of those categories as separated discursively or ideologically. This model asserts the primacy of cognitive ability as a form of visually oriented population management whereby medical seers are not inherently othered from medi-cally seen. This does not undermine the critique of practices of subjugation that have been so well articulated by other historians of science and medicine. Certainly it does not do so with regard to the history of Alzheimer's.

96. As I have argued in the introduction to this book, selfhood is a primary mode of engagement across the humanities and social scientific treatments of Alzheimer's, especially as perceptions of interiority concern personhood. Journalists and historians are fond of pointing out Auguste D.'s clinical state-ment, recorded in Alzheimer's notebooks: "I have lost myself." But what is the relationship between the self of Alzheimer's and the scientific self? Alois Alz-heimer represents more than one "scientific self"; he represents an approach to turn-of-the-century mental performance more broadly. To properly under-stand the historical emergence of mediated personhood and Alzheimer's, one must understand the presumed crisis of selfhood not only via recourse to the experience of the person with the disease but also as a crisis of the scien-tific self that defines, orients, and manages that disease. These visual practices might best be understood as contributive to what Peter Galison and Lorraine Daston call the "scientific self." Drawing on Foucault, the authors argue that after the 1850s, European and American scientists became keenly aware of their own fallibility as investigators. They saw their own subjective nature less as a simple boon to science and more of something to be contained, avoided, or accommodated. But the subjectivity these scientists feared was, in part, I argue, redefined by the objects of their inquiry and their practices of looking. These turn-of-the-century psychiatrists were engaged in widespread practices of classification and institutionalization that engaged in the practice of com-prehending the "scientific self" just as they engaged in practices of organizing the "Alzheimer's self." See Daston and Galison, *Objectivity*, 43–44.

97. See, e.g., Achenbaum, *Crossing Frontiers*, 21–51; Cohen, "Historical Views and Evolution of Concepts"; Katz, *Disciplining Old Age*; Holstein, "Alzheimer's"; Ballenger, *Self, Senility, and Alzheimer's Disease*.

98. Cole, *Journey of Life*, 168.

99. Beard, "On the Decline of the Moral Faculties in Old Age," https://col lections.nlm.nih.gov/bookviewer?PID=nlm:nlmuid-101162285-bk.

100. Beard, *Legal Responsibility in Old Age.*

101. Ballenger, "Biomedical Deconstruction of Senility," 107–9.

102. Beard, *Legal Responsibility in Old Age,* 10.

103. Castellani et al., "Microscopic Investigations," 171.

104. This origin myth and its visual focus are hereby rendered a "proposition," as Bruno Latour would have it, rather than a relative truth. See Harman, *Prince of Networks,* 82–84. As proposition, the origin myth is important not simply because it demonstrates the paradigmatic concerns of a group of scientists that first described Alzheimer's but because it holds a special factish power as both the history and organizing narrative of the disease and notions of truth, visuality, and the brain. Factishes, according to Latour, are neither fact nor fetish; rather, they are both. Factishes exist everywhere there is belief. Their status as both does not distract from their status as one or the other. Factishes are neither a fact that needs no defense nor a fetish that simply acts out the social context of their comprehension. They are both those things, and thus more, dependent on and relative to their position on a network of use and practice. See Latour, *On the Modern Cult of Factish Gods,* 21–22. Treating the plaques and tangles as factishes in this sense allows for a different mode of critique. This methodology seems to pay more respect to the experience of Alzheimer's in all of its contradictions.

105. Berchtold and Cotman, "Evolution in the Conceptualization of Dementia," 182.

106. Huber and Kutschenko, "Medicine in a Neurocentric World."

2. New Media Pioneers

1. Ballenger, *Self, Senility, and Alzheimer's Disease,* 37–38, 197.

2. Lang, "Annual Report of the Trustees of the Westborough State Hospital," 9.

3. In 1916 his position title changed from pathologist to pathologist and director of clinical psychiatry, but this seems to echo a general shift in hospital practice rather than a promotion.

4. See, e.g., Canavan, "A Histological Study." For a related, full-color drawing of the optic nerve of a person with senile dementia, see box 2, folder 8 of the Myrtelle Canavan Papers, Boston Medical Library in the Francis A. Countway Library of Medicine.

5. Box 1, folder 3 of the Myrtelle Canavan Papers.

6. For more on Southard and the relationship between eugenics and psychoanalysis, see Dowbiggin, *Keeping America Sane,* 110–14.

7. Ferraro, "Origin and Formation of Senile Plaques"; Hiroisi and Lee, "Origin of Senile Plaques"; Soniat, "Histogenesis of Senile Plaques."

8. Berrios, "Alzheimer's Disease," 356. For a more comprehensive review, see Ballenger, "Beyond the Characteristic Plaques and Tangles."

9. Terry, "Alzheimer's Disease at Mid-century," 49.

10. Ferraro, "Recent Advances," 268; Margolis, "Senile Cerebral Disease."

11. Boller, "History of Dementia," 11.

12. Neumann and Cohn, "Incidence of Alzheimer's Disease"; Bodian, "A New Method for Staining Nerve Fibers."

13. Riva et al., "Histochemistry," 85.

14. Conn, *Biological Stains*, 11–12.

15. McMenemey, "A Critical Review," 75–76.

16. Greenfield, *Neuropathology*, 484–97; Jervis, "Alzheimer's Disease"; Ferraro and Jervis, "Alzheimer's Disease"; Rothschild, "Alzheimer's Disease"; Newton, "Identity of Alzheimer's Disease"; English, "Alzheimer's Disease"; Ferraro, "Recent Advances"; McMenemey, "A Critical Review."

17. English, "Alzheimer's Disease"; Neumann and Cohn, "Incidence of Alzheimer's Disease"; Malzberg, "Increase of Mental Disease"; Malzberg, "Frequency of Mental Disease"; Malamud and Lowenberg, "Alzheimer's Disease."

18. This was first described in Europe by von Braunmuhl in 1932, but several other case studies were published in that decade. McMenemey et al., "Familial Presenile Dementia."

19. Roth and Morrissey, "Problems in the Diagnosis and Classification of Mental Disorder."

20. Rothschild, "Pathologic Changes in Senile Psychoses"; Rothschild and Sharp, "Origin of Senile Psychoses."

21. See, e.g., Alexander, "Senile Dementia"; Corsellis, *Mental Illness and the Ageing Brain*; Tomlinson et al., "Observations on the Brains of Demented Old People"; Tomlinson et al., "Observations on the Brains of Non-demented Old People."

22. Titford, "A Short History of Histopathology Technique," 107.

23. Terry, "Fine Structure of Neurofibrillary Tangles"; Terry et al., "Ultrastructural Studies"; Kidd, "Paired Helical Filaments"; Kidd, "Alzheimer's Disease." As early as 1959, Alan Cohen and Evan Calkins had shown that amyloid, previously understood to be amorphous, was in fact composed of small fibrils. See Cohen and Calkins, "Electron Microscopic Observations."

24. See Lukiw for this quote in "Alzheimer's Disease," 12. For a good review of important research through the 1980s, see Ulrich, "Histochemistry and Immunohistochemistry of Alzheimer's Disease." A sample of some of the research with the EM includes Suzuki et al., "Chemical Studies on Alzheimer's Disease"; Krigman et al., "Alzheimer's Presenile Dementia"; Shirahama and Cohen, "High-Resolution Electron Microscopic Analysis"; Terry and Peña, "Experimental Production of Neurofibrillary Degeneration"; Miyakawa and Uehara, "Observations of Amyloid Angiopathy"; Miyakawa et al., "Ultrastructure of Capillary Plaque-Like Degeneration"; Wisniewski and Terry,

"Reexamination of the Pathogenesis of the Senile Plaque"; and Wisniewski et al., "Neurofibrillary Pathology."

25. Hirano et al., "Fine Structure of Some Intraganglionic Alterations"; Gibson and Tomlinson, "Numbers of Hirano Bodies."

26. Jardine, *Scenes of Inquiry.*

27. Rasmussen, *Picture Control,* 232–34.

28. Rasmussen, 224.

29. Terry, "Alzheimer's Disease at Mid-century," 59.

30. Robert Terry, interviewed in Katzman and Bick, *Alzheimer Disease,* 23.

31. Margolis describes some of the shift to histochemical research in Alzheimer's in "Senile Cerebral Disease."

32. Hawes et al., "Immunohistochemistry."

33. http://www.moma.org/calendar/exhibitions/2599.

34. See, e.g., Klatzo et al., "Experimental Production"; Woodard, "Alzheimer's Disease in Late Adult Life"; Friede and Magee, "Alzheimer's Disease."

35. Muller and Ciompi, *Senile Dementia.*

36. Khachaturian, "Diagnosis of Alzheimer's Disease," 410.

37. Kay et al., "Old Age Mental Disorders"; Roth et al., "Correlation between Scores for Dementia and Counts of 'Senile Plaques'"; Blessed et al., "Association between Quantitative Measures of Dementia and of Senile Change." See also an interview with Roth in Katzman and Bick, *Alzheimer Disease,* 55–64.

38. Wilson, "Quantifying the Quiet Epidemic."

39. The Newcastle research was corroborated by U.S. researchers doing similar clinically based light microscopy plaque counts. See Farmer et al., "Correlations among Numbers of Neuritic Plaques."

40. For a good early review of these correlative efforts, see Mountjoy, "Number of Plaques and Tangles."

41. Katzman, "Prevalence and Malignancy of Alzheimer Disease." For more on the rise of the Alzheimer's disease movement, see Fox, "From Senility to Alzheimer's Disease," 71–74.

42. Fox, "From Senility to Alzheimer's Disease."

43. Katzman et al., *Alzheimer's Disease,* 265–71, 579.

44. Katzman and Bick, *Alzheimer Disease,* 285–87.

45. Butler, "Is the National Institute on Aging Mission Out of Balance?" 389.

46. Ballenger, *Self, Senility, and Alzheimer's Disease,* 117–18.

47. Ballenger.

48. Chaufan at al., "Medical Ideology as a Double-Edged Sword," 791–92; Lock, *Alzheimer Conundrum,* 41.

49. Fox, "From Senility to Alzheimer's Disease," 89–90.

50. Joint Congressional Subcommittee Hearing, "Impact of Alzheimer's Disease on Nation's Elderly," 1980, https://www.google.com/books/edition/Impact_of_Alzheimer_s_Disease_on_the_Nat/7dbRAAAAMAAJ.

51. Alzheimer's Disease Center et al., *Alzheimer's Disease Q&A,* https://www.google.com/books/edition/Impact_of_Alzheimer_s_Disease_on_the_Nat/UPydVdkF9KIC. Italics in original.

52. Fox, "From Senility to Alzheimer's Disease," 86–87.

53. Van Buren, "Advice to You."

54. Wollin, "Dear Abby."

55. Hendrickson, "A Life Going Mad"; Lerner, *When Illness Goes Public,* 159–79.

56. For more on celebrity and Alzheimer's, see Selberg, "Rhinestone Cowboy."

57. Pear, "How a Single Disease Has Become a Political Cause."

58. Daly, "Reagan Took Up Cause for Mom."

59. Joint Resolution Designating November 1983 as "National Alzheimer's Disease Month," Public Law 98-102 (1983). See https://www.whitehouse.gov/the-press-office/presidential-proclamation-national-alzheimers-disease-awareness-month.

60. Committee on Appropriations, "Hearings," 516. Mace wrote *The 36 Hour Day* in 1981 with Peter Rabins, and it is widely considered one of the most influential care guides ever written, with more than two million copies sold. Johns Hopkins University Press credits it with launching its Consumer Health series. See Birch, "Archives—Thirty Years of 'The 36-Hour Day,'" http://www.hopkinsmedicine.org/news/publications/hopkins_medicine_magazine/archives/winter_2012/thirty_years_of_the_36_hour_day.

61. Committee on Appropriations, "Hearings," 615, 620.

62. Committee on Appropriations, 528–31.

63. Alzheimer's Disease and Related Dementias Services Research Act of 1986, Public Law 99-660 (1986).

64. Boffey, "Alzheimer's Disease."

65. McKhann et al., "Clinical Diagnosis of Alzheimer's Disease," 939.

66. Taylor, "CAT Scans Said to Show Shrunken Hinckley Brain."

67. Kiernan, "Hinckley, Jury Watch 'Taxi Driver' Film."

68. Associated Press, "Hinckley Acquittal Brings Moves to Change Insanity Defense."

69. Rovner, "Scientists Can Explain What Happens to the Brain."

70. Khachaturian, "Diagnosis of Alzheimer's Disease," 412.

71. Grundke-Iqbal, "Microtubule-Associated Protein Tau."

72. Hardy, "A Hundred Years of Alzheimer's Disease Research."

73. Hagner and Borck, "Mindful Practices."

74. This might be understood as a form of "necropolitical" governance in that the person with dementia was most useful to a nation when dead. Histological inquiry was not, perhaps, an explicit exercise in sovereign power. But at this point in time, nationally organized medical research recognized the value of the person with dementia in her death; that is, visual labor serviced a public's health rather than the patient's life. According to Achille Mbembe, for a modern subject to become a subject, he must confront death: "politics is therefore death that lives a human life." Mbembe, "Necropolitics," 14–15.

75. Fuller, "Study of the Neurofibrils in Dementia Paralytica," 459–60.

76. Ballenger, *Self, Senility, and Alzheimer's Disease*, 37.

77. Katzman and Bick, *Alzheimer Disease*, 22.

78. Davidoff and Epstein, *Abnormal Pneumoencephalogram*, 25, 414–16.

79. Menninger, "Encephalography in Alzheimer's Disease"; Romano and Miller, "Clinical and Pneumo-encephalographic Studies"; English, "Alzheimer's Disease," 586; Pacella and Barrera, "Electroencephalography."

80. Wagner, "A Brief History."

81. Huckman et al., "Validity of Criteria"; Albert et al., "CT Density Numbers"; Naeser et al., "Decreased Computerized Tomography Numbers"; Wilson et al., "Computed Tomography in Dementia."

82. Jacobs et al., "Computerized Tomography in Dementia."

83. Katzman et al., *Alzheimer's Disease*, 585.

84. Fleisher et al. "Applications of Neuroimaging," 130.

85. Killiany, "Glimpses of the Living Brain," 512, 515.

86. Littlefield et al., "Functional Brain Imaging," 154.

87. Jagust and D'Esposito, *Imaging the Aging Brain*, 15.

88. Nutt et al., "In Vivo Molecular Imaging Biomarkers."

89. Cohen and Klunk, "Early Detection of Alzheimer's Disease"; Mosconi et al., "Pre-clinical Detection."

90. One of the drawbacks with PiB was that it has a radioactive half-life of only twenty minutes, whereas a compound like florbetapir has almost a two-hour half-life. This is an active area of research. See Yeo et al., "A Systematic Review and Meta-analysis."

91. Talan, "Neuroimaging Tracers."

92. Johnson et al., "Appropriate Use Criteria for Amyloid PET," e9–e10. See also reservations and recommendations for communicating those use criteria with patients in Rabinovici et al., "Testing and Disclosures," and Witte et al., "Clinical Use of Amyloid-Positron Emission Tomography Neuroimaging."

93. Noble and Scarmeas, "Application of PET Imaging to Diagnosis of Alzheimer's Disease," 145. For an overview, see Johnson et al., "Brain Imaging in Alzheimer Disease."

94. Caserta et al., "Normal Brain Aging," 12.

95. Braet and Ratinac, "Creating Next-Generation Microscopists"; Griffiths, "Bringing Electron Microscopy Back into Focus"; Tsien, "Imagining Imaging's Future"; Leapman, "Novel Techniques in Electron Microscopy."

96. Good, "Dementia and Ageing," 166; Fleisher et al., "Applications of Neuroimaging to Disease-Modification Trials."

97. Snyder et al., "Alzheimer's Disease Public–Private Partnerships: Update 2017."

98. This conference took place in 2016. Frontiers Plenary: The White House Frontiers Conference.

99. Foundation for the National Institutes of Health, "Patient Advocacy Groups, Industry and Individuals Join Groundbreaking Public-Private Partnership to Continue Advancing Critical Alzheimer's Disease Research," September 8, 2016, http://www.fnih.org/news/press-releases/critical-alzheimers-disease-research.

100. Weiner and Veitch, "Introduction to Special Issue," 732.

101. Foundation for the National Institutes of Health. See http://adni.loni.usc.edu/news-publications/publications/ and "Data Usage Stats," http://adni.loni.usc.edu/data-samples/adni-data-usage-stats/.

102. Weiner and Veitch, "Overview of Alzheimer's Disease Neuroimaging Initiative," 204. See also Albert, "Detection of Very Early Alzheimer's Disease," s63.

103. http://adni.loni.usc.edu/study-design/background-rationale/. For more on Alzheimer's biomarker development, see Lock, *Alzheimer Conundrum*, 132–55.

104. Markowitz, "There's Such a Thing as Too Much Neuroscience."

105. Weiner et al., "Alzheimer's Disease Neuroimaging Initiative," 209; Mueller et al., "Alzheimer's Disease Neuroimaging Initiative," 870.

106. Alzheimer's Association, "Alzheimer's and Dementia Testing Advances," http://www.alz.org/research/science/earlier_alzheimers_diagnosis.asp.

107. Blendon et al., "Impact of Experience with a Family Member," table 2.

108. Comer, "Renewed Focus."

109. Mueller, "Alzheimer's Disease Neuroimaging Initiative," 871.

110. Belluck and Robbins, "Three F.D.A. Advisers Resign."

111. Jack et al., "Introduction to the Recommendations." A European-based review offered similar reservations in Fletcher et al., "Diagnosing Alzheimer's Disease." See additional pre-ADNI reservations and recommendations for biomarkers in Atkinson et al., "Biomarkers and Surrogate Endpoints," 90.

112. Jones-Davis and Buckholtz, "Impact of ADNI."

113. https://www.whitehouse.gov/BRAIN.

114. For more on U.S. investment into MRI, see Joyce, *Myth of Transparency*, 147.

115. U.S. Department of Health and Human Services, "Obama Adminis-tration Presents National Plan to Fight Alzheimer's Disease," http://www.hhs.gov/news/press/2012pres/05/20120515a.html.

116. Monica Ramirez Basco and Robbie Barbero, "Investing in Research to Help Unlock the Mysteries of the Brain," February 13, 2015, https://www.whitehouse.gov/blog/2015/02/13/investing-research-help-unlock-mysteries-brain.

117. Shen, "Neurotechnology," 26. See also Jonas and Kording, "Could a Neuroscientist Understand a Microprocessor?"

118. Frontiers Plenary, http://www.frontiersconference.org/plenary.

119. It was not surprising that Joe Biden ushered in his 2020 presidential victory with a similar claim about how Alzheimer's fits into a national dream of renewal. He said, "You see, I believe in the possibility of this country. We're always looking ahead, ahead to an America that's freer, more just. Ahead to an America that creates jobs with dignity and respect. Ahead to an America that cures diseases like cancer and Alzheimer's. Ahead to an America that never leaves anyone behind. Ahead to an America that never gives up, never gives in. This is a great nation. And we are a good people. This is the United States of America. And there has never been anything we haven't been able to do when we've done it together." See AP News, "Transcript of President-Elect Joe Biden's Victory Speech."

3. Use It or Lose It

1. BMI Research, "Americas Pharma and Healthcare Insight," 2–3.

2. Because the symptoms of Alzheimer's can vary considerably, a num-ber of drugs not approved to treat Alzheimer's directly are sometimes pre-scribed for what is known as their "off-label" uses. For example, antipsychotic drugs have long been prescribed to treat agitation or aggression in a person with Alzheimer's. They were eventually found to cause an increased risk of death, leading the FDA to create a black box warning for the drugs in 2005. See U.S. Food and Drug Administration, "Postmarket Drug Safety Information for Patients and Providers—Public Health Advisory: Deaths with Antipsychotics in Elderly Patients with Behavioral Disturbances," http://www.fda.gov/drugs/drugsafety/postmarketdrugsafetyinformationforpatientsandproviders/ucm053171. In 2012, Janssen Pharmaceuticals settled a $181 million lawsuit for off-label marketing of their antipsychotic Risperdal in (at the time) the "largest multi-state consumer protection-based pharmaceutical settlement in history." See http://www.ag.ny.gov/press-release/ag-schneiderman-settles-181-million-deceptive-marketing-case-janssen-pharmaceuticals.

3. Cummings et al., "Price of Progress," 331. Compare this to the 19 per-cent success rate of cancer treatments. Cummings et al., "Alzheimer's Disease Drug-Development Pipeline," 2, 6.

4. Elsevier Resource Library, "Alzheimer's Disease Research Insights," 2015, 11, https://www.elsevier.com/research-intelligence/resource-library/alz heimers-disease-research-insights.

5. National Institutes of Health, "Estimates of Funding for Various Research, Condition, and Disease Categories," April 19, 2019, https://report.nih .gov/categorical_spending.aspx.

6. There is some debate. The Marist poll and the Harris Interactive poll reveal Alzheimer's as either the most feared or second most feared, behind cancer.

7. Treichler, *How to Have Theory in an Epidemic*, 315.

8. Alzheimer's Association, "2012 Alzheimer's Disease Facts and Figures Fact Sheet," http://www.alz.org/documents_custom/2012_facts_figures_fact_ sheet.pdf.

9. Governmentality and the "conduct of conduct" were central concerns of much of Foucault's later work. Immediately before his death, he addressed the idea of technologies of the self in more detail. See Foucault, *Technologies of the Self.*

10. With respect to health care, those interests are not always recognizable as official parts of the government. The American health care system is a complicated mixture of private and public providers, regulatory bodies, and insurance, and a kind of neoliberal governmentality operates through all these different actors. The ongoing contentiousness of the Patient Protection and Affordable Care Act, or "Obamacare," is only one recent example of political disagreement over patient rights and responsibilities, but those debates are an American tradition. When we talk about governmentality and health care in this country, then, we need to acknowledge the ways in which the government looks out for the health of its citizens by validating each person's agency but also by outsourcing care and responsibility to a variety of private businesses and organizations. It can be difficult to tell the boundaries of these different private and public actors, and caring for someone with Alzheimer's can involve navigating a dizzying network of choices at different stages of the disease. In fact, the more the federal government gets involved in regulating health care, the more individual patient choice seems to be instrumentalized as part of the system.

11. This process differs from more traditional accounts of risk relationships that orient the disease or the person with it as something entirely "other." Symptoms like memory loss are too rooted in normal behavior, and the social experience is too articulated within familial relationships of aging and love, to be consistently estranged. In contrast, Sander Gilman has argued that the "construction of the image of the patient is thus always a playing out of this desire for a demarcation between ourselves and the chaos represented in culture by disease." Though people living with dementia often encounter a barrage of

harmful stigmas, Gilman's formulation is too simple for Alzheimer's. See Gilman, *Disease and Representation,* 4.

12. Rose, *Politics of Life Itself,* 76.

13. According to Rabinow and Rose, "the concept of biopower seeks to individuate strategies and configurations that combine three dimensions or planes—a form of truth discourse about living beings and an array of authorities considered competent to speak that truth; strategies for intervention upon collective existence in the name of life and health; and modes of subjectification, in which individuals can be brought to work on themselves, under certain forms of authority, in relation to truth discourses, by means of practices of the self, in the name of individual or collective life or health." Rabinow and Rose, "Biopower Today," 203–4.

14. Clarke et al., "Biomedicalization."

15. This kind of discourse fits into what Allen Feldman calls the actuarial gaze: "a visual organization and institutionalization of threat perception and prophylaxis, which crosscuts politics, public health, public safety, policing, urban planning and media practice." See Feldman, "On the Actuarial Gaze," 206.

16. David Shenk, "A Quick Look at Alzheimer's," http://aboutalz.org/. Watch the Pocket Film at http://aboutalz.org/#.

17. Åsberg and Lum, "Picturizing the Scattered Ontologies of Alzheimer's Disease," 114.

18. Alzheimer's Foundation of America, "The Value of Lifestyle Choices for Your Body and Your Brain," 2014, https://www.alzprevention.org/.

19. Dumit, "Pharmaceutical Witnessing," 40.

20. Peterson and Martin, "Tracing the Origins of Success."

21. See Clarke et al. on technoscientific identities in "Biomedicalization," 182.

22. *Dr. Oz Show,* "What's Your Risk for Alzheimer's, Pt. 1," 2011, http://www.doctoroz.com/videos/whats-your-risk-alzheimers-pt-1. His website later posted a five-step plan to combat Alzheimer's in 2012, claiming, "Almost everyone has experienced the life-altering impact of Alzheimer's, either through friends or family. You have the power to help change your and your loved ones' fates by sharing how to stop forgetfulness in its tracks and literally grow your brain so it's stronger than ever."

23. Lest readers underestimate Dr. Oz's influence as a medical authority in the United States, note his May 2012 appearance on the syndicated TV quiz show *Jeopardy* for their celebrity "Power Players Week." According to then host Alex Trebek, a power player is "a man or a woman who through his or her writings or comments in the media are able to influence the way the rest of us feel or think about events in the news." During his mid-show interview, Dr. Oz

said, "We gotta keep up with the science . . . if you can make the right choices, you can control 70% of how you age, that's a lot of power."

24. https://allofus.nih.gov/.

25. Facher, "To Advance Precision Medicine."

26. "Sync for Science," https://www.healthit.gov/topic/sync-science; "Sync for Genes," https://www.healthit.gov/topic/sync-genes.

27. Taylor, "Alzheimer's from the Inside Out."

28. According to the Alzheimer's Association, "just one in seven seniors (16 percent) receives regular cognitive assessments for problems with memory or thinking during routine health checkups, which stands in sharp contrast to regular screening or preventive services for other health factors: blood pressure (91 percent); cholesterol (83 percent), vaccinations (80 percent), hearing or vision (73 percent), diabetes (66 percent) and cancer (61 percent)." See Alzheimer's Association, "2019 Alzheimer's Disease Facts and Figures," 87.

29. Pendlebury, "A 7 Minute Neurocognitive Screening Battery."

30. Nasreddine et al., "Montreal Cognitive Assessment."

31. The Late Show with Stephen Colbert, "Person, Woman, Man, Camera, TV: The Movie," YouTube video, 1:41, July 24, 2020, https://www.youtube.com/watch?v=LhZyHIZpzoM.

32. Parker and Wan, "Trump Keeps Boasting about Passing a Cognitive Test."

33. Lin et al., *Screening for Cognitive Impairment in Older Adults*. See also Langa and Levine, "Diagnosis and Management of Mild Cognitive Impairment."

34. Lock et al., "Genetic Susceptibility and Alzheimer's Disease," 147–48. See also Lock, "Testing for Susceptibility Genes."

35. Cook-Deegan, "Genetics of Alzheimer's Disease."

36. Belluck, "Alzheimer's Stalks a Colombian Family."

37. Fischman, "Alzheimer's Today."

38. Clarke, "Case of the Missing Person."

39. Alzheimer's prevention books are a genre: Carper, *100 Simple Things You Can Do to Prevent Alzheimer's*; Fortanasce, *Anti-Alzheimer's Prescription*; Doraiswamy and Gwyther, *Alzheimer's Action Plan*; Shankle and Amen, *Preventing Alzheimer's*. See also four books by Small and Vorgan: *Memory Bible*; *Memory Prescription*; *Longevity Bible*; and *Alzheimer's Prevention Program*. Prevention tips also come from cognitivevitality.org, *The Doctors* (see http://www.thedoctorstv.com/videos/tips-to-help-defeat-dementia), and *The Dr. Oz Show* (see http://www.doctoroz.com/videos/5-step-alzheimers-prevention-plan).

40. National Institutes of Health, "Independent Panel Finds Insufficient Evidence to Support Preventive Measures for Alzheimer's Disease," April 28, 2010, https://www.nih.gov/news-events/news-releases/independent-panel-finds-insufficient-evidence-support-preventive-measures-alzheimers-disease.

41. National Institute on Aging, "Preventing Alzheimer's Disease: What Do We Know?" https://www.nia.nih.gov/health/preventing-alzheimers-disease -what-do-we-know. See also Tenndstedt and Unverzagt,, "The ACTIVE Study."

42. Jennifer Khan, "An Alzheimer's Researcher Reveals: The Best Ways to Ward Off Dementia," http://www.oprah.com/health/How-to-Ward-Off-De mentia-Alzheimers-Prevention-Program.

43. ADDF, "Who We Are," http://www.alzdiscovery.org/cognitive-vitality/ who-we-are.

44. *Dr. Oz Show,* "What's Your Risk for Alzheimer's, Pt. 1," 2011, http:// www.doctoroz.com/videos/whats-your-risk-alzheimers-pt-1.

45. A sustained optimism, as Lauren Berlant has argued, can be quite cruel. In her book *Cruel Optimism,* Berlant argues that people often live their lives in relationships with unattainable futures; they are unattainable because certain fantasies of the good life can actually prevent the good life from happening. This ethic is true of all sorts of fantasies of self-improvement.

46. Post Typography, "How to Live Longer Better."

47. Institute of Medicine, "Preventing Cognitive Decline and Dementia: A Way Forward," http://nationalacademies.org/hmd/Reports/2017/preventing -cognitive-decline-and-dementia-a-way-forward.aspx.

48. Brain training is only one component of a strong consumer culture around Alzheimer's. The Alzheimer's Association even runs an online store that sells products specifically for people with Alzheimer's and their caregivers: http://www.alzstore.com/.

49. For current claims, see http://ww.lumosity.com/.

50. Simons et al., "Do 'Brain-Training' Programs Work?"; Kable et al., "No Effect of Commercial Cognitive Training."

51. Stanford Center on Longevity, "A Consensus on the Brain Training Industry from the Scientific Community," October 20, 2014. http://longevity3 .stanford.edu/blog/2014/10/15/the-consensus-on-the-brain-training-industry -from-the-scientific-community/.

52. "Cognitive Training Data Response Letter," December 9, 2014, http:// www.cognitivetrainingdata.org/the-controversy-does-brain-training-work/ response-letter/cognitive-training-data-signatories/.

53. See https://www.lumosity.com/hcp.

54. Gamification contributes to emergent practices of self-surveillance con- stitutive of the quantified self and self-improvement. See Whitson, "Foucault's Fitbit."

55. Walz and Deterding, *Gameful World,* 9.

56. Federal Trade Commission, "Lumosity to Pay $2 Million to Settle FTC Deceptive Advertising Charges for Its 'Brain Training' Program," January 5, 2016, https://www.ftc.gov/news-events/press-releases/2016/01/lumosity-pay -2-million-settle-ftc-deceptive-advertising-charges.

57. Stern, "Cognitive Reserve in Ageing and Alzheimer's Disease"; Xu et al., "Cognitive Reserve and Alzheimer's Disease."

58. LeDoux, *Synaptic Self,* 323–24.

59. Postan, "Defining Ourselves," 133.

60. The haphazard, popular, and political diagnosis of public figures is another example of this kind of stigma. After Reagan, Alzheimer's became something of a partisan tool for undermining and shaming your opponent. For example, in the 2020 election, both Biden and Trump were widely accused and suspected of having Alzheimer's (often based on verbal "gaffes"). Dementia stigma was used as a part of meme warfare, and neither side was immune.

61. Nikolas Rose argues that contemporary life is underwritten by a mode of affirmative and optimistic living he calls "ethopolitics . . . self-techniques by which human beings should judge and act upon themselves to make themselves better than they are." The "etho" in this concept is a way of accommodating risk, of living in a responsible relationship to the future. Empathy games are another aspect of that ethical living. Rose, *Politics of Life Itself,* 27.

62. *The Doctors,* "Alzheimer's Disease Health Scare Experiment Reactions," http://www.thedoctorstv.com/videos/alzheimer-s-disease-health-scare-experi ment-reactions.

63. As Dr. Travis made clear in an interview, "the key to our show is that we all have health in common." See O'Hare, "Dr. Travis Stork Reflects on Hitting 1,000 Episodes."

64. Second Wind Dreams, "Virtual Dementia Tour," http://www.second wind.org/virtual-dementia-tour/.

65. Katz, "Virtual Dementia Tour."

66. Katz.

67. Second Wind Dreams, "VDT Return on Investment," https://www.sec ondwind.org/vdtreg-comprehensive-edition.html.

68. The app's creators told me they were trying to find a way to promote this in the United States. See Alzheimer's Research UK, "A Walk through Dementia," http://www.awalkthroughdementia.org/. A company in Australia has also won awards for its virtual empathy experience. See Alzheimer's Australia, "Virtual Dementia Experience Wins International Award for Education and Technology," December 2, 2014, https://vic.fightdementia.org.au/vic/about-us/ media/media-releases/virtual-dementia-experience-wins-international-award -for-education-and-technology.

69. Wasserman, "A Facebook Campaign Simulated Alzheimer's."

70. See also a game by Alexander Tarvet, "Forget-Me-Knot: Gameplay," You-Tube video, 9:36, October 22, 2015. https://www.youtube.com/watch?v=1r3x eIJD-gw.

71. Thomsen, "Ether One."

72. Emily Matchar, "Using Virtual Reality to Walk in the Shoes of Someone with Alzheimer's," http://www.smithsonianmag.com/innovation/using-virtual-reality-walk-shoes-someone-with-alzheimers-180959329/.

4. PET Scans and Polaroids

1. Gubrium and Holstein, "Everyday Visibility of the Aging Body," 224.

2. Featherstone and Wernick, *Images of Aging*.

3. There are, of course, many examples of photographers who try to communicate a more complex account of Alzheimer's and related dementias. The Bob and Diane Fund, for example, offers a yearly cash award to photography that tells "intimate stories of loss, as well as those that point out the urgency of a growing medical crisis for Alzheimer's and/or dementia." Some of those winners conform to popular stereotypes, and others do not. One well worth investigating is the British photographer Paul John Bayfield and his series Keeping Mum. See http://www.bobanddianefund.org/2020-mentorship-grantee.

4. Kitwood, *Dementia Reconsidered*, 7.

5. This is a part of a broader history of wide eyes in visual representations of mental illness. There is also productive research to be done around the question of how the eyes of Alzheimer's relate to other representations of wide eyes in popular culture—fearful eyes in horror movies, for example.

6. Metaphors of seeing and blindness are frequently used as contrasting illustrations of the experiences of people with dementia and their caregivers. For example, this is just a small sample of eye discourse taken from the PBS film *The Forgetting*: "Something I read in the book . . . I'm not dying, I'm just disappearing before your eyes" (patient). "You see that blank look. That's the worst" (caregiver). "It would be like walking into a fog, and not knowing what's there" (patient). "When I'm with her I'm just glad to see her. I just want to see your eyes Mom" (caregiver). An interesting side note to these trends is the way Alzheimer's patients occasionally experience heightened visual acuity as a side effect of their cognitive impairments. As one patient describes his experience with heightened vision, "in a dark time, the eye begins to see." Shenk, *The Forgetting*, 193. This, in turn, leans ironically against the discourse of blindness that is often used to describe the cognitive impairment that accompanies the disease. Even more complicating, many recent studies argue that visual impairment is a symptom of Alzheimer's, and some even suggest that visual tests should be used as a form of screening and tracking the disease. Kirby et al., "Visual Impairment in Alzheimer's Disease," 15.

7. Much of the literature on representations of Alzheimer's addresses stereotypes, selfhood, fear, and symptoms. See Ballenger, *Self, Senility, and Alzheimer's Disease*; Basting, *Forget Memory*; Swinnen, "Dementia in Documentary Film"; and Swinnen, "Ageing in Film," 71–72; Kirkman, "Dementia

in the News"; Kang et al., "Coverage of Alzheimer's Disease"; Van Gorp and Vercruysse, "Frames and Counter-frames"; Cohen-Shalev and Marcus; "An Insider's View of Alzheimer's"; Segers, "Degenerative Dementias"; Wearing, "Dementia and the Biopolitics of the Biopic"; Chivers, *Silvering Screen*, 58–74; and Peel, "Living Death of Alzheimer's." Swinnen and Schweda offer a more comparative perspective in their collection *Popularizing Dementia*.

8. Racine et al., "Contemporary Neuroscience in the Media," 73.

9. As Marita Sturken describes, "popular medical discourse affords viruses all kinds of intentionality, depicting them as 'agents' who change." In Sturken, *Tangled Memories*, 245.

10. *Dr. Oz Show,* "Disease Detectives," 2012, http://www.doctoroz.com/vid eos/dr-oz-s-disease-detectives-pt-4.

11. Margaret Lock deals with this thoroughly in *Alzheimer Conundrum,* but see also Whitehouse and George, *Myth of Alzheimer's.*

12. Beck, "Appeal of the Brain in the Popular Press."

13. Eedgerly, "Oxygen Therapy for Alzheimer's?"

14. Dumit, *Picturing Personhood,* 16, 139.

15. Van Dijck, *Transparent Body,* 6.

16. Wolbarst, *Looking Within,* 7.

17. The 2016 study focused on the "reductive appeal" of neuroscience, but it also concluded that "participants gave neuroscience the highest ratings of any science on the Perceptions of Science scale." See Hopkins et al., "Seductive Allure Is a Reductive Allure," 75.

18. Hook and Farah, "Look Again"; Weisberg et al., "Seductive Allure of Neuroscience Explanations"; Fernandez-Duque, "Superfluous Neuroscience Information."

19. O'Connor et al., "Neuroscience in the Public Sphere"; Dumit, "How (Not) to Do Things with Brain Images"; Dumit, *Picturing Personhood*; Dumit, "Is It Me or My Brain?"

20. Racine et al., "fMRI in the Public Eye."

21. Treichler et al., *Visible Woman,* 5.

22. Rijcke and Beaulieu, "Networked Neuroscience," 146. See also Beaulieu, "Images Are Not the (Only) Truth."

23. Lock, *Alzheimer Conundrum,* 127–28.

24. Sontag, *On Photography,* 155.

25. Marianne Hirsch cites the family photograph's easy accessibility, what she calls an "inclusive, affiliative look." Hirsch, *Familial Gaze,* xiii.

26. This is a relationship that theorists of photography have described in some detail. Roland Barthes famously described the photograph as a kind of "umbilical cord" with the past, a figure that renders it both personal and familial. Barthes, *Camera Lucida,* 81.

27. Andreas Huyssen describes a fundamental shift in Western modernity from the 1980s onward, a shift from concern for "present futures" to a crisis over "present pasts." See Huyssen, *Present Pasts*, 11.

28. Key is a complex interplay between an ideology of self-representation that helps shape the selfie's cultural reception and the material, phatic connectivity implicit in practices of sharing photos. The dominance of informal, ephemeral imagery has led to questions over the value of that imagery as well as its relationship to identity and social agency. Perhaps this is one reason why the digital selfie, so ubiquitous as a contemporary media practice, is also so contested as to its agential value. In response to dismissal of the genre because of its apparent vanity, some critics argue that is not the representational figure that matters but the networked selfie practices that create agency. Gomez Cruz and Thornham, "Selfies beyond Self-Representation," 3.

29. Smith et al., *Alzheimer's for Dummies*.

30. "Strategies for Alzheimer's Caregivers: How Post-it Notes Can Help," https://www.post-it.com/3M/en_US/post-it/ideas/articles/strategies-for-alz heimers-caregivers-how-post-it-notes-can-help/.

31. Munro, "Bear Came over the Mountain," 110–11.

32. Sturken, *Tangled Memories*, 9.

33. Batchen, *Forget Me Not*, 98.

34. Sconce, *Haunted Media*; Skoller, *Making History in Avant-Garde Film*; Andriopoulos, *Possessed*; Andriopoulos, *Ghostly Apparitions*.

35. Barthes, *Camera Lucida*, 92.

36. CBN, "Bring It On," September 7, 2014. http://www1.cbn.com/content/ bring-it-alzheimers-0. See also Moisse and Hopper, "Pat Robertson's Alzheimer's Remark Stuns."

37. Sweeting and Gilhooly, "Dementia and the Phenomenon of Social Death"; Kaufman, "Dementia-Near-Death"; Leibing, "Divided Gazes," 248; Ballenger, *Self, Senility, and Alzheimer's Disease*, 136–37.

38. Kaufman, "Dementia-Near-Death," 27.

39. Margaret Lock describes the many different social factors that shape that moral economy today, concluding that the "debate about what exactly constitutes death, its timing and determination, the technological or ritual orchestration of dying, other parties' competing interests in the body, and the emotional and practical responses of the living to the dying are all moral concerns." Lock, *Twice Dead*, 192.

40. The way Tanzi titles his book is indicative of a larger perspective of the experience of Alzheimer's—as darkness or limited sight. That title joins several others in the darkness/disappearance genre, including Heston and White, *Vanishing Mind*; DeBaggio, *When It Gets Dark*; Thorndike, *Last of His Mind*; Paddock, *A Song of Twilight*; Haugse, *A Long Dark Night*; and Henderson

and Andrews, *Partial View*. These are only a few of the many titles that deploy the theme of darkness or threatened visibility as the dominant aesthetic of Alzheimer's.

41. Yasuda et al., "Effectiveness of Personalised." See also Thomsen and Berntsen, "Cultural Life Script"; Capstick and Ludwin, "Place Memory and Dementia." For a review, see Subramaniam and Woods, "Impact of Individual Reminiscence."

42. *Alzheimer's for Dummies* recommends scrapbooking as a useful activity to keep people with Alzheimer's "occupied" or as an aid in reminiscing. Smith et al., *Alzheimer's for Dummies*, 274, 290. There has also been a recent move to create digital environments for reminiscence therapy. See Subramaniam and Woods, "Towards the Therapeutic Use."

43. National Museums of Liverpool, *My House of Memories* app, https://play .google.com/store/apps/details?id=com.nml.myhouseofmemories.

44. Nayeri, "Museums Fight the Isolation."

45. Minnesota Historical Society, "New App and Training Workshops."

46. Michael Rossato-Bennett, "*Alive Inside Film of Music and Memory Project— Henry's Story*," YouTube video, 1:27, April 13, 2012, https://www.youtube.com/ watch?v=5FWn4JB2YLU.

47. De Hogeweyk, "Living Life as Usual," 5, http://www.hogewey.nl.

48. Glenner, "Your Town Square Visiting Options," https://glenner.org/wp -content/uploads/2019/10/Town-Square-Brochure.pdf.

49. Hurley, "Time-Travel Therapy."

50. NPR, "San Diego Non-profit Builds Village."

51. Powell and Pawlowski, "Dementia Day Care."

52. Rippel, "Life Memoirs."

53. https://storycorps.me/about/the-great-thanksgiving-listen/.

54. https://storycorps.org/about/.

55. Basting, *Forget Memory*, 148.

56. DAI uploaded some of the early educational webinars to YouTube and invited people with and without dementia to watch them. See https://www .youtube.com/user/ameetingoftheminds/videos.

5. Dementia in the Museum

1. https://www.moma.org/collection/works/81006.

2. Italics denote particular verbal emphasis. Ellipses denote a long pause.

3. I use pseudonyms in accounts from my fieldwork. It should be clear that including participant contributions without wholesale interpretation or "translation" is intentional. It is one way to include the perspectives or experiences of people diagnosed with Alzheimer's. Much of my critique in this chapter, however, explicitly addresses institutional and social expectations.

4. My own introduction to the program came in fall 2007 when a colleague who knew of my research introduced me to the program coordinator. After some early exploratory visits, I followed up with more formal research beginning in 2010.

5. MoMA claims that it is not a model for other programs, but it certainly serves as one in the public eye. There are now similar programs around the country at all manner of museums with different kinds of collections.

6. Rosenberg et al., *Meet Me*.

7. MoMA developed an early version of Meet Me with a group called ARTZ, or Artists for Alzheimer's (http://www.imstillhere.org/artz). See Zeisel, *I'm Still Here*, 87–104.

8. MoMA Department of Communications, "The Museum of Modern Art Announces National Expansion of Outreach Program for People Living with Alzheimer's Disease," October 17, 2007, http://press.moma.org/wp-content/press-archives/news/MoMA_Alzheimers_Project_Release.pdf.

9. Hunter, *Museum of Modern Art*, 13.

10. Quoted by D'Harnoncourt, *Museum of Modern Art*, 32.

11. Cohen, *No Aging in India*, xvii.

12. MoMA seems to have stopped using this line. An educator I interviewed was surprised to hear of its use. According to John Zeisel, ARTZ creative director Sean Caulfield created the line as an "active and creative name objective." Zeisel, *I'm Still Here*, 88.

13. Sturken, *Tourists of History*, 9.

14. Peter Whitehouse and William Deal have argued that "Alzheimer's disease is a particularly postmodern condition." See Whitehouse and Deal, "Situated beyond Modernity," 1314.

15. Wasson, *Museum Movies*, 96.

16. Morgan, "From Modernist Utopia to Cold War Reality," 151.

17. Greider, "In Museums."

18. Martin, *Bipolar Expeditions*, 143.

19. Generally, I limited my detailed note taking to discrete moments in between our time with each artwork. Occasionally I would take notes more actively, but I found that this practice drew the attention of those around me, and I did not wish to distract from the activities at hand. After I completed the session, I sometimes relied on my own memory to transcribe what I encountered on the visit. The accuracy of my own transcripts, then, is clearly reliant on the very practices and abilities I was there to investigate. I find this practice not only acceptable but also contributive to the ambiguity of the subject I am trying to describe.

20. For a valuable comparative exercise, readers may wish to refer to the subsection "Experience" of the MoMA publication, which offers a similarly

structured, albeit more celebratory account of the Meet Me experience. Some of it contradicts notably with my own account. See Rosenberg et al., *Meet Me,* 19–52.

21. Fackelmann, "Alzheimer's Program Is One from the Art."

22. Abraham, *When Words Have Lost Their Meaning,* 90.

23. John Zeisel of ARTZ disagrees. He in fact identifies a number of particular paintings at MoMA as more apt to be "understood" or "partially understood" by someone with Alzheimer's. See Zeisel, *I'm Still Here,* 92–93, 100.

24. Kirby et al., "Visual Impairment in Alzheimer's Disease."

25. A woman during another session was once so hostile to others' comments, so aggressively disruptive, that she immediately controlled the mood and tenor of the session's conversation. She left the session after the second painting, and the change in tone was immediate and evident. Everyone then got along very well, feedback increased, and participants seemed happy.

26. Rosenberg et al., *Meet Me,* 83.

27. ARTZ, http://www.imstillhere.org/artz.

28. Rosenberg et al., *Meet Me,* 59.

29. Leibing, "Entangled Matters," 179.

6. Dementia on the Canvas

1. These interventions fit into a broader trend that reorients personhood in social practices, embodiment, or community. For a contemporary review of how art approaches selfhood in dementia research, see Caddell and Clare, "Interventions."

2. Meulenberg and Gibson, "De Kooning's Dementia," 1838.

3. Shimamura and Palmer, *Aesthetic Science.*

4. Miller and Hou, "Portraits of Artists"; Mendez, "Dementia as a Window."

5. Rankin et al., "A Case-Controlled Study of Altered Visual Art Production"; Gretton and Ffytche, "Art and the Brain."

6. Art therapy can also designate a model of psychotherapy or psychoanalysis, but I use the term here to refer to that professional standard of practice that locates therapeutic benefit or other positive outcomes in the creation of art.

7. Safar and Press, "Art and the Brain"; Ehresman, "From Rendering to Remembering."

8. Kahn-Denis, "Art Therapy with Geriatric Dementia Clients"; Stewart, "Art Therapy and Neuroscience Blend"; Kinney and Rentz, "Observed Well-Being"; Rusted et al., "A Multi-centre Randomized"; Phillips et al., "Effects of a Creative Expression." For reviews, see Beard, "Art Therapies and Dementia Care," and Cowl and Gaugler, "Efficacy of Creative Arts Therapy."

9. Chancellor et al., "Art Therapy for Alzheimer's Disease and Other Dementias."

10. Beard, "Art Therapies," 638; Medeiros and Basting, "Shall I Compare Thee," 351.

11. Broderick, "Arts Practices in Unreasonable Doubt?"

12. George et al., "Impact of Participation in TimeSlips."

13. Fritsch et al., "Impact of TimeSlips."

14. Creativity is a difficult concept to define, one certainly dependent on the context of its use. In a review of the research on art therapy and dementia, Crystal Ehresmen says that "for simplicity," she refers to creativity as "the process that goes into creating any novel product or piece of visual artwork." Ehresmen, "From Rendering," 8.

15. Abraham, *When Words Have Lost Their Meaning,* 90.

16. Indeed, even when art therapy deemphasizes individuality, it reauthorizes selfhood within "intersubjectivity" or "community" practice. Wexler, *Art and Disability,* 173–203.

17. Robinson, "How to Escape Education's Death Valley," https://www.ted .com/talks/ken_robinson_how_to_escape_education_s_death_valley.

18. Malchiodi, *Art Therapy Sourcebook,* 65.

19. National Center for Creative Aging, "Who We Are," http://www.creative aging.org/about-ncca-o.

20. Given the overwhelming interest in neuroculture in all areas of the academy, this is a myth that we help condition "in the co-construction of the very neurocultural problems and prospects, hopes and fears, concerns and anxieties, we profess to study." See Williams et al., "Neuroculture," 75.

21. Signal vs Noise, "William Utermohlen's Self-Portraits," http://37signals .com/svn/.

22. *Huffington Post,* "William Utermohlen's Self-Portraits."

23. Andrew Purcell, "Self-Portraits of a Declining Brain," January 2012, http://www.newscientist.com/blogs/culturelab/2012/01/self-portraits-declin ing-brain.html.

24. Grady, "Self-Portraits Chronicle a Descent into Alzheimer's."

25. Associated Press, "Artist Paints His Struggle with Alzheimer's."

26. This is not just a strategy for popular reception; according to Margaret Lock, Myriad Genetics sponsored a 2008 exhibition of Utermohlen's work in conjunction with an international Alzheimer's conference held in Chicago that adopted a similar strategy of retrospective, before-and-after display. See Lock, *Alzheimer Conundrum,* 244.

27. Crutch et al., "Some Workmen Can Blame Their Tools," 2132.

28. Crutch and Rossor, "Artistic Changes in Alzheimer's Disease," 148.

29. Siebers, *Disability Aesthetics,* 15.

30. *Huffington Post,* "William Utermohlen's Self-Portraits."

31. O'Neill, "Art of the Demographic Dividend," 1829.

32. Graw, "Value of Painting."

33. Maurer and Prvulovic, "Paintings of an Artist," 244.

34. Of course, we need not limit this account to one country, as this is an orientation with capitalism more broadly. These are ideologically structured narratives that are often coded as natural or human. However, as I have actively argued in this book, the narrative of Alzheimer's in the United States harnesses presupposed universals like these in the defense of its own practical and ethical solutions.

35. Gullette, *Aged by Culture*, 16, 143.

36. Stephen Katz provides a helpful reading of dementia, progress, and memorial ethics through some different accounts of modernity in "Embodied Memory."

37. McLean, *Person in Dementia*, 54.

38. Storr, "At Last Light"; Espinel, "De Kooning's Late Colours and Forms"; Meulenberg and Gibson, "De Kooning's Dementia"; Stewart, "De Kooning's Dementia"; Kontos, "Painterly Hand."

39. Defending the relational aspects of selfhood, Kate McFadden and Anne Basting have argued that "although cultural stereotypes envision creative people working alone, creativity and the arts are fundamentally social, for the product of creative endeavor is nearly always shared with others." As this case study shows, this is not always the case—or at least it begs a more complex account. See McFadden and Basting, "Healthy Aging Persons and Their Brains," 153.

40. Clark et al., "Painting from Memory."

41. Storr, "At Last Light."

42. Thomas, "Shaping de Kooning's Legacy."

43. Quoted in Thomas.

44. Clark et al., "Painting from Memory," 3.

45. Rosenberg et al., *Meet Me*, 68.

46. Meulenberg and Gibson, "De Kooning's Dementia," 1838.

47. Moulier-Boutang, *Cognitive Capitalism*, 56–57.

48. Kurant et al., "Do We Need a Lab?" 250.

49. Martin, *Bipolar Expeditions*, 243.

50. Nelson, "Invention of Creativity," 68.

51. Medeiros and Basting, "Shall I Compare Thee," 351.

52. This is often known as little "c" and big "C" creativity.

7. Loved Ones

1. Genova, *Still Alice*, 292.

2. Genova originally wrote a less hopeful ending for the book, with Alice's husband crying alone in a coffee shop after getting news of a failed drug trial. In a Goodreads Q&A, Genova wrote that her literary agent asked her to change

the ending (presumably to be more positive) before Simon and Schuster agreed to publish it. Goodreads, "Ask Lisa Genova!" August 22, 2011, https://www.goodreads.com/topic/show/636127-still-alice-question; Bogel, "The Controversial Ending(s) of Still Alice."

3. National Academies of Sciences, Engineering, and Medicine, "Families Caring for an Aging America," https://nam.edu/families-caring-for-an-aging-america/.

4. As of 2016, Medicare provides professional care planning for people newly diagnosed with Alzheimer's, and some states offer care training for home care providers and—in some cases—limited funding for long-term care. Another important step has been the Caregiver Advise, Record, Enable (CARE) Act, new legislation passed in many states that aims to help facilitate and monitor home health care. When a dependent leaves a hospital, the law requires the hospital to register and provide training for the caregiver. The idea is not to let dependents and caregivers slip through the cracks, leaving them without the resources for adequate care.

5. Ahmed, "In the Name of Love," 19.

6. Taylor, "On Recognition."

7. Cohen, "Politics of Care," 338.

8. Alyssa Newcomb, "Glen Campbell Reveals He Has Alzheimer's," http://abcnews.go.com/Entertainment/music-legend-glen-campbell-reveals-alzheimers/story?id=13906837.

9. Ayers, "Oscars 2015."

10. Fineman, "Masking Dependency," 228.

11. See Metzl and Kirkland, *Against Health,* and Kipnis, *Against Love,* for interrogations of the normativity of health and love, respectively.

12. For some relevant attempts to define love and its capacities, see Fromm, *Art of Loving;* Secomb, *Philosophy and Love;* Hardt and Negri, *Commonwealth;* Berlant, *Desire/Love.* For a debate between Hardt and Berlant on the subject, see nomorepotlucks, "No One Is Sovereign in Love: A Conversation between Lauren Berlant and Michael Hardt," May 2011, http://nomorepotlucks.org/site/no-one-is-sovereign-in-love-a-conversation-between-lauren-berlant-and-michael-hardt/.

13. Cohen, *Thinking about Dementia,* 14

14. Reagan, "Letter to My Fellow Americans"; Gordon, "In Poignant Public Letter."

15. Charlton Heston once described Nancy and Ronald Reagan's relationship as "the greatest love affair in the history of the American Presidency." See Russell, "Greatest Love Affair."

16. BBC News, "End of a Love Story," June 5, 2004, http://news.bbc.co.uk/2/hi/americas/265714.stm.

17. Finn, "From Rock Videos to an Alzheimer's Stamp."

18. U.S. Postal Service, "Alzheimer's Semipostal Fundraising Stamp Dedicated Today," November 30, 2017. https://about.usps.com/news/national-releases/2017/pr17_076.htm.

19. Hendrix, "A Pain Vast and Personal."

20. Hendrix.

21. Alzheimer's Association, "2021 Alzheimer's Disease Facts and Figures," 36–37. For more on costs associated with dementia care, see Jutkowitz et al., "Societal and Family."

22. Conversely, one study found that "lonely individuals were more than twice as likely to develop an AD-like dementia syndrome than were those who were not lonely, even after controlling for level of social isolation." See Wilson et al., "Loneliness and Risk of Alzheimer Disease."

23. Alzheimer's Association, "2021 Alzheimer's Disease Facts and Figures," 36–49; see also Reinhard et al., "Home Alone."

24. This issue was rooted in confusion over which group was the intended recipient of the money, and it led to a countersuit for copyright infringement. See Sachdev, "Alzheimer's Charities Fight over Money."

25. Jensen, "HBO Documentaries."

26. Even the most progressive of Alzheimer's advocates support this kind of narrative: Anne Basting argues that we need to reform cultures of Alzheimer's by looking for new ways to make meaning and to "fill the void" left by fear of meaninglessness "as we wait for scientists to bring us a cure, or at the very least, clear steps for prevention." In Basting, *Forget Memory*, 69–70.

27. Post, "Stumbling on Joy," 249.

28. Kitwood, *Dementia Reconsidered*; Woodward, *Between Remembering and Forgetting*; Killick, "Learning Love from People with Dementia," 54–56.

29. Hendrie et al., "NIH Cognitive and Emotional Health Project," 15.

30. Oprah Winfrey Network, "B. Smith on Living for the Moment with Alzheimer's."

31. Flegenheimer, "Tale of Love and Illness Ends in Deaths."

32. A group of Australian researchers found that one in six caregivers of a family member with dementia have seriously considered suicide. See O'Dwyer et al., "Suicidal Ideation." They also found homicidal ideation a "real and significant phenomenon among family carers of people with dementia." See O'Dwyer et al., "Homicidal Ideation." For popular and practical reflections on homicide, suicide, and dementia, see Cohen "Preventing the Unthinkable," and Marquardt, "Elderly Murder-Suicide."

33. Obama, "National Alzheimer's Disease Awareness Month, 2009."

34. Hughes et al., *Dementia*; Leibing, "Divided Gazes."

35. Taylor, *Alzheimer's from the Inside Out*, 146.

36. Take, for example, the issue of proxy consent and participation in research. Frequently people with Alzheimer's are unable to give consent because of the way the disease affects self-awareness and decision-making abilities. Because of this, a proxy is often used to give consent on their behalf. There is a range of potential surrogate participation, including double informed consent, which involves obtaining consent from the proxy and confirmation of that decision from the person with Alzheimer's. This "allows persons with dementia to participate and upholds the ethical principle of autonomy or self determination." Beck and Shue, "Surrogate Decision-making," S14. Regardless of the caliber of proxy decision, because the proxy is frequently the primary caregiver, these proxy decisions can place an enormous strain on these relationships. As B. Lynn Beattie argues, "the proxy is in an unenviable position, at times caught between justifiable persuasion and undue influence." Beattie, "Consent in Alzheimer's Disease Research," S28.

37. The biographical film is conducive to the subject of Alzheimer's. See Swinnen, "Dementia in Documentary Film," 113–14; Wearing, "Dementia and the Biopolitics of the Biopic."

38. In 2012 *U.S. Weekly* put *The Notebook* at the top of its list of the best romance movies ever made. See *U.S. Weekly*, "30 Most Romantic Movies of All Time."

39. Williams, "For Winslet."

40. In a large study aimed at describing the experience of informal, familial Alzheimer's caregivers, "caregiving, although difficult, was met with a sense of commitment flowing from the quality of the relationship at earlier times." See Butcher et al., "Experience of Caring for a Family Member," 49.

41. Liao, "Personhood and the Ethics of Dementia," 466.

42. This narrative rebounded on a national scale as U.S. Supreme Court justice Sandra Day O'Connor had a similar, well-publicized experience caring for her husband.

43. Philley, "Away from Her," 20–22.

44. Critics were enamored with the precociousness of the ingénue writer/ director, applauding the maturity of her work despite her young age. Polley claimed that she wanted to make a movie about Alzheimer's that didn't need to show people in their youth—presumably referencing movies about Alzheimer's like *Iris* or *The Notebook*: "It's like we need to justify making a movie about people who are older. There's something that rubs me the wrong way about that." Torrance, "Director Shows Deft Touch." While that is a noble ethic, Polley fails to recognize that the actors themselves bring images of youth with them in the guise of their own acting oeuvre. As Philley writes in his commentary, "*Away from Her* has much to say to the generation that remembers Julie Christie in *Doctor Zhivago* 42 years ago, and can now see her in a dramatically different context." Philley, "Away from Her," 22.

45. Workforce for Older Americans, "Retooling for an Aging America," 124.

46. Wolff et al., "Family Caregivers," 1028.

47. Boris and Klein, "Laws of Care."

48. Boris and Klein, "Organizing the Carework Economy," 193.

49. Boris and Klein, 208.

50. Popular representations of paid care workers in care facilities follow the same patterns. See, for example, the films *Age Old Friends*, *The Savages*, and *Win Win*.

51. Structural inequality pervades all relationships of dependency and care, but Alzheimer's heightens the failure of independence and selfhood—qualities that so strongly underwrite personhood in the United States. Conversely, recognition of that personhood as failure heightens the ideology and expectation of independence imposed on the caregiver. For more, see the notion of the "Independent Man" in Feder Kittay and Feder's introduction to *Subject of Care*, 1–5. In the face of the expectation of independence, Feder Kittay proposes a corrective, relational model of personhood based on the "capacity to be in certain relationships with other persons, to sustain contact with other persons, to shape one's own world and the world of others, and to have a life that another person can conceive of as an imaginative possibility for him- or herself." In Feder Kittay, "When Caring Is Just," 266.

52. Feder Kittay, *Love's Labor*, 132–34.

53. For more on this genealogy of affect, see Berlant, "Intimacy"; Clough and Halley, *Affective Turn*; Stewart, *Ordinary Affects*; and Gregg and Seigworth, *Affect Theory Reader*. For its legacies in feminist and queer theory, see Ahmed, *Promise of Happiness*; Berlant, *Female Complaint*; Berlant, *Cruel Optimism*; Illouz, *Consuming the Romantic Utopia*; Sedgwick, "A Dialogue on Love"; Sedgwick, *Touching Feeling*.

54. Staiger et al., "Introduction," 6.

55. Hoad, "Three Poems and a Pandemic," 148. I acknowledge the existence of research on the bioethics of other diseases that might inform an extended version of this essay. In particular, I recognize the overlaps between HIV/AIDS and issues of love, care, death, and concordant problems with national policy, identity, and visibility. But it is not my intention to make this work comparative, and I am somewhat insecure with the politics of a pathological solidarity, despite my reflection on this source.

56. Dean, *Governmentality*, 167–68.

57. Berlant, *Female Complaint*, 35.

58. This dualism between love and cognition is heightened by the careers of the many cinematic characters who get Alzheimer's: college professors. The first narrative feature to focus on Alzheimer's, *Do You Remember Love* (see http://

www.emmys.com/shows/do-you-remember-love), features a poetry professor, while *Still Alice* features a linguistics professor.

59. Michael Reagan (@ReaganWorld), "#Alzheimers is not a comedy," Twitter, April 28, 2016, https://twitter.com/ReaganWorld/status/7258580655 39432449?ref_src=twsrc%5Etfw.

60. Kroll, "Will Ferrell Pulls Out of Ronald Reagan Movie."

Epilogue

1. https://adage.com/video/google-loretta.

2. Valinsky, "Google's Super Bowl Ad: People Shed Tears for 'Loretta,'" https://www.cnn.com/2020/02/03/business/google-super-bowl-ad-loretta -trnd/index.html.; Sparks, "Google's Super Bowl."

3. Alison Kafer makes this point more broadly for disability: "The task, then, is not so much to refuse the future as to imagine disability and disability futures otherwise, as part of other, alternate temporalities that do not cast disabled people out of time, as the sign of the future of no future." See Kafer, *Feminist, Queer, Crip*, 34. This is a critical practice that seeks to show how individuals and groups experience time differently. Time itself is not universal but is lived differently through divergent social logics and material environments—what Sarah Sharma has called "differential temporalities." See Sharma, *In the Meantime*, 14.

4. A more pragmatic approach might be to deemphasize representational capacity as the primary logic of aging. Within her treatment of "prognosis time," Jasbir Puar has called for a shift in disability politics, arguing for a "push for a broader politics of debility that destabilizes the seamless production of abled-bodies in relation to disability." See Puar, "Prognosis Time," 166–67. That critical step might be helpful for rethinking the dichotomies that so frequently structure the experience of Alzheimer's at the same time that it pays heed to a universalizing embrace of the disease. In other words, the shift from disability to debility might decenter those identitarian claims so injurious to people living with Alzheimer's without losing sight of the variable, individual experiences of the disease. To conceive of a cognitive, mediatic debilitation, it is necessary to identify these feedback loops between cognitive ability and cognitive infrastructures. Rather than understanding disability as outside of or othered by these systems, it is better to show how disablement is inherent to everyday life as a consequence of media integration. Given that Alzheimer's has no cure, has no known cause, and is actively felt, feared, and futured, it is possible to conceive of it not only as a disease but as a debilitating national condition. Ablement and disablement are swept up in a broader experience of everyday cognitive life.

5. Perhaps a critique of cognitive labor can help academic work about Alzheimer's acknowledge the mode of production of which it is a part. The

university is an excellent place for a conversation like this not simply because our work is ostensibly "about" cognitive ability but also because the university is the contemporary battleground for the fight over representation's value. As academic laborers, we should have something to say about the stakes of education and its instrumentalizing practices. If one considers the university a battleground, it is less a place for the production of cognitive capacity and more a place for pragmatic critique. As George Caffentzis and Silvia Federici succinctly argue, "as was the factory, so now is the university." Caffentzis and Federici, "Notes on the Edu-Factory," 125. See also Price, *Mad at School,* and Chen, "Brain Fog."

6. Canguilhem, *The Normal and the Pathological,* 286.

Bibliography

Abraham, Ruth. *When Words Have Lost Their Meaning*. Westport, Conn.: Praeger, 2005.

Achenbaum, W. Andrew. *Crossing Frontiers: Gerontology Emerges as a Science*. New York: Cambridge University Press, 1995.

Achenbaum, W. Andrew. *Older Americans, Vital Communities: A Bold Vision for Societal Aging*. Baltimore: Johns Hopkins University Press, 2005.

Addison, Heather. "Transcending Time: Jean Harlow and Hollywood's Narrative of Decline." *Journal of Film and Video* 57, no. 4 (2005): 32–46.

Adelman, Richard C. "The Alzheimerization of Aging." *The Gerontologist* 35 (August 1995): 526–32.

Aguayo, Joseph. "Charcot and Freud: Some Implications of Late 19th Century French Psychiatry and Politics for the Origin of Psychoanalysis." *Psychoanalysis and Contemporary Thought* 9 (1986): 223–60.

Ahmed, Sara. "In the Name of Love." *Borderlands* 2, no. 3 (2003): 1–41.

Ahmed, Sara. *The Promise of Happiness*. Durham, N.C.: Duke University Press Books, 2010.

Akin, Charlotte. *The Long Road Called Goodbye: Tracing the Course of Alzheimer's*. Omaha, Neb.: Creighton University Press, 2000.

Albert, Marilyn. "Detection of Very Early Alzheimer's Disease through Neuroimaging." *Alzheimer Disease and Associated Disorders* 17, Suppl. 2 (2003): s63–65.

Albert, Marilyn S., Steven T. DeKosky, Dennis Dickson, Bruno Dubois, Howard H. Feldman, Nick C. Fox, Anthony Gamst, et al. "The Diagnosis of Mild Cognitive Impairment due to Alzheimer's Disease: Recommendations from the National Institute on Aging–Alzheimer's Association Workgroups on

Diagnostic Guidelines for Alzheimer's Disease." *Alzheimer's and Dementia* 7, no. 3 (2011): 270–79.

Albert, Marilyn, Margaret A. Naeser, Harvey L. Levine, and Arthur J. Garvey. "CT Density Numbers in Patients with Senile Dementia of the Alzheimer's Type." *Archives of Neurology* 41, no. 12 (1984): 1264–69.

Alberti, Samuel J. M. M. *Morbid Curiosities Medical Museums in Nineteenth-Century Britain.* Oxford: Oxford University Press, 2011.

Alexander, D. A. "'Senile Dementia': A Changing Perspective." *British Journal of Psychiatry: Journal of Mental Science* 121, no. 561 (1972): 207–14.

Alford, L. B. "An Analysis of Fourteen Cases of Senile Dementia Showing Neither Atrophic nor Arteriosclerotic Cerebral Changes at Autopsy." *Journal of Nervous and Mental Disease* 46, no. 2 (1917): 100–114.

Ally, Brandon A. "Using EEG and MEG to Understand Brain Physiology in Alzheimer's Disease and Related Dementias." In *The Handbook of Alzheimer's Disease and Other Dementias,* edited by Andrew E. Budson and Neil W. Kowall, 575–603. London: Wiley-Blackwell, 2011.

Alper, Meryl. *Giving Voice: Mobile Communication, Disability, and Inequality.* Cambridge, Mass.: MIT Press, 2017.

Alzheimer, Alois. "Concerning a Unique Disease of the Cerebral Cortex," translated by Clifford Saper and Herbert Horst. In *Alzheimer: 100 Years and Beyond,* edited by M. Jucker, K. Beyreuther, C. Haass, and R. M. Nitsch, 3–11. Berlin: Springer, 2006.

Alzheimer, Alois. "On Certain Peculiar Diseases of Old Age." Translated by Hans Forstl and Raymond Levy. *History of Psychiatry,* no. ii (1991): 71–101.

Alzheimer, Alois. "The Present Status of Our Knowledge of the Pathological Histology of the Cortex in the Psychoses." Translated by Henry Cotton. *American Journal of Psychiatry* 1, no. 1 (1913): 175–205.

Alzheimer's and Dementia. "Alzheimer's Association Update." 10, no. 4 (2014): 509–10.

Alzheimer's Association. "2011 Alzheimer's Disease Facts and Figures." *Alzheimer's and Dementia* 7, no. 2 (2011): 208–44.

Alzheimer's Association. "2012 Alzheimer's Disease Facts and Figures." *Alzheimer's and Dementia* 8 (2012): 131–68.

Alzheimer's Association. "2013 Alzheimer's Disease Facts and Figures." *Alzheimer's and Dementia* 12, no. 4 (2013). http://www.alz.org/facts/overview.asp.

Alzheimer's Association. "2019 Alzheimer's Disease Facts and Figures." *Alzheimer's and Dementia* 15, no. 3 (2019): 321–87.

Alzheimer's Association. "2021 Alzheimer's Disease Facts and Figures." *Alzheimer's and Dementia* 17, no. 3 (2021). https://www.alz.org/alzheimers-dementia/facts-figures.

Alzheimer's Disease Center, Albert Einstein College of Medicine, and National Institute on Aging. *Alzheimer's Disease Q&A.* Washington, D.C.: U.S. Department of Health, Education, and Welfare, 1980.

Amaducci, L. A., W. A. Rocca, and B. S. Schoenberg. "Origin of the Distinction between Alzheimer's Disease and Senile Dementia: How History Can Clarify Nosology." *Neurology* 36 (November 1986): 1497–99.

Anderson, Nancy. "Facing Animals in the Laboratory: Lessons of Nineteenth-Century Medical School Microscopy Manuals." In *Educated Eye: Visual Culture and Pedagogy in the Life Sciences,* edited by Nancy A. Anderson and Michael R. Dietrich, 44–67. Hanover, N.H.: Dartmouth College Press, 2012.

Andriopoulos, Stefan. *Ghostly Apparitions: German Idealism, the Gothic Novel, and Optical Media.* New York: Zone Books, 2013.

Andriopoulos, Stefan. *Possessed: Hypnotic Crimes, Corporate Fiction, and the Invention of Cinema.* Chicago: University of Chicago Press, 2008.

Anoop, A., Pradeep K. Singh, Reeba S. Jacob, and Samir K. Maji. "CSF Biomarkers for Alzheimer's Disease Diagnosis." *International Journal of Alzheimer's Disease* 2010 (June 23, 2010): 606802.

Arledge, Elizabeth, dir. *The Forgetting.* PBS, 2004.

Åsberg, Cecilia, and Jennifer Lum. "PharmAD-Ventures: A Feminist Analysis of the Pharmacological Imaginary of Alzheimer's Disease." *Body and Society* 15, no. 4 (2009): 95–117.

Åsberg, Cecilia, and Jennifer Lum. "Picturizing the Scattered Ontologies of Alzheimer's Disease: Towards a Materialist Feminist Approach to Visual Technoscience Studies." *European Journal of Women's Studies* 17, no. 4 (2010): 323–45.

Ashida, Sato, Laura M. Koehly, J. S. Roberts, Clara A. Chen, Susan Hiraki, and Robert C. Green. "Disclosing the Disclosure: Factors Associated with Communicating the Results of Genetic Susceptibility Testing for Alzheimer's Disease." *Journal of Health Communication* 14, no. 8 (2009): 768–84.

Associated Press. "Artist Paints His Struggle with Alzheimer's." MSNBC, March 11, 2006. http://www.nbcnews.com/id/11752410/ns/health-alzhei mers_disease/t/artist-paints-his-struggle-alzheimers/.

Associated Press. "Hinckley Acquittal Brings Moves to Change Insanity Defense." *New York Times,* June 24, 1982, sec. U.S. http://www.nytimes .com/1982/06/24/us/hinkley-acquittal-brings-moves-to-change-insanity -defense.html.

Associated Press. "Transcript of President-Elect Joe Biden's Victory Speech." *AP News,* November 7, 2020. https://apnews.com/article/election-2020-joe -biden-religion-technology-race-and-ethnicity-2b961c70bc72c2516046bff d378e95de.

Atkinson, Arthur J., Wayne A. Colburn, Victor G. DeGruttola, David L. DeMets, Gregory J. Downing, Daniel F. Hoth, John A. Oates, et al. "Biomarkers and Surrogate Endpoints: Preferred Definitions and Conceptual Framework." *Clinical Pharmacology and Therapeutics* 69, no. 3 (2001): 89–95.

Atteveldt, Nienke M. van, Sandra I. van Aalderen-Smeets, Carina Jacobi, and Nel Ruigrok. "Media Reporting of Neuroscience Depends on Timing, Topic and Newspaper Type." *PLoS ONE* 9, no. 8 (2014): 104780.

August, Bille, dir. *A Song for Martin*. Sweden: Drama, Music, Romance, 2001.

Ayers, Mike. "Oscars 2015: The Story behind Glen Campbell's 'I'm Not Gonna Miss You.'" *WSJ* (blog), February 19, 2015. http://blogs.wsj.com/speakeasy/2015/02/19/oscars-2015-the-story-behind-glen-campbells-im-not-gonna-miss-you/.

Backhaus, Peter. *Communication in Elderly Care Cross-Cultural Perspectives*. London: Continuum, 2011.

Balke, Friedrich. "'Can Thought Go On without a Body?' On the Relationship between Machines and Organisms in Media Philosophy." *Cultural Studies* 30, no. 4 (2016): 610–29.

Ball, M. J. "Topographic Distribution of Neurofibrillary Tangles and Granulovacuolar Degeneration in Hippocampal Cortex of Aging and Demented Patients: A Quantitative Study." *Acta Neuropathologica* 42, no. 2 (1978): 73–80.

Ballenger, Jesse F. "Beyond the Characteristic Plaques and Tangles: Mid Twentieth Century U.S. Psychiatry and the Fight against Senility." In *Concepts of Alzheimer Disease: Biological, Clinical, and Cultural Perspectives*, edited by Peter J. Whitehouse, Konrad Maurer, and Jesse F. Ballenger. Baltimore: Johns Hopkins University Press, 2003.

Ballenger, Jesse F. "The Biomedical Deconstruction of Senility and the Persistent Stigmatization of Old Age in the United States." In *Thinking about Dementia: Culture, Loss, and the Anthropology of Senility*, edited by Lawrence Cohen and Annette Leibing, 106–20. New Brunswick, N.J.: Rutgers University Press, 2006.

Ballenger, Jesse F. *Self, Senility, and Alzheimer's Disease in Modern America: A History*. Baltimore: Johns Hopkins University Press, 2006.

Banet-Weiser, Sarah. *Authentic TM Politics and Ambivalence in a Brand Culture*. New York: New York University Press, 2012.

Barnes, Deborah E., and Kristine Yaffe. "The Projected Effect of Risk Factor Reduction on Alzheimer's Disease Prevalence." *The Lancet Neurology* 10, no. 9 (2011): 819–28.

Barrett, Albert. "A Case of Alzheimer's Disease with Unusual Neurological Disturbances." *Journal of Nervous and Mental Disease* 40, no. 6 (1913): 361–74.

Barthes, Roland. *Camera Lucida: Reflections on Photography*. 1st American ed. New York: Hill and Wang, 1981.

Barusch, Amanda Smith. *Love Stories of Later Life: A Narrative Approach to Understanding Romance*. New York: Oxford University Press, 2008.

Basting, Anne Davis. *Forget Memory: Creating Better Lives for People with Dementia*. Baltimore: Johns Hopkins University Press, 2009.

Batchen, Geoffrey. *Forget Me Not: Photography and Remembrance*. New York: Princeton Architectural Press, 2004.

Batchen, Geoffrey. *Photography Degree Zero: Reflections on Roland Barthes's Camera Lucida*. Cambridge, Mass.: MIT Press, 2009.

Bayley, John. *Iris and Her Friends: A Memoir of Memory and Desire*. New York: W. W. Norton, 2000.

Beach, Thomas. "The History of Alzheimer's Disease: Three Debates." *Journal of the History of Medicine and Allied Sciences* 42 (1987): 327–49.

Beard, George Miller. *Legal Responsibility in Old Age: Based on Researches into the Relation of Age to Work: Read before the Medico-Legal Society of the City of New York at the Regular Meeting of the Society, March, 1873; Republished with Notes and Additions from the Transactions of the Society*. New York, 1874.

Beard, George. *The Problems of Insanity*. New York: New York Medico-Legal Society, 1880.

Beard, Renée L. "Advocating Voice: Organisational, Historical and Social Milieux of the Alzheimer's Disease Movement." *Sociology of Health and Illness* 26, no. 6 (2004): 797–819.

Beard, Renée L. "Art Therapies and Dementia Care: A Systematic Review." *Dementia* 11, no. 5 (2011): 633–56.

Beattie, B. L. "Consent in Alzheimer's Disease Research: Risk/Benefit Factors." *Canadian Journal of Neurological Sciences* 34, Suppl. 1 (2007): S27–31.

Beaulieu, Anne. "Images Are Not the (Only) Truth: Brain Mapping, Visual Knowledge, and Iconoclasm." *Science, Technology, and Human Values* 27, no. 1 (2002): 53–86.

Beck, Cornelia, and Valorie Shue. "Surrogate Decision-Making and Related Issues." *Alzheimer Disease and Associated Disorders* 17, Suppl. 1 (2003): S12–16.

Beck, Diane M. "The Appeal of the Brain in the Popular Press." *Perspectives on Psychological Science* 5, no. 6 (2010): 762–66.

Beckmann, H., K. Maurer, and P. Riederer, eds. *Alzheimer's Disease: Epidemiology, Neuropathology, Neurochemistry, and Clinics*. New York: Springer, 1990.

Belluck, Pam. "Alzheimer's Stalks a Colombian Family." *New York Times*, June 1, 2010, sec. Health. http://www.nytimes.com/2010/06/02/health/02alzheimers.html.

Belluck, Pam, and Rebecca Robbins. "Three F.D.A. Advisers Resign over Agency's Approval of Alzheimer's Drug." *New York Times*, June 10, 2021.

https://www.nytimes.com/2021/06/10/health/aduhelm-fda-resign-alzhei
mers.html.

Bennett, Jane. *Vibrant Matter: A Political Ecology of Things*. Durham, N.C.: Duke University Press, 2010.

Benoit, Cecilia, and Helga Hallgrimsdóttir. *Valuing Care Work: Comparative Perspectives*. Toronto: University of Toronto Press, 2011.

Berchtold, N. C., and C. W. Cotman. "Evolution in the Conceptualization of Dementia and Alzheimer's Disease: Greco-Roman Period to the 1960s." *Neurobiology of Aging* 19, no. 3 (1998): 173–89.

Beresford, Peter, and Jasna Russo. "Supporting the Sustainability of Mad Studies and Preventing Its Co-option." *Disability and Society* 31, no. 2 (2016): 270–74.

Berge, Ann F. La. "Debate as Scientific Practice in Nineteenth-Century Paris: The Controversy over the Microscope." *Perspectives on Science* 12, no. 4 (2004): 424–53.

Berge, Ann La. "The History of Science and the History of Microscopy." *Perspectives on Science* 7, no. 1 (1999): 111.

Berlant, Lauren, ed. *Compassion: The Culture and Politics of an Emotion*. New York: Routledge, 2004.

Berlant, Lauren Gail. *Cruel Optimism*. Durham, N.C.: Duke University Press, 2011.

Berlant, Lauren. *Desire/Love*. New York: Punctum Books, 2012.

Berlant, Lauren Gail. *The Female Complaint: The Unfinished Business of Sentimentality in American Culture*. Durham, N.C.: Duke University Press, 2008.

Berlant, Lauren. "Intimacy: A Special Issue." *Critical Inquiry* 24, no. 2 (1998): 281–88.

Berlant, Lauren Gail. "Nearly Utopian, Nearly Normal: Post-Fordist Affect in 'La Promesse' and 'Rosetta.'" *Public Culture* 19, no. 2 (2007): 273–301.

Berlant, Lauren Gail. *The Queen of America Goes to Washington City: Essays on Sex and Citizenship*. Durham, N.C.: Duke University Press, 1997.

Berrios, G. E. "Alzheimer's Disease: A Conceptual History." *International Journal of Geriatric Psychiatry* 5, no. 6 (1990): 355–65.

Berrios, G. E., and H. L. Freeman. "Alzheimer and His Time." In *Alzheimer's and the Dementias*, edited by G. E. Berrios, H. L. Freeman, and H. L'Etang, 29–55. London: Royal Society of Medicine, 1991.

Berrios, G. E., and H. L. Freeman. "Dementia before the Twentieth Century." In *Alzheimer's and the Dementias*, edited by G. E. Berrios, H. L. Freeman, and H. L'Etang, 27. London: Royal Society of Medicine, 1991.

Berrios, German, Rogelio Luque, and Jose Villagran. "Schizophrenia: A Conceptual History." *International Journal of Psychology and Psychological Therapy* 3, no. 2 (2003): 111–40.

Bérubé, Michael. "Representation." In *Keywords for Disability Studies,* edited by Rachel Adams and David Serlin, 151–55. New York: New York University Press, 2015.

Bick, Katherine L. "The Early Story of Alzheimer Disease." In *Alzheimer Disease,* edited by Robert Terry, Robert Katzman, Katherine L. Bick, and Sangram Sisodia, 2nd ed., 1–9. Philadelphia: Lippincott Williams Wilkins, 1999.

Bick, Katherine L., Luigi Amaducci, Giancarlo Pepeu, and Alois Alzheimer, eds. *The Early Story of Alzheimer's Disease: Translation of the Historical Papers.* New York: Liviana Press, 1987.

Bish, Randy. "For Those Who Doubt the Existence of Angels." *Pittsburgh Tribune-Review,* October 7, 2010.

Blay, Sergio Luís, and Érica Toledo Pisa Peluso. "Public Stigma: The Community's Tolerance of Alzheimer Disease." *American Journal of Geriatric Psychiatry* 18, no. 2 (2010): 163–71.

Bleckner, Jeff, dir. *Do You Remember Love.* United States: Dave Bell Associates, 1985. DVD.

Blendon, Robert J., John M. Benson, Elizabeth M. Wikler, Kathleen J. Weldon, Jean Georges, Matthew Baumgart, and Beth A. Kallmyer. "The Impact of Experience with a Family Member with Alzheimer's Disease on Views about the Disease across Five Countries." *International Journal of Alzheimer's Disease* 2012 (2012).

Blessed, G., B. E. Tomlinson, and Martin Roth. "The Association between Quantitative Measures of Dementia and of Senile Change in the Cerebral Grey Matter of Elderly Subjects." *British Journal of Psychiatry* 114, no. 512 (1968): 797–811.

Block, Stefan Merrill. *The Story of Forgetting: A Novel.* New York: Random House, 2008.

Blum, Alan. "The Enigma of the Brain and Its Place as Cause, Character and Pretext in the Imaginary of Dementia." *History of the Human Sciences* 25, no. 4 (2012): 108–24.

Blumer, Alder. "The History of Use of the Term 'Dementia.'" *American Journal of Psychiatry* 63, no. 3 (1907): 337–47.

BMI Research. "Americas Pharma and Healthcare Insight—October 2016." *Business Monitor International,* October 2016.

Bodian, David. "A New Method for Staining Nerve Fibers and Nerve Endings in Mounted Paraffin Sections." *Anatomical Record* 65, no. 1 (1936): 89–97.

Boffey, Philip. "Alzheimer's Disease: Families Are Bitter." *New York Times,* May 7, 1985, sec. C.

Bogel, Anne. "The Controversial Ending(s) of Still Alice." *Modern Mrs Darcy* (blog), March 2, 2015. https://modernmrsdarcy.com/controversial-endings -still-alice/.

Bogousslavsky, Julien, and François Boller. *Neurological Disorders in Famous Artists*. New York: Karger, 2005.

Boller, François. "History of Dementia." In *Handbook of Clinical Neurology*, edited by C. Duyckaerts and I. Litvan, 89:3–13. New York: Elsevier, 2008.

Bond, Anthony, Joanna Woodall, T. J. Clark, L. J. Jordanova, Joseph Leo Koerner, National Portrait Gallery, and Art Gallery of New South Wales. *Self Portrait: Renaissance to Contemporary*. London: National Portrait Gallery, 2005.

Bonneau, Georges-Pierre, Thomas Ertl, and Gregory M. Nielson. *Scientific Visualization: The Visual Extraction of Knowledge from Data*. Berlin: Springer, 2006.

Bonner, Thomas. *Becoming a Physician: Medical Education in Great Britain, France, Germany, and the United States, 1750–1945*. New York: Oxford University Press, 1995.

Boris, Eileen, and Jennifer Klein. "Laws of Care: The Supreme Court and Aides to Elderly People." *Dissent* 54, no. 4 (2007): 5–7.

Boris, Eileen, and Jennifer Klein. "Organizing the Carework Economy: When the Private Becomes Public." In *Rethinking U.S. Labor History: Essays on the Working-Class Experience*, edited by Donna T. Haverty-Stacke and Daniel J. Walkowitz, 1756–2009. New York: Continuum, 2010.

Bowen, David M., Carolyn B. Smith, Pamela White, and Alan N. Davison. "Neurotransmitter-Related Enzymes and Indices of Hypoxia in Senile Dementia and Other Abiotrophies." *Brain* 99, no. 3 (1976): 459–96.

Boym, Svetlana. *The Future of Nostalgia*. New York: Basic Books, 2001.

Bracegirdle, Brian. "The History of Histology: A Brief Survey of Sources." *History of Science* 15, no. 2 (1977): 77–101.

Bracegirdle, Brian. *A History of Microscopical Technique*. Ithaca, N.Y.: Cornell University Press, 1978.

Braet, F., and K. Ratinac. "Creating Next-Generation Microscopists: Structural and Molecular Biology at the Crossroads." *Journal of Cellular and Molecular Medicine* 11, no. 4 (2007): 759–63.

Brandeis University. "Seeing Alzheimer's Amyloids with Electron Microscopy for First Time." *ScienceDaily*, May 13, 2008. https://www.sciencedaily.com/releases/2008/05/080512170723.htm.

Broderick, Sheelagh. "Arts Practices in Unreasonable Doubt? Reflections on Understandings of Arts Practices in Healthcare Contexts." *Arts and Health* 3, no. 2 (2011): 95–109.

Brown, Julie K. *Health and Medicine on Display: International Expositions in the United States, 1876–1904*. Cambridge, Mass.: MIT Press, 2009.

Brown, William J., and Michael D. Basil. "Media Celebrities and Public Health: Responses to 'Magic' Johnson's HIV Disclosure and Its Impact on AIDS Risk and High-Risk Behaviors." *Health Communication* 7, no. 4 (1995): 345.

Budson, Andrew E., and Neil W. Kowall, eds. *The Handbook of Alzheimer's Disease and Other Dementias*. Wiley-Blackwell Handbooks of Behavioral Neuroscience 14. Malden, Mass.: Wiley-Blackwell, 2011.

Burke, Lucy. "Introduction: Thinking about Cognitive Impairment." *Journal of Literary and Cultural Disability Studies* 2, no. 1 (2008): i–iv.

Burnham, John C. *How the Idea of Profession Changed the Writing of Medical History*. Vol. 18. London: Wellcome Institute for the History of Medicine, 1998.

Burnham, John C., William McGuire, Sigmund Freud, and C. G. Jung. *Jelliffe, American Psychoanalyst and Physician*. Chicago: University of Chicago Press, 1983.

Burr, Charles W. "Insanity in the Aged." *International Clinics* 17, no. 2 (1907): 231.

Butcher, Howard Karl, Patricia A. Holkup, and Kathleen Coen Buckwalter. "The Experience of Caring for a Family Member with Alzheimer's Disease." *Western Journal of Nursing Research* 23 (2001): 33–55.

Butler, Robert. "Age-ism: Another Form of Bigotry." *Gerontologist* 9, no. 4 (1969): 243–46.

Butler, Robert N. "Is the National Institute on Aging Mission out of Balance?" *The Gerontologist* 39, no. 4 (1999): 389–91.

Butterfield, Herbert. *The Whig Interpretation of History*. London: G. Bell, 1951.

Buxton, William. *Patronizing the Public*. Lanham, Md.: Lexington Books, 2009.

Caddell, Lisa S., and Linda Clare. "Interventions Supporting Self and Identity in People with Dementia: A Systematic Review." *Aging and Mental Health* 15, no. 7 (2011): 797–810.

Caffentzis, George, and Silvia Federici. "Notes on the Edu-Factory and Cognitive Capitalism." In *Toward a Global Autonomous University*, 125–31. Brooklyn, N.Y.: Autonomedia, 2009.

Campbell, Glen, and Julian Raymond. "Not Gonna Miss You," *"I'll Be Me"* Soundtrack. Big Machine Records, 2015. CD.

Canavan, Myrtelle. "A Histological Study of the Optic Nerves in a Random Series of Insane Hospital Cases." *Journal of Nervous and Mental Disease* 43 (1916): 217–30.

Canguilhem, Georges. *The Normal and the Pathological*. New York: Zone Books, 1989.

Capstick, Andrea, and Katherine Ludwin. "Place Memory and Dementia: Findings from Participatory Film-Making in Long-Term Social Care." *Health and Place* 34 (July 2015): 157–63.

Carlson, Licia. *The Faces of Intellectual Disability: Philosophical Reflections*. Apparent 1st ed. Bloomington: Indiana University Press, 2009.

Carper, Jean. *100 Simple Things You Can Do to Prevent Alzheimer's and Age-Related Memory Loss*. New York: Little, Brown, 2010.

Cartwright, Lisa. *Screening the Body: Tracing Medicine's Visual Culture*. Minneapolis: University of Minnesota Press, 1995.

Casamajor, Louis. "Alzheimer, Alois: A Contribution to the Knowledge of the Pathological Neurologia and Its Relation to the Degeneration Process in Nervous Tissues." *Neurological Bulletin* 1, no. 11–12 (1918): 449.

Caserta, Maria, Yvonne Bannon, Francisco Fernandez, Brian Giunta, Mike Schoenberg, and Jun Tan. "Normal Brain Aging: Clinical, Immunological, Neuropsychological, and Neuroimaging Features." In *International Review of Neurobiology: Neurobiology of Dementia*, edited by Alireza Minagar, 84:1–19. Amsterdam: Academic Press, 2009.

Cassavetes, Nick, dir. *The Notebook*. New Line Cinema, 2004. DVD.

Castellani, Rudy J., B. A. Alexiev, D. Phillips, G. Perry, and M. A. Smith. "Microscopic Investigations in Neurodegenerative Diseases." In *Modern Research and Educational Topics in Microscopy*, edited by A. Mendez-Vilas and J. Diaz, 171–82. Badajoz, Spain: Formatex, 2007.

Castellani, Rudy J., Hyoung-Gon Lee, Xiongwei Zhu, Akihiko Nunomura, George Perry, and Mark A. Smith. "Neuropathology of Alzheimer Disease: Pathognomonic but Not Pathogenic." *Acta Neuropathologica* 111, no. 6 (2006): 503–9.

Castellani, Rudy J., George Perry, and Mark A. Smith. "Is Alzheimer's Disease a Myth? When Is Disease a Disease?" *Current Alzheimer Research* 6, no. 1 (2009): 82.

Chamberlin, J. Edward, and Sander L. Gilman. *Degeneration: The Dark Side of Progress*. New York: Columbia University Press, 1985.

Chancellor, Bree, Angel Duncan, and Anjan Chatterjee. "Art Therapy for Alzheimer's Disease and Other Dementias." *Journal of Alzheimer's Disease* 39, no. 1 (2014): 1–11.

Charcot, J. M., and Christopher G. Goetz. *Charcot, the Clinician, the Tuesday Lessons: Excerpts from Nine Case Presentations on General Neurology Delivered at the Salpêtrière Hospital in 1887–88 by Jean-Martin Charcot*. New York: Raven Press, 1987.

Chaufan, Claudia, Brooke Hollister, Jennifer Nazareno, and Patrick Fox. "Medical Ideology as a Double-Edged Sword: The Politics of Cure and Care in the Making of Alzheimer's Disease." *Social Science and Medicine* 74, no. 5 (2012): 788–95.

Chen, Chaomei. *Mapping Scientific Frontiers: The Quest for Knowledge Visualization*. London: Springer, 2003.

Chen, Mel Y. "Brain Fog: The Race for Cripistemology." *Journal of Literary and Cultural Disability Studies* 8, no. 2 (2014): 171–84.

Chess, Eric. "For Early Signs of Dementia, Check Bank Accounts, Not Biomarkers." *STAT* (blog), December 5, 2019. https://www.statnews.com/2019/12/05/dementia-early-warning-check-bank-accounts-not-biomarkers/.

Childs, Donald J. *Modernism and Eugenics: Woolf, Eliot, Yeats and the Culture of Degeneration.* Cambridge: Cambridge University Press, 2001.

Chivers, Sally. *The Silvering Screen: Old Age and Disability in Cinema.* Toronto: University of Toronto Press, 2011.

Christen, Yves, and Patricia Smith Churchland. *Neurophilosophy and Alzheimer's Disease.* Research and Perspectives in Alzheimer's Disease 13. Berlin: Springer, 1992.

Chun, Wendy Hui Kyong. *Programmed Visions Software and Memory.* Cambridge, Mass.: MIT Press, 2011.

Cipriani, Gabriele, Cristina Dolciotti, Lucia Picchi, and Ubaldo Bonuccelli. "Alzheimer and His Disease: A Brief History." *Neurological Sciences* 32, no. 2 (2010): 275–79.

Clark, George, Frederick H. Kasten, and H. J. Conn. *History of Staining.* Baltimore: Williams and Wilkins, 1983.

Clark, T. J., Caroline Tanner, and Lauren White. "Painting from Memory." *Occasional Papers of the Doreen B. Townsend Center for the Humanities,* no. 5 (1996).

Clarke, Adele, Laura Mamo, Jennifer Ruth Fosket, Jennifer R. Fishman, and Janet K. Shim. *Biomedicalization: Technoscience, Health, and Illness in the U.S.* Durham, N.C.: Duke University Press, 2010.

Clarke, Adele, Janet K. Shim, Laura Mamo, Jennifer Ruth Fosket, and Jennifer R. Fishman. "Biomedicalization: Technoscientific Transformations of Health, Illness, and U.S. Biomedicine." *American Sociological Review* 68, no. 2 (2003): 161–94.

Clarke, Juanne N. "The Case of the Missing Person: Alzheimer's Disease in Mass Print Magazines 1991–2001." *Health Communication* 19, no. 3 (2006): 269–76.

Clough, Patricia Ticineto, and Jean Halley, eds. *The Affective Turn: Theorizing the Social.* 1st ed. Durham, N.C.: Duke University Press, 2007.

Coe, Fredric. "'A Sudden Lift of Wings': Poetry and Prose about Alzheimer's Disease." *Perspectives in Biology and Medicine* 54, no. 1 (2011): 106–14.

Cohen, Alan S., and Evan Calkins. "Electron Microscopic Observations on a Fibrous Component in Amyloid of Diverse Origins." *Nature* 183, no. 4669 (1959): 1202–3.

Cohen, Ann D., and William E. Klunk. "Early Detection of Alzheimer's Disease Using PiB and FDG PET." *Neurobiology of Disease* 72, Part A (2014): 117–22.

Cohen, Donna. "Preventing the Unthinkable: Get Rid of Guns and Other Deadly Weapons in Your Home." *Care ADvantage,* Fall/Winter 2014–15.

Cohen, Donna, and Carl Eisdorfer. *The Loss of Self: A Family Resource for the Care of Alzheimer's Disease and Related Disorders.* New York: W. W. Norton, 2001.

Cohen, Gene. "Historical Views and Evolution of Concepts." In *Alzheimer's Disease*, edited by Barry Reisberg, 29–33. New York: Free Press, 1983.

Cohen, Gene. "Research on Creativity and Aging: The Positive Impact of the Arts on Health and Illness." *Generations* 30, no. 1 (2006): 7–15.

Cohen, Lawrence. *No Aging in India: Alzheimer's, the Bad Family, and Other Modern Things*. Berkeley: University of California Press, 1998.

Cohen, Lawrence. "Politics of Care." *Medical Anthropology Quarterly* 22, no. 4 (2008): 336–39.

Cohen, Lawrence, and Annette Leibing, eds. *Thinking about Dementia: Culture, Loss, and the Anthropology of Senility*. New Brunswick, N.J.: Rutgers University Press, 2006.

Cohen-Shalev, Amir, and Esther-Lee Marcus. "An Insider's View of Alzheimer: Cinematic Portrayals of the Struggle for Personhood." *International Journal of Ageing and Later Life* 7, no. 2 (2013): 73–96.

Cole, Thomas. *The Journey of Life: A Cultural History of Aging in America*. Cambridge: Cambridge University Press, 1992.

Coleman, Raymond. "The Impact of Histochemistry—a Historical Perspective." *Acta Histochemica* 102, no. 1 (2000): 5–14.

Collins, Allan. "Why Cognitive Science." *Cognitive Science* 1, no. 1 (1977): 1–2.

Comer, Ben. "Renewed Focus on Alzheimer's Could Help New Drugs to Market." *Medical Marketing and Media,* December 16, 2010.

Committee on the Future Health Care Workforce for Older Americans. *Retooling for an Aging America*. Washington, D.C.: National Academies Press, 2008.

Compain, Frederic, dir. *Glassy-Eyed: William Utermohlen, Vision from within Alzheimer's Disease*. Icarus, 2010. DVD.

Conn, H. J. *Biological Stains: A Handbook on the Nature and Uses of the Dyes Employed in the Biological Laboratory*. 3rd ed. Geneva, N.Y.: W. F. Humphrey Press, 1936.

Conn, H. J., and Lloyd Arnold. *The History of Staining; with Contributions from Lloyd Arnold (and Others)*. Geneva, N.Y.: Biotech, 1948.

Cook-Deegan, Robert Mullan. "The Genetics of Alzheimer's Disease: Some Future Implications." In *Concepts of Alzheimer Disease: Biological, Clinical, and Cultural Perspectives,* edited by Peter J. Whitehouse, Konrad Maurer, and Jesse F. Ballenger, 321. Baltimore: Johns Hopkins University Press, 2000.

Coole, Diana, and Samantha Frost, eds. *New Materialisms: Ontology, Agency, and Politics*. Durham, N.C.: Duke University Press, 2010.

Coopmans, Catelijne, Janet Vertesi, Michael E. Lynch, and Steve Woolgar. Introduction to *Representation in Scientific Practice Revisited,* edited by Catelijne Coopmans, Janet Vertesi, and Michael E. Lynch, 1–12. Cambridge, Mass.: MIT Press, 2014.

Corsellis, J. A. *Mental Illness and the Ageing Brain*. Oxford: Oxford University Press, 1962.

Couldry, Nick, and Andreas Hepp. "Conceptualizing Mediatization: Contexts, Traditions, Arguments: Editorial." *Communication Theory* 23, no. 3 (2013): 191–202.

Cowl, Andrielle L., and Joseph E. Gaugler. "Efficacy of Creative Arts Therapy in Treatment of Alzheimer's Disease and Dementia: A Systematic Literature Review." *Activities, Adaptation, and Aging* 38, no. 4 (2014): 281–330.

Crary, Jonathan. *Techniques of the Observer: On Vision and Modernity in the Nineteenth Century*. Cambridge, Mass.: MIT Press, 1990.

Cronin-Golomb, Alice, and Patrick R. Hof. *Vision in Alzheimer's Disease*. Vol. 34. Basel: Karger, 2004.

Crutch, Sebastian J., Ron Isaacs, and Martin N. Rossor. "Some Workmen Can Blame Their Tools: Artistic Change in an Individual with Alzheimer's Disease." *Lancet* 357, no. 9274 (2001): 2129–33.

Crutch, Sebastian J., and Martin N. Rossor. "Artistic Changes in Alzheimer's Disease." *International Review of Neurobiology* 74 (2006): 147–61.

Cummings, Jeffrey L., Travis Morstorf, and Kate Zhong. "Alzheimer's Disease Drug-Development Pipeline: Few Candidates, Frequent Failures." *Alzheimer's Research and Therapy* 6, no. 4 (2014): 37.

Cummings, Jeffrey, Carl Reiber, and Parvesh Kumar. "The Price of Progress: Funding and Financing Alzheimer's Disease Drug Development." *Alzheimer's and Dementia: Translational Research and Clinical Interventions* 4 (January 1, 2018): 330–43.

Dahm, Ralf. "Alois Alzheimer and the Beginnings of Research into Alzheimer's Disease." In *Alzheimer: 100 Years and Beyond,* edited by M. Jucker, K. Beyreuther, C. Haass, and R. M. Nitsch, 49. Berlin: Springer, 2006.

Daly, Michael. "Reagan Took Up Cause for Mom." *Daily News* (New York), June 9, 2004, sec. News.

Daniels, Katherine J., Angela L. Lamson, and Jennifer Hodgson. "An Exploration of the Marital Relationship and Alzheimer's Disease: One Couple's Story." *Families Systems Health* 25, no. 2 (2007): 162.

Daston, Lorraine, and Peter Galison. *Objectivity*. New York: Zone Books, 2007.

Davidoff, Leo M., and Bernard S. Epstein. *The Abnormal Pneumoencephalogram*. Philadelphia: Lea and Febiger, 1950.

Daviglus, Martha L., Carl C. Bell, Wade Berrettini, Phyllis E. Bowen Jr., Connolly E. Sander, Nancy Jean Cox, Jacqueline M. Dunbar-Jacob, et al. "National Institutes of Health State-of-the-Science Conference Statement: Preventing Alzheimer Disease and Cognitive Decline." *Annals of Internal Medicine* 153, no. 3 (2010): 176–81.

Davis, Lennard J., ed. *The Disability Studies Reader*. 4th ed. New York: Routledge, 2013.

Davis, Lennard J. "Editorial: Disability-Visuality." *Journal of Visual Culture* 5, no. 2 (2006): 131–36.

Davis, Lennard. *The End of Normal: Identity in a Biocultural Era*. Ann Arbor: University of Michigan Press, 2014.

Davis, Lennard J. *Enforcing Normalcy: Disability, Deafness, and the Body*. New York: Verso, 1995.

Davis, Lennard J., and Michael Bérubé. *Bending Over Backwards: Disability, Dismodernism and Other Difficult Positions*. 1st ed. New York: New York University Press, 2002.

Deacon, David, and James Stanyer. "Mediatization: Key Concept or Conceptual Bandwagon?" *Media, Culture, and Society* 36, no. 7 (2014): 1032–44.

Deacon, David, and James Stanyer. "'Mediatization and' or 'Mediatization of'? A Response to Hepp et al." *Media, Culture, and Society* 37, no. 4 (2015): 655–57.

Dean, Mitchell. *Governmentality: Power and Rule in Modern Society*. London: Sage, 1999.

DeBaggio, Thomas. *Losing My Mind: An Intimate Look at Life with Alzheimer's*. New York: Free Press, 2002.

Decker, Hannah. "How Kraepelinian Was Kraepelin? How Kraepelinian Are the Neo-Kraepelinians?—From Emil Kraepelin to DSM-III." *History of Psychiatry*, September 18, 2007.

DeKosky, S. T., and J. H. Growdon. "The Human Alzheimer Disease Project: Answering the Call." *JAMA Neurology* 73, no. 4 (2016): 373–74.

Delbo, Charlotte. *Days and Memory*. Marlboro, Vt.: Marlboro Press, 1990.

D'Harnoncourt, Rene. *The Museum of Modern Art*. New York: Art in America, 1964.

Dickerson, Bradford C. "Molecular Neuroimaging of the Dementias." In *The Handbook of Alzheimer's Disease and Other Dementias*, edited by Andrew E. Budson and Neil W. Kowall, 557–74. London: Wiley-Blackwell, 2011.

Dillman, Rob J. M. "Alzheimer Disease: Epistemological Lessons from History?" In *Concepts of Alzheimer's Disease: Biological, Clinical, and Cultural Perspectives*, edited by Peter J. Whitehouse, Konrad Maurer, and Jesse F. Ballenger, 129–57. Baltimore: Johns Hopkins University Press, 2000.

Doraiswamy, P. Murali, and Lisa Gwyther. *The Alzheimer's Action Plan*. New York: St. Martin's Press, 2008.

Dorfman, Natalia. "The Age of Alzheimer's." *Medical Marketing and Media*, August 1, 2006.

Dowbiggin, Ian Robert. *Keeping America Sane: Psychiatry and Eugenics in the United States and Canada, 1880–1940*. Ithaca, N.Y.: Cornell University Press, 1997.

Duckworth, K., J. H. Halpern, R. K. Schutt, and C. Gillespie. "Use of Schizophrenia as a Metaphor in US Newspapers." *Psychiatric Services* 54, no. 10 (2003): 1402–4.

Dumit, Joseph. "How (Not) to Do Things with Brain Images." In *Representation in Scientific Practice Revisited,* edited by Catelijne Coopmans, Janet Vertesi, and Michael E. Lynch, 291–313. Cambridge, Mass. MIT Press, 2014.

Dumit, Joseph. "Is It Me or My Brain? Depression and Neuroscientific Facts." *Journal of Medical Humanities* 24, no. 1 (2003): 35–47.

Dumit, Joseph. "Pharmaceutical Witnessing: Drugs for Life in an Era of Direct-to-Consumer Advertising." In *Technologized Images, Technologized Bodies: Anthropological Approaches to a New Politics of Vision,* edited by P. Harvey, J. Edwards, and P. Wade, 37–63. Oxford: Berghahn, 2010.

Dumit, Joseph. *Picturing Personhood: Brain Scans and Biomedical Identity.* Princeton, N.J.: Princeton University Press, 2004.

Duyckaerts, Charles, and Jean-Jacques Hauw. "Of Stains and Brains: A Brief Account of How Microscopic and Clinical Observations Contributed to the Understanding of Alzheimer's Disease." In *Alzheimer: 100 Years and Beyond,* edited by M. Jucker, K. Beyreuther, C. Haass, and R. M. Nitsch, 109–13. Berlin: Springer, 2006.

Eckholm, Erik. "Robertson Stirs Passions with Suggestion to Divorce an Alzheimer's Patient." *New York Times,* September 17, 2011.

Edwards, David. *Art Therapy.* London: Sage, 2004.

Eedgerly. "Oxygen Therapy for Alzheimer's?" *Alzheimers and Dementia* (blog), January 23, 2012. http://www.alznorcalblog.org/2012/01/23/oxygen-therapy-alzheimers/.

Ehresman, Crystal. "From Rendering to Remembering: Art Therapy for People with Alzheimer's Disease." *International Journal of Art Therapy* 19, no. 1 (2014): 43–51.

Ellard, Kristen. "The Struggle for Identity: Issues and Debates in the Emerging Specialty of American Psychiatry from the Late 19th Century to Post-WWII." *Human Architecture* 4, no. 1/2 (2006): 227–64.

Ellcessor, Elizabeth. *Restricted Access: Media, Disability, and the Politics of Participation.* New York: New York University Press, 2016.

Ellena, Eric, and Berna Huebner. *I Remember Better When I Paint.* Films Media Group, 2009. Internet resource and film.

Ellis, Katie, and Gerard Goggin. *Disability and the Media.* Key Concerns in Media Studies 9. Houndmills, U.K.: Palgrave Macmillan, 2015.

Ellis, Katie, and Mike Kent. *Disability and New Media.* New York: Routledge, 2011.

English, W. H. "Alzheimer's Disease: Its Incidence and Recognition." *Psychiatric Quarterly* 16, no. 1 (1942): 91–106.

English, W. H. "Alzheimer's Disease: Review of the Literature and Report of One Case." *Psychiatric Quarterly* 14, no. 3 (1940): 583–94.

Engstrom, Eric. "Researching Dementia in Imperial Germany: Alois Alzheimer and the Economies of Psychiatric Practice." *Culture Medicine Psychiatry* 31 (2007): 405–13.

Ernaux, Annie, and Tanya Leslie. *I Remain in Darkness*. 1st Seven Stories Press ed. New York: Seven Stories Press, 1999.

Espinel, Carlos Hugo. "De Kooning's Late Colours and Forms: Dementia, Creativity, and the Healing Power of Art." *The Lancet* 347, no. 9008 (1996): 1096–98.

Eyre, Richard, dir. *Iris*. Miramax, 2001. DVD.

Facher, Lev. "To Advance Precision Medicine, NIH Turns to Long-Mistreated Communities." *STAT* (blog), September 22, 2017. https://www.statnews.com/2017/09/22/nih-precision-medicine-all-of-us/.

Fackelmann, Kathleen. "Alzheimer's Program Is One from the Art." *USA Today*, October 16, 2007. http://www.usatoday.com/news/health/2007-10-16-alzheimers-art_N.htm.

Faircloth, Christopher A. *Aging Bodies: Images and Everyday Experience*. Walnut Creek, Calif.: AltaMira Press, 2003.

Farah, Martha J., and Andrea S. Heberlein. "Personhood and Neuroscience: Naturalizing or Nihilating?" *American Journal of Bioethics* 7, no. 1 (2007): 37–48.

Farmer, Peter M., Arthur Peck, and Robert D. Terry. "Correlations among Numbers of Neuritic Plaques, Neurofibrillary Tangles, and the Severity of Senile Dementia: 135." *Journal of Neuropathology* 35, no. 3 (1976): 367.

Fazio, Sam. *The Enduring Self in People with Alzheimer's: Getting to the Heart of Individualized Care*. Baltimore: Health Professions Press, 2008.

Featherstone, Mike, and Andrew Wernick, eds. *Images of Aging*. London: Routledge, 1995.

Feder Kittay, Eva. "When Caring Is Just and Justice Is Caring: Justice in Mental Retardation." In *The Subject of Care: Feminist Perspectives on Dependency*, edited by Eva Feder Kittay and Ellen K. Feder, 257–76. Feminist Constructions 9. Lanham, Md.: Rowman and Littlefield, 2002.

Feder Kittay, Eva, and Ellen K. Feder, eds. Introduction to *The Subject of Care: Feminist Perspectives on Dependency*, 1–12. Feminist Constructions 9. Lanham, Md.: Rowman and Littlefield, 2002.

Feffer, Stuart. "Ernst Abbe, Carl Zeiss, and the Transformation of Microscopical Optics." In *Scientific Credibility and Technical Standards in 19th and Early 20th Century Germany and Britain*, edited by J. Z. Buchwald, 23–66. Cornwall, U.K.: Kluwer, 1996.

Feldman, Allen. "On the Actuarial Gaze." *Cultural Studies* 19, no. 2 (2005): 203–26.

Feldman, Ilana, and Miriam Ticktin. *In the Name of Humanity: The Government of Threat and Care.* Durham N.C.: Duke University Press, 2010.

Fernandez-Duque, Diego, Jessica Evans, Colton Christian, and Sara D. Hodges. "Superfluous Neuroscience Information Makes Explanations of Psychological Phenomena More Appealing." *Journal of Cognitive Neuroscience* 27, no. 5 (2014): 926–44.

Ferraro, Armando. "The Origin and Formation of Senile Plaques." *Archives of Neurology and Psychiatry* 25, no. 5 (1931): 1042.

Ferraro, Armando. "Recent Advances and Progressive Trend of Neuro-pathology in Psychiatry." *Psychiatric Quarterly* 19 (1945): 267–82.

Ferraro, Armando, and George A. Jervis. "Alzheimer's Disease." *Psychiatric Quarterly* 15, no. 1 (1941): 3–16.

Filley, Christopher M. "Caregivers Take Center Stage in 'The Savages': The Savages. Directed by Tamara Jenkins. Searchlight Pictures 2007." *Neurology Today* 8, no. 3 (2008): 20.

Fineman, Martha. "Masking Dependency: The Political Role of Family Rhetoric." In *The Subject of Care: Feminist Perspectives on Dependency,* edited by Eva Feder Kittay and Ellen K. Feder, 215–44. Feminist Constructions 9. Lanham, Md.: Rowman and Littlefield, 2002.

Finger, Stanley. *Minds behind the Brain: A History of the Pioneers and Their Discoveries.* Oxford: Oxford University Press, 2004.

Finn, Robin. "From Rock Videos to an Alzheimer's Stamp." *New York Times,* October 31, 2008.

Fischman, Josh. "Alzheimer's Today." *U.S. News and World Report,* December 11, 2006.

Flegenheimer, Matt. "Tale of Love and Illness Ends in Deaths." *New York Times,* March 30, 2012. http://www.nytimes.com/2012/03/31/us/love-that-endured-alzheimers-ends-in-2-deaths.html.

Fleisher, Adam S., Michael Donohue, Kewei Chen, James B. Brewer, and Paul S. Aisen. "Applications of Neuroimaging to Disease-Modification Trials in Alzheimer's Disease." *Behavioural Neurology* 21, no. 1 (2009): 129–36.

Fletcher, Lydia C. B., Katie E. Burke, Paul L. Caine, Natasha L. Rinne, Charlotte A. Braniff, Hannah R. Davis, Kathryn A. Miles, and Claire Packer. "Diagnosing Alzheimer's Disease: Are We Any Nearer to Useful Biomarker-Based, Non-Invasive Tests?" *GMS Health Technology Assessment* 9 (2013): Article 1.

Flexner, Abraham. *Medical Education in the United States and Canada: A Report to the Carnegie Foundation for the Advancement of Teaching.* New York: Carnegie Foundation for the Advancement of Teaching, 1910.

Folino, Lauren. "Roche Launches First-Ever Early-Stage Alzheimer's Awareness Website." *Medical Marketing,* September 21, 2011.

Fortanasce, Vincent. *The Anti-Alzheimer's Prescription: The Science-Proven Plan to Start at Any Age.* New York: Gotham Books, 2008.

Foucault, Michel. *The Birth of the Clinic: An Archaeology of Medical Perception.* Translated by Alan Sheridan. New York: Vintage Books, 1973.

Foucault, Michel. *History of Madness.* Edited by Jean Khalfa. London: Routledge, 2009.

Foucault, Michel. "Of Other Spaces." In *The Visual Culture Reader,* 2nd ed., edited by Nicholas Mirzoeff, 229–42. London: Routledge, 2002.

Foucault, Michel. *Psychiatric Power: Lectures at the Collège de France, 1973–74.* Edited by Jacques Lagrange. New York: Palgrave Macmillan, 2006.

Foucault, Michel. *Society Must Be Defended: Lectures at the Collège de France, 1975–76.* Edited by Mauro Bertani and Alessandro Fontana. New York: Picador, 2003.

Foucault, Michel. *Technologies of the Self: A Seminar with Michel Foucault.* Edited by Luther H. Martin, Huck Gutman, and Patrick H. Hutton. Amherst: University of Massachusetts Press, 1988.

Fox, Daniel M., and Christopher Lawrence. *Photographing Medicine: Images and Power in Britain and America since 1840.* Vol. 21. New York: Greenwood Press, 1988.

Fox, Jacob H., Jordan L. Topel, and Michael S. Huckman. "Use of Computerized Tomography in Senile Dementia." *Journal of Neurology, Neurosurgery, and Psychiatry* 38, no. 10 (1975): 948–53.

Fox, Patrick. "From Senility to Alzheimer's Disease: The Rise of the Alzheimer's Disease Movement." *Milbank Quarterly* 67, no. 1 (1989): 58–102.

Frackowiak, Richard S. J. *Imaging Neuroscience.* Oxford: Oxford University Press, 2003.

Franzen, Jonathan. "My Father's Brain: What Alzheimer's Takes Away." *New Yorker,* September 10, 2001.

Freeman, H. L. "Social Aspects of Alzheimer's Disease." In *Alzheimer's and the Dementias,* edited by G. E. Berrios, H. L. Freeman, and H. L'Etang, 57–68. London: Royal Society of Medicine, 1991.

Freeman, Joseph T. *Aging: Its History and Literature.* New York: Human Sciences Press, 1979.

Freeman, Joseph T. "Nascher: Excerpts from His Life, Letters, and Works." *The Gerontologist* 1, no. 1 (1961): 17–26.

Friede, Reinhard L., and Kenneth R. Magee. "Alzheimer's Disease: Presentation of a Case with Pathologic and Enzymatic-Histochemical Observations." *Neurology* 12, no. 3 (1962): 213–22.

Friesen, Norm, and Theo Hug. "After the Mediatic Turn: McLuhan's Training of the Senses and Media Pedagogy Today." In *Medialität und Realität,* edited by Johannes Fromme, Stefan Iske, and Winfried Marotzki, 83–101. Wiesbaden, Germany: VS Verlag für Sozialwissenschaften, 2011.

Fritsch, Thomas, Jung Kwak, Stacey Grant, Josh Lang, Rhonda R. Montgomery, and Anne D. Basting. "Impact of TimeSlips, a Creative Expression Intervention Program, on Nursing Home Residents with Dementia and Their Caregivers." *The Gerontologist* 49, no. 1 (2009): 117–27.

Fromm, Erich. *The Art of Loving.* 15th Anniversary ed. New York: Harper Perennial Modern Classics, 2006.

Fuller, Solomon. "Alzheimer's Disease: Senium Praecox—The Report of a Case and Review of Published Cases." *Journal of Nervous and Mental Disease* 39, no. 7 (1912): 440–55.

Fuller, Solomon. "Alzheimer's Disease: Senium Praecox—The Report of a Case and Review of Published Cases." *Journal of Nervous and Mental Disease* 39, no. 8 (1912): 536–57.

Fuller, Solomon Carter. "Amyloid Degeneration of the Brain in Two Cases of General Paresis." *American Journal of Insanity* 70, no. 4 (1914): 323–57.

Fuller, Solomon. "Errata." *American Journal of Psychiatry* 68, no. 3 (1912): 522.

Fuller, Solomon. "Histopathological Alterations in the Cellular Neuroglia and Fibrillary Mesoblastic Components of the Cerebral Cortical Interstitium." *Boston Medical and Surgical Journal* 190, no. 8 (1924): 314–22.

Fuller, Solomon Carter. "A Phenomenon Observed in the Blood of Morphinomaniacs." *New England Medical Gazette* 34, no. 6 (1899): 241–50.

Fuller, Solomon Carter. "Photomicrographs for Illustrating Histological Objects." *Medical Student* 13, no. 6 (1901): 80–84.

Fuller, Solomon. "A Study of the Miliary Plaques Found in Brains of the Aged." *American Journal of Psychiatry* 68, no. 2 (1911): 147–219.

Fuller, Solomon. "Study of the Neurofibrils in Dementia Paralytica, Dementia Senilis, Chronic Alcoholism, Cerebral Lues, and Microcephalic Idiocy." *American Journal of Psychiatry* 63, no. 4 (1907): 415–81.

Fuller, Solomon Carter, and Henry Klopp. "An Examination of Three Thousand One Hundred and Forty Admissions to Westborough State Hospital with Reference to the Frequency of Involution Melancholia (Kraepelin's Melancholia)." *Journal of the American Institute of Homeopathy* 4, no. 7 (1912): 855–59.

Fuller, Solomon, and Henry Klopp. "Further Observations on Alzheimer's Disease." *American Journal of Insanity* 69, no. 1 (1912): 17–29.

Gaines, Atwood D., and Eric T. Juengst. "Origin Myths in Bioethics: Constructing Sources, Motives and Reason in Bioethic(s)." *Culture, Medicine, and Psychiatry* 32, no. 3 (2008): 303–27.

Gaines, Atwood D., and Peter J. Whitehouse. "Building a Mystery: Alzheimer's Disease, Mild Cognitive Impairment, and Beyond." *Philosophy, Psychiatry, and Psychology* 13, no. 1 (2006): 61–74, 89, 91.

Garland-Thomson, Rosemarie. "Disability Studies: A Field Emerged." *American Quarterly* 65, no. 4 (2013): 915–26.

Garland-Thomson, Rosemarie. *Staring: How We Look.* 1st ed. Oxford: Oxford University Press, 2009.

Gavrus, Delia. "Men of Dreams and Men of Action: Neurologists, Neurosurgeons, and the Performance of Professional Identity, 1920–1950." *Bulletin of the History of Medicine* 85, no. 1 (2011): 57–92.

Genova, Lisa. *Still Alice.* New York: Simon and Schuster, 2007.

George, Daniel R., Heather L. Stuckey, Caroline F. Dillon, and Megan M. Whitehead. "Impact of Participation in TimeSlips, a Creative Group-Based Storytelling Program, on Medical Student Attitudes toward Persons with Dementia: A Qualitative Study." *The Gerontologist* 51, no. 5 (2011): 699–703.

George, Danny, and Peter Whitehouse. "The Classification of Alzheimer's Disease and Mild Cognitive Impairment." In *Treating Dementia: Do We Have a Pill for It?*, edited by Jesse F. Ballenger, Peter J. Whitehouse, Constantine G. Lyketsos, Peter V. Rabins, and Jason Karlawish, 5–24. Baltimore: Johns Hopkins University Press, 2009.

George, Daniel, Peter Whitehouse, and Jesse F. Ballenger. "The Evolving Classification of Dementia: Placing the DSM-V in a Meaningful Historical and Cultural Context and Pondering the Future of 'Alzheimer's.'" *Culture, Medicine, and Psychiatry* 35, no. 3 (2011): 417–35.

Gibson, Peter H., and B. E. Tomlinson. "Numbers of Hirano Bodies in the Hippocampus of Normal and Demented People with Alzheimer's Disease." *Journal of the Neurological Sciences* 33, no. 1–2 (1977): 199–206.

Giddens, Anthony. *Modernity and Self-Identity: Self and Society in the Late Modern Age.* Cambridge: Polity Press, 1991.

Gillick, Muriel R. *Tangled Minds: Understanding Alzheimer's Disease and Other Dementias.* New York: Dutton, 1998.

Gilman, Sander L. *The Case of Sigmund Freud: Medicine and Identity at the Fin de Siècle.* Baltimore: Johns Hopkins University Press, 1993.

Gilman, Sander L. *Difference and Pathology: Stereotypes of Sexuality, Race, and Madness.* Ithaca, N.Y.: Cornell University Press, 1985.

Gilman, Sander L. *Disease and Representation: Images of Illness from Madness to AIDS.* Ithaca, N.Y.: Cornell University Press, 1988.

Gilman, Sander L. *Picturing Health and Illness: Images of Identity and Difference.* Baltimore: Johns Hopkins University Press, 1995.

Gilman, Sander L. *Seeing the Insane.* Lincoln: University of Nebraska Press, 1982.

Glenner. "Town Square." *The George G. Glenner Alzheimer's Family Centers, Inc.* (blog), June 25, 2019. https://glenner.org/town-square/.

Goedert, Michel. "Oskar Fischer and the Study of Dementia." *Brain* 132, no. 4 (2009): 1102–11.

Goedert, Michel, and Bernardino Ghetti. "Alois Alzheimer: His Life and Times." *Brain Pathology* 17, no. 1 (2007): 57–62.

Goetz, Christopher G. "Visual Art in the Neurologic Career of Jean-Martin Charcot." *Archives of Neurology* 48, no. 4 (1991): 421–25.

Goggin, Gerard, and Christopher Newell. *Digital Disability: The Social Construction of Disability in New Media*. Lanham, Md.: Rowman and Littlefield, 2003.

Gómez, Edgar, and Helen Thornham. "Selfies beyond Self-Representation: The (Theoretical) f(r)Ictions of a Practice." *Journal of Aesthetics and Culture* 7, no. 1 (2015).

Gooblar, Jonathan, and Brian Carpenter. "Print Advertisements for Alzheimer's Disease Drugs: Informational and Transformational Features." *American Journal of Alzheimer's Disease and Other Dementias* 28, no. 4 (2013): 355–62.

Good, Catriona. "Dementia and Ageing." *British Medical Bulletin* 65 (2003): 159–68.

Goodey, C. F. *A History of Intelligence and "Intellectual Disability": The Shaping of Psychology in Early Modern Europe*. Farnham, U.K.: Ashgate, 2011.

Gordon, Michael R. "In Poignant Public Letter, Reagan Reveals That He Has Alzheimer's." *New York Times*, November 6, 1994, sec. U.S. https://www.ny times.com/1994/11/06/us/in-poignant-public-letter-reagan-reveals-that -he-has-alzheimer-s.html.

Grady, Denise. "Self-Portraits Chronicle a Descent into Alzheimer's." *New York Times*, October 24, 2006. http://www.nytimes.com/2006/10/24/health/ 24alzh.html.

Grady, Denise, Beatrice De Gea, Nick Harbaugh, Nancy Donaldson, and Soo-Jeong Kang. "When Illness Makes a Spouse a Stranger." *New York Times*, May 5, 2012.

Graeber, M. B., S. Kösel, S. Egensperger, E. Grasbon-Frodl, U. Muller, K. Bisel, P. Hoff, H. J. Moller, P. Mehraein, and K. Fujisawa. "Rediscovery of the Case Described by Alois Alzheimer in 1911: Historical, Histological and Molecular Genetic Analysis." *Neurogenetics* 1 (1997): 73–80.

Graeber, M. B., S. Kösel, E. Grasbon-Frodl, H. J. Möller, and P. Mehraein. "Histopathology and APOE Genotype of the First Alzheimer Disease Patient, Auguste D." *Neurogenetics* 1, no. 1 (1998): 223–28.

Graeber, M. B., and P. Mehraein. "Reanalysis of the First Case of Alzheimer's Disease." *European Archives of Clinical Neuroscience* 249, Suppl. 3 (1999): 10–13.

Graff-Radford, Neill R., Lilah, M. Besser, Julia E. Crook, Walter A. Kukull, and Dennis W. Dickson. "Neuropathologic Differences by Race from the National Alzheimer's Coordinating Center." *Alzheimer's and Dementia* 12, no. 6 (2016): 669–77.

Graham, Judith. "Loneliness as a Health Threat: New Campaign Raises Awareness." *STAT* (blog), November 16, 2016. https://www.statnews.com/2016/11/16/loneliness-health/.

Grasel, Elmar, Jens Wiltfang, and Johannes Kornhuber. "Non-drug Therapies for Dementia: An Overview of the Current Situation with Regard to Proof of Effectiveness." *Dementia and Geriatric Cognitive Disorders* 15, no. 3 (2003): 115–25.

Graw, Isabelle. "The Value of Painting: Notes on Unspecificity, Indexicality and Highly Valuable Quasi- Persons." In *Joy Forever: The Political Economy of Social Creativity*, edited by Michal Kozlowski, Agnieszka Kurant, Janek Sowa, Krystian Szadkowski, and Kuba Szreder, 65–73. London: MayFly Books, 2014.

Greenfield, J. Godwin. *Neuropathology*. London: E. Arnold, 1958.

Gregg, Melissa. *Cultural Studies' Affective Voices*. New York: Palgrave Macmillan, 2006.

Gregg, Melissa, and Gregory J. Seigworth, eds. *The Affect Theory Reader*. Durham, N.C.: Duke University Press, 2010.

Greider, Linda. "In Museums, Those with Alzheimer's Find Themselves Again." *AARP Bulletin*, October 2, 2009. http://www.aarp.org/health/brain-health/info-10-2009/in_museums_those_with_alzheimer_s_find_themselves_again.html.

Gretton, Cosima, and Dominic H. Ffytche. "Art and the Brain: A View from Dementia." *International Journal of Geriatric Psychiatry* 29, no. 2 (2014): 111–26.

Griffiths, Gareth. "Bringing Electron Microscopy Back into Focus for Cell Biology." *Trends in Cell Biology* 11, no. 4 (2001): 153–54.

Gross, Jane. *A Bittersweet Season*. New York: Knopf, 2011.

Grossberg, Lawrence. *Caught in the Crossfire: Kids, Politics, and America's Future*. Boulder, Colo.: Paradigm, 2005.

Grossberg, Lawrence. "Does Cultural Studies Have Futures? Should It? (Or What's the Matter with New York?): Cultural Studies, Contexts, and Conjunctures." *Cultural Studies* 20, no. 1 (2006): 1–32.

Grossman, Lev. "*Time*'s Person of the Year: You." *Time*, December 25, 2006.

Grundke-Iqbal, I., K. Iqbal, M. Quinlan, Y. C. Tung, M. S. Zaidi, and H. M. Wisniewski. "Microtubule-Associated Protein Tau: A Component of Alzheimer Paired Helical Filaments." *Journal of Biological Chemistry* 261, no. 13 (1986): 6084–89.

Gubrium, Jaber. *Oldtimers and Alzheimer's: The Descriptive Organization of Senility*. Greenwich, Conn.: JAI Press, 1986.

Gubrium, Jaber, and James Holstein. "The Everyday Visibility of the Aging Body." In *Aging Bodies: Images and Everyday Experience*, edited by Christopher A. Faircloth, 205–28. Walnut Creek, Calif.: AltaMira Press, 2003.

Guinn, David. "Mental Competence, Caregivers, and the Process of Consent: Research Involving Alzheimer's Patients or Others with Decreasing Mental Capacity." *Cambridge Quarterly of Healthcare Ethics* 11, no. 3 (2002): 230–45.

Gullette, Margaret Morganroth. *Aged by Culture*. Chicago: University of Chicago Press, 2004.

Hacking, Ian. *Representing and Intervening: Introductory Topics in the Philosophy of Natural Science*. Cambridge: Cambridge University Press, 1983.

Hagner, Michael. "Cultivating the Cortex in German Neuroanatomy." *Science in Context* 14, no. 4 (2001): 541.

Hagner, Michael, and Cornelius Borck. "Mindful Practices: On the Neurosciences in the Twentieth Century." *Science in Context* 14, no. 4 (2001): 507.

Haller, Beth A. *Representing Disability in an Ableist World: Essays on Mass Media*. Louisville, Ky.: Advocado Press, 2010.

Halpern, Orit. *Beautiful Data: A History of Vision and Reason since 1945*. Illustrated ed. Durham, N.C.: Duke University Press, 2015.

Hammond, John. *The Camera Lucida in Art and Science*. Bristol, U.K.: Adam Hilger, 1987.

Hansen, Mark B. N. "Media Theory." *Theory, Culture, and Society* 23, no. 2–3 (2006): 297–306.

Hardt, Michael, and Antonio Negri. *Commonwealth*. Cambridge, Mass.: Belknap Press of Harvard University Press, 2009.

Hardy, John. "A Hundred Years of Alzheimer's Disease Research." *Neuron* 52, no. 1 (2006): 3–13.

Harlin, Renny, dir. *Deep Blue Sea*. Warner Bros., 1999. DVD.

Harman, Graham. *Prince of Networks: Bruno Latour and Metaphysics*. Prahran, Vic.: Re.press, 2009.

Harrington, Anne. *Medicine, Mind, and the Double Brain: A Study in Nineteenth-Century Thought*. Princeton, N.J.: Princeton University Press, 1987.

Haskins, Ekaterina. "'Put Your Stamp on History': The USPS Commemorative Program *Celebrate the Century* and Postmodern Collective Memory." *Quarterly Journal of Speech* 89, no. 1 (2003): 1–18.

Haugse, John. *Heavy Snow: My Father's Disappearance into Alzheimer's*. Deerfield Beach, Fla.: Health Communications, 1999.

Hawes, D., C. R. Taylor, and R. Cote. "Immunohistochemistry." In *Modern Surgical Pathology*, edited by N. Weidner, R. Cote, S. Suster, and L. Weiss, 1:57–80. Philadelphia: Saunders, 2003.

Hawkes, Peter W., and John C. H. Spence. *Science of Microscopy*. New York: Springer, 2007.

Hayles, N. Katherine. "Cognition Everywhere: The Rise of the Cognitive Nonconscious and the Costs of Consciousness." *New Literary History* 45, no. 2 (2014): 199–220.

Hayles, N. Katherine. "Cognitive Assemblages: Technical Agency and Human Interactions." *Critical Inquiry* 43, no. 1 (2016): 32–55.

Heinz, T. "Evolution of the Silver and Gold Stains in Neurohistology." *Biotechnic and Histochemistry* 80, no. 5–6 (2005): 211.

Henderson, Cary Smith, Jackie Henderson Main, Ruth D. Henderson, and Nancy Andrews. *Partial View: An Alzheimer's Journal*. Dallas, Tex.: Southern Methodist University Press, 1998.

Hendrickson, Paul. "A Life Going Mad: Daughter Crusades against Alzheimer's That Killed Rita Hayworth." *St. Petersburg Times* (Florida), April 17, 1989.

Hendrie, Hugh C., Marilyn S. Albert, Meryl A. Butters, Sujuan Gao, David S. Knopman, Lenore J. Launer, Kristine Yaffe, Bruce N. Cuthbert, Emmeline Edwards, and Molly V. Wagster. "The NIH Cognitive and Emotional Health Project: Report of the Critical Evaluation Study Committee." *Alzheimer's and Dementia* 2, no. 1 (2006): 12–32.

Hendrix, Steve. "A Pain Vast and Personal, Writ Small." *Washington Post*, October 23, 2008.

Hentschel, Klaus. *Visual Cultures in Science and Technology: A Comparative History*. Oxford: Oxford University Press, 2014.

Hepp, Andreas, Stig Hjarvard, and Knut Lundby. "Mediatization: Theorizing the Interplay between Media, Culture and Society." *Media, Culture, and Society* 37, no. 2 (2015): 314–24.

Heston, Leonard L., Leonard L. Heston, and June A. White. *The Vanishing Mind: A Practical Guide to Alzheimer's Disease and Other Dementias*. New York: W. H. Freeman, 1991.

Hinckley, David. "'The Alzheimer's Project': An Unflinching Look at a Brain Stealer." *New York Daily News*, May 8, 2009. https://www.nydailynews.com/entertainment/tv-movies/alzheimer-project-unflinching-brain-stealer-article-1.410361.

Hind, H. Lloyd, and W. Brough Randles. *Handbook of Photomicrography*. New York: Routledge, 1913.

Hirano, Asao, Herbert M. Dembitzer, Leonard T. Kurland, and H. M. Zimmerman. "The Fine Structure of Some Intraganglionic Alterations." *Journal of Neuropathology and Experimental Neurology* 27, no. 2 (1968): 167–82.

Hiroisi, S., and C. C. Lee. "Origin of Senile Plaques." *Archives of Neurology and Psychiatry* 35, no. 4 (1936): 827–39.

Hirsch, Marianne, ed. *The Familial Gaze*. 1st ed. Hanover, N.H.: Dartmouth College Press, 1999.

Hirsch, Marianne. *Family Frames: Photography, Narrative, and Postmemory*. Cambridge, Mass.: Harvard University Press, 1997.

Hoad, Neville. "Three Poems and a Pandemic." In *Political Emotions: New Agendas in Communication*, edited by Janet Staiger, Janet Cvetkovich, and Ann Reynolds, 134–50. New York: Routledge, 2010.

Hoch, August. "The Dementia of Cerebral Aterio-sclerosis." *Psychiatric Bulletin of the New York State Hospitals* 9 (1916): 306–15.

Holmes, William. "A New Method for the Impregnation of Nerve Axons in Mounted Paraffin Sections." *Journal of Pathology and Bacteriology* 54, no. 1 (1942): 132–36.

Holstein, Martha. "Aging, Culture, and the Framing of Alzheimer Disease." In *Concepts of Alzheimer's Disease: Biological, Clinical, and Cultural Perspectives,* edited by Peter J. Whitehouse, Konrad Maurer, and Jesse F. Ballenger, 158–80. Baltimore: Johns Hopkins University Press, 2000.

Holstein, Martha. "Alzheimer's Disease and Senile Dementia, 1885–1920: An Interpretive History of Disease Negotiation." *Journal of Aging Studies* 11, no. 1 (1997): 1–13.

Holtzmann-Kevles, Bettyann. *Naked to the Bone: Medical Imaging in the Twentieth Century.* New Brunswick, N.J.: Rutgers University Press, 1997.

Hook, Cayce J., and Martha J. Farah. "Look Again: Effects of Brain Images and Mind–Brain Dualism on Lay Evaluations of Research." *Journal of Cognitive Neuroscience* 25, no. 9 (2013): 1397–1405.

Hopkins, Emily J., Deena Skolnick Weisberg, and Jordan C. V. Taylor. "The Seductive Allure Is a Reductive Allure: People Prefer Scientific Explanations That Contain Logically Irrelevant Reductive Information." *Cognition* 155 (October 2016): 67–76.

Horn, Eva. "Editor's Introduction: 'There Are No Media.'" *Grey Room,* October 1, 2007, 6–13.

Huber, Lara, and Lara Kutschenko. "Medicine in a Neurocentric World: About the Explanatory Power of Neuroscientific Models in Medical Research and Practice." *Medicine Studies* 1 (2009): 307–13.

Huberman, Georges Didi. *Invention of Hysteria.* Cambridge, Mass.: MIT Press, 2003.

Huckman, Michael S., Jacob Fox, and Jordan Topel. "The Validity of Criteria for the Evaluation of Cerebral Atrophy by Computed Tomography." *Radiology* 116, no. 1 (1975): 85–92.

Huffington Post. "William Utermohlen's Self-Portraits of His Decline from Alzheimer's Disease." February 10, 2012, sec. Arts. http://www.huffington post.com/2012/02/09/william-utermohlens-self-portraits_n_1265712 .html.

Hughes, Julian C., Stephen J. Louw, and Steven R. Sabat. *Dementia: Mind, Meaning, and the Person.* Oxford: Oxford University Press, 2006.

Hughes, T., K. Tyler, D. Danner, and A. Carter. "African American Caregivers: An Exploration of Pathways and Barriers to a Diagnosis of Alzheimer's Disease for a Family Member with Dementia." *Dementia* 8, no. 1 (2009): 95–116.

Hunter, Sam. *The Museum of Modern Art, New York: The History and the Collection.* New York: Abradale Press/H. N. Abrams in association with the Museum of Modern Art, New York, 1984.

Hurd, Michael D., Paco Martorell, Adeline Delavande, Kathleen J. Mullen, and Kenneth M. Langa. "Monetary Costs of Dementia in the United States." *New England Journal of Medicine* 368, no. 14 (2013): 1326–34.

Hurley, Amanda Kolson. "Time-Travel Therapy." *The Atlantic,* December 12, 2016. https://www.theatlantic.com/magazine/archive/2017/01/time-travel -therapy/508787/.

Huyssen, Andreas. *After the Great Divide Modernism, Mass Culture, Postmodernism.* Bloomington: Indiana University Press, 1986.

Huyssen, Andreas. *Present Pasts: Urban Palimpsests and the Politics of Memory.* Stanford, Calif.: Stanford University Press, 2003.

Hydén, Lars-Christer, and Jens Brockmeier. *Health, Illness and Culture: Broken Narratives.* New York: Routledge, 2008.

Illouz, Eva. *Consuming the Romantic Utopia: Love and the Cultural Contradictions of Capitalism.* Berkeley: University of California Press, 1997.

Innes, Anthea, and Karen Hatfield. *Healing Arts Therapies and Person-Centered Dementia Care.* London: Jessica Kingsley, 2002.

Jablensky, Assen. "Living in a Kraepelinian World: Kraepelin's Impact on Modern Psychiatry." *History of Psychiatry* 19 (September 2007): 381–88.

Jack, Clifford R., Jr., Marilyn S. Albert, David S. Knopman, Guy M. McKhann, Reisa A. Sperling, Maria C. Carrillo, Bill Thies, and Creighton H. Phelps. "Introduction to the Recommendations from the National Institute on Aging–Alzheimer's Association Workgroups on Diagnostic Guidelines for Alzheimer's Disease." *Alzheimer's and Dementia* 7, no. 3 (2011): 257–62.

Jacobs, Lawrence, William Kinkel, Frank Painter, Joseph Murawski, and Reid R. Heffner. "Computerized Tomography in Dementia with Special Reference to Changes in Size of Normal Ventricles during Aging and Normal Pressure Hydrocephalus." In *Alzheimer's Disease: Senile Dementia and Related Disorders,* edited by Robert Katzman, Robert D. Terry, and Katherine L. Bick, 241–46. New York: Raven Press, 1978.

Jäger, Ludwig, Erika Linz, and Irmela Schneider. *Media, Culture, and Mediality: New Insights into the Current State of Research.* Berlin: transcript, 2014.

Jagust, William, and Mark D'Esposito. *Imaging the Aging Brain.* New York: Oxford University Press, 2009.

Jardine, Nicholas. *The Scenes of Inquiry.* Oxford: Clarendon Press, 2000.

Jarman, Michelle, and Alison Kafer. "Guest Editors' Introduction: Growing Disability Studies—Politics of Access, Politics of Collaboration." *Disability Studies Quarterly* 34, no. 2 (2014).

Jaworska, Agnieszka. "Respecting the Margins of Agency: Alzheimer's Patients and the Capacity to Value." *Philosophy and Public Affairs* 28, no. 2 (1999): 105–38.

Jeffreys, Mark. "The Visible Cripple (Scars and Other Disfiguring Displays Included)." In *Disability Studies: Enabling the Humanities,* edited by Sharon L. Snyder, Brenda J. Brueggemann, and Rosemarie G. Thomson, 31–39. New York: Modern Language Association of America, 2002.

Jelliffe, Smith Ely. "Obituaries: Alois Alzheimer." *Journal of Nervous and Mental Disease* 44 (1916): 475–77.

Jelliffe, Smith Ely. "Pathology: Die Colloidentartung des Gehirns" (Colloid Degeneration of the Brain). *Journal of Nervous and Mental Disease* 25, no. 7 (1898): 565.

Jelliffe, Smith Ely, and William A. White. "The Modern Treatment of Nervous and Mental Diseases." *JAMA* 61, no. 10 (1913): 792–93.

Jellinger, K. A. "Alzheimer 100: Highlights in the History of Alzheimer Research." *Journal of Neural Transmission* 113, no. 11 (2006): 1603–23.

Jellinger, Kurt A. "Alzheimer's Disease: A Challenge for Modern Neuropathobiology." *Acta Neuropathologica* 118, no. 1 (2009): 1–3.

Jenkins, Tamara, dir. *The Savages.* 20th Century Fox, 2007. DVD.

Jensen, Elizabeth. "HBO Documentaries Put Alzheimer's Disease under a Microscope." *New York Times,* May 1, 2009. http://www.nytimes.com/2009/05/03/arts/television/03jens.html.

Jervis, George A. "Alzheimer's Disease." *Psychiatric Quarterly* 11 (1937): 5–18.

Johnson, Keith A., Nick C. Fox, Reisa A. Sperling, and William E. Klunk. "Brain Imaging in Alzheimer Disease." *Cold Spring Harbor Perspectives in Medicine* 2, no. 4 (2012): a006213.

Johnson, Keith A., Satoshi Minoshima, Nicolaas I. Bohnen, Kevin J. Donohoe, Norman L. Foster, Peter Herscovitch, Jason H. Karlawish, et al. "Appropriate Use Criteria for Amyloid PET: A Report of the Amyloid Imaging Task Force, the Society of Nuclear Medicine and Molecular Imaging, and the Alzheimer's Association." *Journal of Nuclear Medicine* 54, no. 3 (2013): 476–90.

Johnson, Keith A., Satoshi Minoshima, Nicolaas I. Bohnen, Kevin J. Donohoe, Norman L. Foster, Peter Herscovitch, Jason H. Karlawish, et al. "Update on Appropriate Use Criteria for Amyloid PET Imaging: Dementia Experts, Mild Cognitive Impairment, and Education. Amyloid Imaging Task Force of the Alzheimer's Association and Society for Nuclear Medicine and Molecular Imaging." *Alzheimer's and Dementia* 9, no. 4 (2013): e106–9.

Johnson, Merri Lisa, and Robert McRuer. "Cripistemologies: Introduction." *Journal of Literary and Cultural Disability Studies* 8, no. 2 (2014): 127–47.

Jonas, Eric, and Konrad Paul Kording. "Could a Neuroscientist Understand a Microprocessor?" *PLOS Computational Biology* 13, no. 1 (2017): e1005268.

Jones, Caroline A., and Peter Galison, eds. *Picturing Science, Producing Art.* New York: Routledge, 1998.

Jones, Jeffrey M., and Joni L. Jones. "Famous Forgetters: Notable People and Alzheimer's Disease." *American Journal of Alzheimer's Disease and Other Dementias* 25, no. 2 (2010): 116–18.

Jones, Meg Leta. *Ctrl + Z: The Right to Be Forgotten.* New York: New York University Press, 2016.

Jones-Davis, Dorothy M., and Neil Buckholtz. "The Impact of ADNI: What Role Do Public–Private Partnerships Have in Pushing the Boundaries of Clinical and Basic Science Research on Alzheimer's Disease?" *Alzheimer's and Dementia* 11, no. 7 (2015): 860–64.

Jordanova, L. J. *Defining Features: Scientific and Medical Portraits 1660–2000.* London: Reaktion Books, 2000.

Jordanova, L. J. "Medicine and Genres of Display." In *Visual Display: Culture beyond Appearances,* edited by Lynne Cooke and Peter Woollen, 202–17. New York: New Press, 1995.

Joyce, Kelly A. *Magnetic Appeal: MRI and the Myth of Transparency.* Ithaca, N.Y.: Cornell University Press, 2008.

Juan, Joaquin De, and Rosa M. Perez-Canaveras. "How We Teach Recognizing Images in Histology." In *Science Technology and Education of Microscopy: An Overview,* edited by Mendez-Vilas, 787–94. Badajoz, Spain: Formatex, 2003.

Jutkowitz, Eric, Robert L. Kane, Joseph E. Gaugler, Richard F. MacLehose, Bryan Dowd, and Karen M. Kuntz. "Societal and Family Lifetime Cost of Dementia: Implications for Policy." *Journal of the American Geriatrics Society* 65, no. 10 (2017): 2169–75.

Kable, Joseph W., M. Kathleen Caulfield, Mary Falcone, Mairead McConnell, Leah Bernardo, Trishala Parthasarathi, Nicole Cooper, et al. "No Effect of Commercial Cognitive Training on Neural Activity during Decision-Making." *Journal of Neuroscience* 37, no. 31 (2017): 7390–402.

Kafer, Alison. *Feminist, Queer, Crip.* 1st ed. Bloomington: Indiana University Press, 2013.

Kahn-Denis, Kathleen B. "Art Therapy with Geriatric Dementia Clients." *Art Therapy* 14, no. 3 (1997): 194–99.

Kang, Seok, Sherice Gearhart, and Hyuhn-Suhck Bae. "Coverage of Alzheimer's Disease from 1984 to 2008 in Television News and Information Talk Shows in the United States: An Analysis of News Framing." *American Journal of Alzheimer's Disease and Other Dementias* 25, no. 8 (2010): 687–97.

Kantor, Sybil. *Alfred H. Barr, Jr., and the Intellectual Origins of the Museum of Modern Art.* Cambridge, Mass.: MIT Press, 2002.

Kaplan, Mary. *Solomon Carter Fuller: Where My Caravan Has Rested.* Lanham, Md.: University Press of America, 2005.

Kaplan, Mary, and Alfred Henderson. "Solomon Carter Fuller, M.D. (1872–1953): American Pioneer in Alzheimer's Disease Research." *Journal of the History of the Neurosciences* 9, no. 3 (2000): 250–61.

Kastenbaum, Robert, David D. Van Tassel, and Thomas R. Cole. *Handbook of the Humanities and Aging.* New York: Springer, 1992.

Katz, Marina. "'Virtual Dementia Tour' Leaves Participants Frustrated but Sympathetic." *ABC News,* June 29, 2009. https://abcnews.go.com/Prime time/AlzheimersNews/story?id=7961176.

Katz, Renée S., and Therese A. Johnson. *When Professionals Weep: Emotional and Countertransference Responses in End-of-Life Care.* New York: Routledge, 2006.

Katz, Stephen. *Disciplining Old Age: The Formation of Gerontological Knowledge.* Charlottesville: University Press of Virginia, 1996.

Katz, Stephen. "Embodied Memory: Ageing, Neuroculture, and the Genealogy of Mind." In *Interdisciplinary Studies in the Humanities.* Vol. 4. Stanford, Calif.: Stanford University Press, 2012.

Katzman R. "The Prevalence and Malignancy of Alzheimer Disease: A Major Killer." *Archives of Neurology* 33, no. 4 (1976): 217–18.

Katzman, Robert, and Katherine L. Bick. *Alzheimer Disease: The Changing View.* Burlington, Vt.: Academic Press, 2000.

Katzman, Robert, Robert D. Terry, and Katherine L. Bick, eds. *Alzheimer's Disease: Senile Dementia and Related Disorders.* New York: Raven Press, 1978.

Kaufman, Sharon R. *And a Time to Die: How American Hospitals Shape the End of Life.* New York: Scribner, 2005.

Kaufman, Sharon R. "Dementia-Near-Death and 'Life Itself.'" In *Thinking about Dementia: Culture, Loss, and the Anthropology of Senility,* edited by Lawrence Cohen and Annette Leibing, 23–42. New Brunswick, N.J.: Rutgers University Press, 2006.

Kay, D. W. K., P. Beamish, and Martin Roth. "Old Age Mental Disorders in Newcastle upon Tyne." *British Journal of Psychiatry* 110, no. 465 (1964): 146–58.

Keller, Evelyn Fox. "The Biological Gaze." In *FutureNatural: Nature, Science, Culture,* edited by George Robertson, 107–21. New York: Routledge, 1996.

Khachaturian, Zaven. "A Chapter in the Development on Alzheimer's Disease Research: A Case Study of Public Policies on the Development and Funding of Research Program." In *Alzheimer: 100 Years and Beyond,* edited by M. Jucker, K. Beyreuther, C. Haass, and R. M. Nitsch, 63–86. Berlin: Springer, 2006.

Khachaturian, Zaven. "Diagnosis of Alzheimer's Disease: Two-Decades of Progress." *Journal of Alzheimer's Disease* 9, Suppl. 3 (2006): 409–15.

Kidd, Michael. "Alzheimer's Disease: An Electron Microscopical Study." *Brain* 87, no. 2 (1964): 307–20.

Kidd, M. "Paired Helical Filaments in Electron Microscopy of Alzheimer's Disease." *Nature* 197, no. 4863 (1963): 192–93.

Kiernan, Laura. "Hinckley, Jury Watch 'Taxi Driver' Film." *Washington Post,* May 29, 1982.

Killiany, Ronald J. "Glimpses of the Living Brain with Alzheimer's Disease." In *The Handbook of Alzheimer's Disease and Other Dementias,* edited by Andrew E. Budson and Neil W. Kowall, 505–34. Malden, Mass.: Wiley-Blackwell, 2011.

Killick, John. "Learning Love from People with Dementia." In *Between Remembering and Forgetting: The Spiritual Dimensions of Dementia,* 1st ed., edited by James Woodward, 52–58. New York: Mowbray, 2010.

Kim, Scott, Christopher Cox, and Eric Caine. "Impaired Decision-Making Ability in Subjects with Alzheimer's Disease and Willingness to Participate in Research." *American Journal of Psychiatry* 159 (2002): 797–802.

Kinney, Jennifer M., and Clarissa A. Rentz. "Observed Well-Being among Individuals with Dementia: Memories in the Making, an Art Program, versus Other Structured Activity." *American Journal of Alzheimer's Disease and Other Dementias* 20, no. 4 (2005): 220–27.

Kipnis, Laura. *Against Love: A Polemic.* New York: Pantheon Books, 2003.

Kirby, Elizabeth, Stephan Bandelow, and Eef Hogervorst. "Visual Impairment in Alzheimer's Disease: A Critical Review." *Journal of Alzheimer's Disease* 21, no. 1 (2010): 15–34.

Kirkman, Allison M. "Dementia in the News: The Media Coverage of Alzheimer's Disease." *Australasian Journal on Ageing* 25, no. 2 (2006): 74–79.

Kittay, Eva Feder. *Love's Labor: Essays on Women, Equality, and Dependency.* Essays on Women, Equality, and Dependency 17. New York: Routledge, 1999.

Kittay, Eva Feder, and Licia Carlson, eds. *Cognitive Disability and Its Challenge to Moral Philosophy.* 1st ed. Chichester, U.K.: Wiley-Blackwell, 2010.

Kittler, Friedrich. *Gramophone, Film, Typewriter.* Translated by Geoffrey Winthrop-Young and Michael Wutz. 1st ed. Stanford, Calif.: Stanford University Press, 1999.

Kitwood, T. M. *Dementia Reconsidered: The Person Comes First.* Philadelphia: Open University Press, 1997.

Klatzo, Igor, Henryk Wiśniewski, and Eugene Streicher. "Experimental Production of Neurofibrillary Degeneration." *Journal of Neuropathology and Experimental Neurology* 24, no. 2 (1965): 187–99.

Klunk, William, and Chester Mathis. "Imaging the Pathology of Alzheimer's Disease: Building on a Century-Old Blueprint." In *Alzheimer: 100 Years and Beyond,* edited by M. Jucker, K. Beyreuther, C. Haass, and R. M. Nitsch, 399–403. Berlin: Springer, 2006.

Kontos, Pia C. "Embodied Selfhood: An Ethnographic Exploration of Alzheimer's Disease." In *Thinking about Dementia: Culture, Loss, and the Anthropology of Senility*, edited by Lawrence Cohen and Annette Leibing, 195–217. New Brunswick, N.J.: Rutgers University Press, 2006.

Kontos, Pia C. "'The Painterly Hand': Embodied Consciousness and Alzheimer's Disease." *Journal of Aging Studies* 17, no. 2 (2003): 151–70.

Korczyn, Amos D. "Commentary on 'Recommendations from the National Institute on Aging-Alzheimer's Association Workgroups on Diagnostic Guidelines for Alzheimer's Disease.'" *Alzheimer's and Dementia* 7, no. 3 (2011): 333–34.

Kraepelin, Emil. "The Loss of Three German Investigators, Alzheimer, Brodmann, Nissl." *Journal of Nervous and Mental Disease* 55, no. 2 (1922): 91–102.

Krell-Roesch, Janina, Prashanthi Vemuri, Anna Pink, Rosebud O. Roberts, Gorazd B. Stokin, Michelle M. Mielke, Teresa J. H. Christianson, et al. "Association between Mentally Stimulating Activities in Late Life and the Outcome of Incident Mild Cognitive Impairment, with an Analysis of the APOE E4 Genotype." *JAMA Neurology* 74, no. 3 (2017): 332–38.

Krigman, M. R., R. G. Feldman, and K. Bensch. "Alzheimer's Presenile Dementia: A Histochemical and Electron Microscopic Study." *Laboratory Investigation* 14 (April 1965): 381–96.

Kroeker, Allan, dir. *Age-Old Friends.* HBO, 1989.

Kroll, Justin. "Will Ferrell Pulls Out of Ronald Reagan Movie after Outcry from Family." *Variety* (blog), April 29, 2016. http://variety.com/2016/film/news/will-ferrell-ronald-reagan-movie-controversy-1201763542/.

Kudlick, Catherine J. "Disability History: Why We Need Another 'Other.'" *American Historical Review* 108, no. 3 (2003): 763–93.

Kuppers, Petra. "Crip Time." *Tikkun* 29, no. 4 (2014): 29–30.

Kurant, Agnieszka, Janek Sowa, and Krystian Szadkowski. "Do We Need a Lab? Capture, Exploitation and Resistance in Contemporary Creative Communities." In *Joy Forever: The Political Economy of Social Creativity*, edited by Michal Kozlowski, Agnieszka Kurant, Janek Sowa, Krystian Szadkowski, and Kuba Szreder. N.p.: MayFly Books, 2014.

Lamy, C., C. Duyckaerts, P. Delaere, Ch. Payan, J. Fermanian, V. Poulain, and J. J. Hauw. "Comparison of Seven Staining Methods for Senile Plaques and Neurofibrillary Tangles in a Prospective Series of 15 Elderly Patients." *Neuropathology and Applied Neurobiology* 15, no. 6 (1989): 563–78.

Landsberg, Alison. *Prosthetic Memory: The Transformation of American Remembrance in the Age of Mass Culture.* New York: Columbia University Press, 2004.

Lane, Christopher. *Shyness: How Normal Behavior Became a Sickness.* New Haven, Conn.: Yale University Press, 2007.

Lang, Walter. *Annual Report of the Trustees of the Westborough State Hospital.* 1919. Francis A. Countway Library of Medicine, Boston.

Langa, Kenneth M., Eric B. Larson, Eileen M. Crimmins, Jessica D. Faul, Deborah A. Levine, Mohammed U. Kabeto, and David R. Weir. "A Comparison of the Prevalence of Dementia in the United States in 2000 and 2012." *JAMA Internal Medicine* 177, no. 1 (2016): 51–58.

Langa, Kenneth M., and Deborah A. Levine. "The Diagnosis and Management of Mild Cognitive Impairment: A Clinical Review." *JAMA* 312, no. 23 (2014): 2551.

Langdon, F. W. "Biological Aspects of Dementia Praecox." *American Journal of Psychiatry* 73, no. 4 (1917): 681–92.

Lanska, D. J. "The Role of Technology in Neurologic Specialization in America." *Neurology* 48, no. 6 (1997): 1722–28.

Latour, Bruno. *On the Modern Cult of Factish Gods.* Durham, N.C.: Duke University Press, 2010.

Latour, Bruno. *We Have Never Been Modern.* Cambridge, Mass.: Harvard University Press, 1993.

Latour, Bruno, and Steve Woolgar. *Laboratory Life: The Social Construction of Scientific Facts.* Beverly Hills, Calif.: Sage, 1979.

Leapman, Richard. "Novel Techniques in Electron Microscopy." *Current Opinion in Neurobiology* 14, no. 5 (2004): 591–98.

Lears, T. J. Jackson. "From Salvation to Self-Realization: Advertising and the Therapeutic Roots of Consumer Culture, 1880–1930." In *The Culture of Consumption: Critical Essays in American History 1880–1980,* edited by Richard Wightman Fox and T. J. Jackson Lears, 3–38. New York: Pantheon, 1983.

LeDoux, Joseph. *Synaptic Self: How Our Brains Become Who We Are.* New York: Penguin Books, 2003.

Leibing, Annette. "Divided Gazes: Alzheimer's Disease, the Person within, and Death in Life." In *Thinking about Dementia: Culture, Loss, and the Anthropology of Senility,* edited by Annette Leibing and Lawrence Cohen, 240–68. New Brunswick, N.J.: Rutgers University Press, 2006.

Leibing, Annette. "Entangled Matters: Alzheimer's, Interiority, and the 'Unflattening' of the World." *Culture, Medicine, and Psychiatry* 32, no. 2 (2008): 177–93.

Lemke, T. "New Materialisms: Foucault and the 'Government of Things.'" *Theory, Culture, and Society* 32, no. 4 (2015): 3–25.

Lerner, Barron H. *When Illness Goes Public: Celebrity Patients and How We Look at Medicine.* Baltimore: Johns Hopkins University Press, 2006.

Levine, Carol, and Thomas H. Murray. *The Cultures of Caregiving: Conflict and Common Ground among Families, Health Professionals, and Policy Makers.* Baltimore: Johns Hopkins University Press, 2004.

Liao, Solomon. "Personhood and the Ethics of Dementia: Iris." In *The Picture of Health: Medical Ethics and the Movies,* edited by Henri G. Colt, Silvia Quadrelli, and Lester D. Friedman, 527. New York: Oxford University Press, 2011.

Lin, Jennifer S., Elizabeth O'Connor, Rebecca C. Rossom, Leslie A. Perdue, Brittany U. Burda, Matthew Thompson, and Elizabeth Eckstrom. *Screening for Cognitive Impairment in Older Adults: An Evidence Update for the U.S. Preventive Services Task Force.* U.S. Preventive Services Task Force Evidence Syntheses, Formerly Systematic Evidence Reviews. Rockville, Md.: Agency for Healthcare Research and Quality, 2013. http://www.ncbi.nlm.nih.gov/books/NBK174643/.

Lindemann, Hilde. "Holding Well, Wrongly, Clumsily." In *Cognitive Disability and Its Challenges to Moral Philosophy,* edited by Licia Carlson and Eva F. Kittay, 161–69. Malden, Mass.: Wiley-Blackwell, 2010.

Linker, Beth. "On the Borderland of Medical and Disability History: A Survey of the Fields." *Bulletin of the History of Medicine* 87, no. 4 (2013): 499–535.

Linton, Simi. *Claiming Disability: Knowledge and Identity.* New York: New York University Press, 1998.

Littlefield, Melissa, and Jenell Johnson, eds. *The Neuroscientific Turn.* Ann Arbor: University of Michigan Press, 2012.

Littlefield, Melissa, Jenell Johnson, and Susan Fitzpatrick, eds. "Functional Brain Imaging: Neuro-Turn or Wrong Turn?" In *The Neuroscientific Turn,* 180–98. Ann Arbor: University of Michigan Press, 2012.

Lock, Margaret. *The Alzheimer Conundrum: Entanglements of Dementia and Aging.* Princeton, N.J.: Princeton University Press, 2015.

Lock, Margaret. "Testing for Susceptibility Genes: A Cautionary Tale." In *Disclosure Dilemmas: Ethics of Genetic Prognosis after the "Right to Know/Not to Know" Debate,* edited by Christoph Rehmann-Sutter and Hansjakob Müller, 65–84. London: Ashgate, 2009.

Lock, Margaret. *Twice Dead: Organ Transplants and the Reinvention of Death.* Berkeley: University of California Press, 2001.

Lock, Margaret, Julia Freeman, Gillian Chilibeck, Briony Beveridge, and Miriam Padolsky. "Susceptibility Genes and the Question of Embodied Identity." *Medical Anthropology Quarterly* 21, no. 3 (2007): 256–76.

Lock, Margaret, Stephanie Lloyd, and Janalyn Prest. "Genetic Susceptibility and Alzheimer's Disease: The Penetrance and Uptake of Genetic Knowledge." In *Thinking about Dementia: Culture, Loss, and the Anthropology of Senility,* edited by Lawrence Cohen and Annette Leibing, 123–54. New Brunswick, N.J.: Rutgers University Press, 2006.

Lockett, Betty A. *Aging, Politics, and Research: Setting the Federal Agenda for Research on Aging.* New York: Springer, 1983.

Longmore, Paul K. *Why I Burned My Book and Other Essays on Disability.* 1st ed. Philadelphia: Temple University Press, 2003.

Lowry, Brian. "The Alzheimer's Project." *Variety*, May 6, 2009.

Ludmerer, Kenneth Marc. *Time to Heal: American Medical Education from the Turn of the Century to the Era of Managed Care*. Oxford: Oxford University Press, 1999.

Luhrmann, Tanya. *Of Two Minds: The Growing Disorder in American Psychiatry*. New York: Knopf, 2000.

Lukiw, Walter J. "Alzheimer's Disease—100 Years of Research: A Historical Perspective." In *Alzheimer's Disease Research Trends*, edited by A. P. Chan, 11–15. New York: Nova Biomedical, 2008.

Lundby, Knut. *Mediatization: Concept, Changes, Consequences*. New York: Peter Lang, 2009.

Lunt, Peter, and Sonia Livingstone. "Is 'Mediatization' the New Paradigm for Our Field? A Commentary on Deacon and Stanyer (2014, 2015) and Hepp, Hjarvard and Lundby (2015)." *Media, Culture, and Society* 38, no. 3 (2016): 462–70.

Lyketsos, Constantine G. "Commentary on 'Recommendations from the National Institute on Aging–Alzheimer's Association Workgroups on Diagnostic Guidelines for Alzheimer's Disease.' New Criteria for a New Era." *Alzheimer's and Dementia* 7, no. 3 (2011): 328–29.

Lyketsos, Constantine G., Oscar Lopez, Beverly Jones, Annette L. Fitzpatrick, John Breitner, and Steven DeKosky. "Prevalence of Neuropsychiatric Symptoms in Dementia and Mild Cognitive Impairment." *JAMA* 288, no. 12 (2002): 1475–83.

Lynch, Michael E., and Steve Woolgar, eds. *Representation in Scientific Practice*. Cambridge, Mass.: MIT Press, 1990.

Lynes, Russell. *Good Old Modern*. New York: Atheneum, 1973.

Mace, Nancy, and Peter V. Rabins. *The 36-Hour Day: A Family Guide to Caring for Persons with Alzheimer Disease, Related Dementing Illnesses, and Memory Loss in Later Life*. Baltimore: Johns Hopkins University Press, 1999.

Mack, J. L., and Peter Whitehouse. "Quality of Life in Dementia: State of the Art—Report of the International Working Group for Harmonization of Dementia Drug Guidelines and the Alzheimer's Society Satellite Meeting." *Alzheimer Disease and Associated Disorders* 15, no. 2 (2001): 59–62.

Maffly, Brian. "Visual Arts: 'Alzheimer's from the Inside Out.'" *Salt Lake Tribune*, October 27, 2008. http://archive.sltrib.com/story.php?ref=/entertainment/ci_10815055.

Magner, Lois N. *A History of Medicine*. 2nd ed. Boca Raton, Fla.: Taylor and Francis, 2005.

Magoun, Horace Winchell, and Louise H. Marshall. *American Neuroscience in the Twentieth Century: Confluence of the Neural, Behavioral, and Communicative Streams*. Lisse, The Netherlands: A. A. Balkema, 2003.

Malabou, Catherine. *What Should We Do with Our Brain?* New York: Fordham University Press, 2008.

Malamud, William, and K. Lowenberg. "Alzheimer's Disease: A Contribution to Its Etiology and Classification." *Archives of Neurology and Psychiatry* 21, no. 4 (1929): 805–27.

Malchiodi, Cathy. *Art Therapy Sourcebook.* 2nd ed. New York: McGraw-Hill Education, 2007.

Malzberg, Benjamin. "The Frequency of Mental Disease: A Study of Trends in New York State." *Acta Psychiatrica Scandinavica* 39, no. 1 (1963): 19–30.

Malzberg, Benjamin. "The Increase of Mental Disease." *Psychiatric Quarterly* 17, no. 3 (1943): 488–507.

Margolis, G. "Senile Cerebral Disease: A Critical Survey of Traditional Concepts Based upon Observations with Newer Technics." *Laboratory Investigation* 8, no. 2 (1959): 335–70.

Markowitsch, Hans J. *Intellectual Functions and the Brain: An Historical Perspective.* Seattle, Wash.: Hogrefe and Huber, 1992.

Markowitz, John C. "There's Such a Thing as Too Much Neuroscience." *New York Times,* October 14, 2016. http://www.nytimes.com/2016/10/15/opinion/theres-such-a-thing-as-too-much-neuroscience.html.

Marquardt, Elizabeth. "Elderly Murder-Suicide: Should We Praise Old Men Who Kill Their Wives and Themselves?" *Huffington Post,* April 9, 2012. http://www.huffingtonpost.com/elizabeth-marquardt/elderly-murder-suicide_b_1402935.html.

Marsh, Aaron, and Steve Brown. "Family Caregiving: The Issue of Our Time." *Caring* 30, no. 5 (2011): 22–30.

Martin, Emily. *Bipolar Expeditions: Mania and Depression in American Culture.* Princeton, N.J.: Princeton University Press, 2007.

Martin, Emily. *The Woman in the Body.* Boston: Beacon Press, 1992.

Martin, Joseph B. "The Integration of Neurology, Psychiatry, and Neuroscience in the 21st Century." *American Journal of Psychiatry* 159, no. 5 (2002): 695–704.

Martin, Richard. "Gone but Not Forsaken." *Tampa Bay Times,* October 17, 2011.

Massey, Irving. *The Neural Imagination.* Austin: University of Texas Press, 2009.

Maurer, Konrad. "The History of Alois Alzheimer's First Case Auguste D.: How Did the Eponym 'Alzheimer's Disease' Come into Being?" In *Alzheimer: 100 Years and Beyond,* edited by M. Jucker, K. Beyreuther, C. Haass, and R. M. Nitsch, 13–34. Berlin: Springer, 2006.

Maurer, Konrad, and Ulrike Maurer. *Alzheimer: The Life of a Physician and the Career of a Disease.* New York: Columbia University Press, 2003.

Maurer, K., and D. Prvulovic. "Paintings of an Artist with Alzheimer's Disease: Visuoconstructural Deficits during Dementia." *Journal of Neural Transmission* 111, no. 3 (2004): 235–45.

Maurer, Konrad, Stephan Volk, and Hector Gerbaldo. "Auguste D.: The History of Alois Alzheimer's First Case." In *Concepts of Alzheimer's Disease: Biological, Clinical, and Cultural Perspectives*, edited by Peter J. Whitehouse, Konrad Maurer, and Jesse F. Ballenger, 5–29. Baltimore: Johns Hopkins University Press, 2000.

Maurer, K., S. Volk, and H. Gerbaldo. "Auguste D and Alzheimer's Disease." *The Lancet* 349 (1997): 1546–49.

Mayeda, Elizabeth Rose, M. Maria Glymour, Charles P. Quesenberry, and Rachel A. Whitmer. "Inequalities in Dementia Incidence between Six Racial and Ethnic Groups over 14 Years." *Alzheimer's and Dementia* 12, no. 3 (2016): 216–24.

Mayer-Schönberger, Viktor. *Delete: The Virtue of Forgetting in the Digital Age.* With a new afterword by the author. Princeton, N.J.: Princeton University Press, 2011.

Mbembe, Achille. "Necropolitics." *Public Culture* 15, no. 1 (2003): 11–40.

McCarthy, Tom, dir. *Win Win.* Fox Searchlight, 2011.

McFadden, Susan H., and Anne D. Basting. "Healthy Aging Persons and Their Brains: Promoting Resilience through Creative Engagement." *Clinics in Geriatric Medicine* 26, no. 1 (2010): 149–61.

McGaffin, C. G. "An Anatomical Analysis of Seventy Cases of Senile Dementia." *American Journal of Psychiatry* 66, no. 4 (1910): 649–56.

McIntyre, Maura. "Love Stories about Caregiving and Alzheimer's Disease: A Performative Methodology." *Journal of Health Psychology* 13, no. 2 (2008): 213–25.

McKhann, G., D. Drachman, M. Folstein, R. Katzman, D. Price, and E. M. Stadlan. "Clinical Diagnosis of Alzheimer's Disease: Report of the NINCDS-ADRDA Work Group under the Auspices of Department of Health and Human Services Task Force on Alzheimer's Disease." *Neurology* 34, no. 7 (1984): 939–44.

McKhann, Guy M., David S. Knopman, Howard Chertkow, Bradley T. Hyman, Clifford R. Jack, Claudia H. Kawas, William E. Klunk, et al. "The Diagnosis of Dementia due to Alzheimer's Disease: Recommendations from the National Institute on Aging–Alzheimer's Association Workgroups on Diagnostic Guidelines for Alzheimer's Disease." *Alzheimer's and Dementia* 7, no. 3 (2011): 263–69.

McLean, Athena. *The Person in Dementia: A Study in Nursing Home Care in the US.* Peterborough, Ont.: Broadview Press, 2007.

McLuhan, Marshall. *Understanding Media: The Extensions of Man.* New York: McGraw-Hill, 1964.

McMenemey, W. H. "A Critical Review: Dementia in Middle Age." *Journal of Neurology and Psychiatry* 4, no. 1 (1941): 48–79.

McMenemey, W. H. "Alzheimer's Disease: A Report of Six Cases." *Journal of Neurology and Psychiatry* 3, no. 3 (1940): 211–40.

McMenemey, W. H., C. Worster-Drought, J. Flind, and H. G. Williams. "Familial Presenile Dementia: Report of a Case with Clinical and Pathological Features of Alzheimer's Disease." *Journal of Neurology and Psychiatry* 2, no. 4 (1939): 293–302.

McRuer, Robert. *Crip Theory: Cultural Signs of Queerness and Disability*. New York: New York University Press, 2006.

McRuer, Robert. "Disability Nationalism in Crip Times." *Journal of Literary and Cultural Disability Studies* 4, no. 2 (2010): 163–78.

McRuer, Robert, and Merri Lisa Johnson. "Proliferating Cripistemologies: A Virtual Roundtable." *Journal of Literary and Cultural Disability Studies* 8, no. 2 (2014): 149–69.

Medeiros, Kate de, and Anne Basting. "'Shall I Compare Thee to a Dose of Donepezil?' Cultural Arts Interventions in Dementia Care Research." *The Gerontologist* 54, no. 3 (2014): 344–53.

Mehta, Kala M., and Gwen W. Yeo. "Systematic Review of Dementia Prevalence and Incidence in United States Race/Ethnic Populations." *Alzheimer's and Dementia* 13, no. 1 (2017): 72–83.

Melvin, Tessa. "New Center Fights Big Killer of the Aged." *New York Times*, December 6, 1981, sec. 11.

Mendez, Mario F. "Dementia as a Window to the Neurology of Art." *Medical Hypotheses* 63, no. 1 (2004): 1–7.

Méndez-Vilas, A., and J. Diaz. *Modern Research and Educational Topics in Microscopy*. Badajoz, Spain: Formatex, 2007.

Menninger, William C. "Encephalography in Alzheimer's Disease." *Radiology* 23, no. 6 (1934): 695–99.

Mersch, Dieter. "Meta/Dia: Two Approaches to the Medial." In *Media Transatlantic: Developments in Media and Communication Studies between North American and German-Speaking Europe*, edited by Norm Friesen, 153–80. Berlin: Springer International, 2016.

Mervis, Jeffrey. "Obama's Science Advisers Look at Reform of Schools." *Science* 326, no. 5953 (2009): 654.

Merzenich, Michael. *Soft-Wired: How the New Science of Brain Plasticity Can Change Your Life*. 2nd ed. San Francisco: Parnassus, 2013.

Metzl, Jonathan, and Anna Kirkland, eds. *Against Health: How Health Became the New Morality*. New York: New York University Press, 2010.

Meulenberg, Frans, and Peter H. Gibson. "De Kooning's Dementia." *The Lancet* 347, no. 9018 (1996): 1838.

Meyer, Adolf. "Henry A. Cotton." *American Journal of Psychiatry* 90 (1934): 921–23.

Mialet, Hélène. *Hawking Incorporated: Stephen Hawking and the Anthropology of the Knowing Subject.* Chicago: University of Chicago Press, 2012.

Miller, Bruce L., and Craig E. Hou. "Portraits of Artists: Emergence of Visual Creativity in Dementia." *Archives of Neurology* 61, no. 6 (2004): 842–44.

Millett, Ann. "Cultural Commentary: Staring Back and Forth—The Photographs of Kevin Connolly." *Disability Studies Quarterly* 28, no. 3 (2008).

Mills, Charles, and Mary Shiveley. "Preliminary Report, Clinical and Pathological, of a Case of Progressive Dementia." *American Journal of Psychiatry* 54, no. 2 (1897): 211.

Mills, Mara. "Deaf Jam: From Inscription to Reproduction to Information." *Social Text* 28, no. 102 (2010): 35–58.

Mills, Mara. "On Disability and Cybernetics: Helen Keller, Norbert Wiener, and the Hearing Glove." *Differences* 22, no. 2–3 (2011): 74–111.

Mills, Mara. "Trained Judgment, Intervention, and the Biological Gaze: How Charles Minot Saw Senescence." In *Educated Eye: Visual Culture and Pedagogy in the Life Sciences,* edited by Nancy A. Anderson and Michael R. Dietrich, 14–43. Hanover, N.H.: Dartmouth College Press, 2012.

Minnesota Historical Society. "New App and Training Workshops Harness the Power of Museums to Better the Lives of Americans Living with Dementia." *Minnesota Historical Society* (blog), September 20, 2018. https://www .mnhs.org/media/kits/houseofmemories.

Mirzoeff, Nicholas. *The Right to Look: A Counterhistory of Visuality.* Durham, N.C.: Duke University Press, 2011.

Mitchell, David T. "Narrative Prosthesis." In *Disability Studies: Enabling the Humanities,* edited by Sharon L. Snyder, Brenda J. Brueggemann, and Rosemarie G. Thomson, 15–30. New York: Modern Language Association of America, 2002.

Mitchell, W. J. T. *Picture Theory: Essays on Verbal and Visual Representation.* Chicago: University of Chicago Press, 1994.

Mitchell, W. J. T. "There Are No Visual Media." In *Media Art Histories,* edited by Oliver Grau, 395–406. Cambridge, Mass.: MIT Press, 2007.

Mitchell, W. J. T. *What Do Pictures Want? The Lives and Loves of Images.* Chicago: University of Chicago Press, 2005.

Mitchell, W. J. T., and Mark B. N. Hansen, eds. *Critical Terms for Media Studies.* Chicago: University of Chicago Press, 2010.

Miyakawa, Taihei, Shiro Sumiyoshi, Eiichi Murayama, and Motonori Deshimaru. "Ultrastructure of Capillary Plaque-like Degeneration in Senile Dementia." *Acta Neuropathologica* 29, no. 3 (1974): 229–36.

Miyakawa, T., and Y. Uehara. "Observations of Amyloid Angiopathy and Senile Plaques by the Scanning Electron Microscope." *Acta Neuropathologica* 48, no. 2 (1979): 153–56.

Mizuno, Yoshikuni, Abraham Fisher, and Israel Hanin. *Mapping the Progress of Alzheimer's and Parkinson's Disease.* Vol. 51. New York: Kluwer Academic/ Plenum, 2002.

Moisse, Katie. "Alzheimer's Disease: Music Brings Patients 'Back to Life.'" *Good Morning America,* April 12, 2012. http://abcnews.go.com/Health/Alz heimersCommunity/alzheimers-disease-music-brings-patients-back-life/ story?id=16117602.

Moisse, Katie, and Jessica Hopper. "Pat Robertson's Alzheimer's Remark Stuns." *ABC News,* September 16, 2011. http://abcnews.go.com/Health/Alz heimersCommunity/pat-robertson-alzheimers-makes-divorce/story?id=14 526660.

Mol, Annemarie. *The Body Multiple: Ontology in Medical Practice.* Durham, N.C.: Duke University Press, 2002.

Mol, Annemarie, Ingunn Moser, and Jeannette Pols, eds. *Care in Practice: On Tinkering in Clinics, Homes, and Farms.* Bielefeld, Germany: transcript, 2010.

Moller, H. J., and M. B. Graeber. "Johann F.: The Historical Relevance of the Case for the Concept of Alzheimer Disease." In *Concepts of Alzheimer's Disease: Biological, Clinical, and Cultural Perspectives,* edited by Peter J. White-house, Konrad Maurer, and Jesse F. Ballenger, 30–46. Baltimore: Johns Hopkins University Press, 2000.

Moore, Jeffrey. *The Memory Artists.* London: Weidenfeld and Nicolson, 2004.

Morgan, Carol. "From Modernist Utopia to Cold War Reality: A Critical Moment in Museum Education." In *The Museum of Modern Art at Mid-century: Continuity and Change,* edited by John Elderfield, 151–73. New York: Museum of Modern Art, 1995.

Morley, John E. "A Brief History of Geriatrics." *Journals of Gerontology* 59A, no. 11 (2004): 1132–52.

Morris, David B. *Illness and Culture in the Postmodern Age.* Berkeley: University of California Press, 1998.

Mosconi, Lisa, Valentina Berti, Lidia Glodzik, Alberto Pupi, Susan De Santi, and Mony J. de Leon. "Pre-clinical Detection of Alzheimer's Disease Using FDG-PET, with or without Amyloid Imaging." *Journal of Alzheimer's Disease* 20, no. 3 (2010): 843–54.

Moser, Ingunn. "Making Alzheimer's Disease Matter: Enacting, Interfering and Doing Politics of Nature." *Geoforum* 39, no. 1 (2008): 98–110.

Moulier-Boutang, Yann. *Cognitive Capitalism.* 1st ed. Cambridge: Polity, 2012.

Mountjoy, C. Q. "Number of Plaques and Tangles, Loss of Neurons: Their Correlation with Deficient Neurotransmitter Synthesis and the Degree of

Dementia." In *Histology and Histopathology of the Aging Brain,* edited by Jürg Ulrich, 74–89. Interdisciplinary Topics in Gerontology 5. New York: Karger, 1988.

Mrak, Robert E. "The Big Eye in the 21st Century: The Role of Electron Microscopy in Modern Diagnostic Neuropathology." *Journal of Neuropathology and Experimental Neurology* 61, no. 12 (2002): 1027–39.

Mueller, Susanne G., Michael W. Weiner, Leon J. Thal, Ronald C. Petersen, Clifford Jack, William Jagust, John Q. Trojanowski, Arthur W. Toga, and Laurel Beckett. "The Alzheimer's Disease Neuroimaging Initiative." *Neuroimaging Clinics of North America* 15, no. 4 (2005): 869–77.

Muller, Ch., and L. Ciompi. *Senile Dementia: Clinical and Therapeutic Aspects.* 1st ed. Berlin: Hans Huber, 1968.

Munro, Alice. "The Bear Came over the Mountain." *New Yorker,* December 27, 1999.

Murray, Stuart. "Autism and the Contemporary Sentimental: Fiction and the Narrative Fascination of the Present." *Literature and Medicine* 25, no. 1 (2006): 24–45.

Musumeci, Giuseppe. "The Old and the New Concepts of Histochemistry." *Journal of Histology and Histopathology* 2, no. 1 (2015): 10.

Myrtelle Canavan Papers. Boston Medical Library, Francis A. Countway Library of Medicine, Boston.

Naeser, M. A., C. Gebhardt, and H. L. Levine. "Decreased Computerized Tomography Numbers in Patients with Presenile Dementia. Detection in Patients with Otherwise Normal Scans." *Archives of Neurology* 37, no. 7 (1980): 401–9.

Naftali, Raz. "The Aging Brain Observed in Vivo." In *Cognitive Neuroscience of Aging,* edited by Roberto Cabeza, Lars Nyberg, and Denise Park, 17–53. Oxford: Oxford University Press, 2004.

Naglie, Gary, David Hogan, Murray Krahn, B. Lynn Beattie, Sandra Black, Chris MacKnight, Morris Freedman, et al. "Predictors of Patient Self-Ratings of Quality of Life in Alzheimer Disease: Cross-Sectional Results from the Canadian Alzheimer's Disease Quality of Life Study." *American Journal of Geriatric Psychiatry* 19, no. 10 (2011): 881–90.

Nandy, Kalidas, and Ira Sherwin. *The Aging Brain and Senile Dementia: Proceedings of the Symposium on the Aging Brain and Senile Dementia Held in Boston, Massachusetts, June 2–4, 1976.* Advances in Behavioral Biology 8. New York: Plenum Press, 1977.

Naoumenko, Julia, and Irwin Feigin. "A Stable Silver Solution for Axon Staining in Paraffin Sections." *Journal of Neuropathology and Experimental Neurology* 26, no. 4 (1967): 669–73.

Nascher, I. L. *Geriatrics: The Diseases of Old Age and Their Treatment.* P. Blakiston's Son & Co, 1914.

Nascher, I. L. *The Wretches of Povertyville: A Sociological Study of the Bowery.* Chicago: J. J. Lanzit, 1909.

Nasreddine, Ziad S., Natalie A. Phillips, Valérie Bédirian, Simon Charbonneau, Victor Whitehead, Isabelle Collin, Jeffrey L. Cummings, and Howard Chertkow. "The Montreal Cognitive Assessment, MoCA: A Brief Screening Tool for Mild Cognitive Impairment." *Journal of the American Geriatrics Society* 53, no. 4 (2005): 695–99.

National Institute of Mental Health. *Neuroimaging and Mental Illness: A Window into the Brain—Frequently Asked Questions about Brain Scans.* Bethesda, Md.: U.S. Department of Health and Human Services, 2009. http://purl .access.gpo.gov/GPO/LPS125935.

National Institute on Aging. *The Alzheimer's Project.* HBO, 2011. https://www .nia.nih.gov/alzheimers/alzheimers-project-hbo.

National Institutes of Health. *Aging: Alzheimer's Disease.* Bethesda, Md.: National Institutes of Health, 2012.

Nayeri, Farah. "Museums Fight the Isolation and Pain of Dementia." *New York Times,* March 11, 2018, sec. Arts. https://www.nytimes.com/2018/03/11/ arts/dementia-national-museums-liverpool.html.

Nelkin, Dorothy, and Laurence Tancredi. *Dangerous Diagnostics: The Social Power of Biological Information.* New York: Basic Books, 1989.

Nelson, Camilla. "The Invention of Creativity: The Emergence of a Discourse." *Cultural Studies Review* 16, no. 2 (2010): 49–74.

Nelson, James Lindemann. "Alzheimer's Disease and Socially Extended Mentation." In *Cognitive Disability and Its Challenges to Moral Philosophy,* edited by Licia Carlson and Eva F. Kittay, 225–36. Malden, Mass.: Wiley-Blackwell, 2010.

Neumann, M., and R. Cohn. "Incidence of Alzheimer's Disease in a Large Mental Hospital: Relation to Senile Psychosis and Psychosis with Cerebral Arteriosclerosis." *Archives of Neurology and Psychiatry* 69, no. 5 (1953): 615–36.

New England Journal of Medicine. "Solomon Carter Fuller—1872–1953." 250, no. 3 (1954): 127.

New England Society of Psychiatry. "Proceedings." *American Journal of Psychiatry* 64, no. 3 (1908): 573–82.

Newton, R. D. "The Identity of Alzheimer's Disease and Senile Dementia and Their Relationship to Senility." *Journal of Mental Science* 94 (1948): 225–49.

Nicholls, Richard. "Iris Murdoch, Novelist and Philosopher, Is Dead." *New York Times,* February 9, 1999.

Nielson, Gregory M., H. Hagen, and Heinrich Müller. *Scientific Visualization: Overviews, Methodologies, and Techniques.* Los Alamitos, Calif.: IEEE Computer Society Press, 1997.

Noble, James M., and Nikolaos Scarmeas. "Application of PET Imaging to Diagnosis of Alzheimer's Disease and Mild Cognitive Impairment." In

International Review of Neurobiology: Neurobiology of Dementia, edited by Alireza Minagar, 84:133–49. Amsterdam: Academic Press, 2009.

Noda, U. "A Study of Nissl's Staebchenzellen in the Cerebral Cortex of General Paresis, Senile Dementia, Epilepsy, Glioma, Tuberculous Meningitis and Delirium Tremens." *Journal of Nervous and Mental Disease* 53, no. 3 (1921): 162–215.

Noll, Richard. *American Madness.* Cambridge, Mass.: Harvard University Press, 2011.

Noyes, Brigg B., Robert D. Hill, Bret L. Hicken, Marilyn Luptak, Randall Rupper, Nancy K. Dailey, and Byron D. Bair. "Review: The Role of Grief in Dementia Caregiving." *American Journal of Alzheimer's Disease and Other Dementias* 25 (2010): 9–17.

NPR. "San Diego Non-profit Builds Village to Help Alzheimer's Patients Cope." *All Things Considered,* January 17, 2017. https://www.npr.org/2017/01/17/510301337/san-diego-non-profit-builds-village-to-help-alzheimers-patients-cope.

Nutt, R., L. J. Vento, and M. H. T. Ridinger. "In Vivo Molecular Imaging Biomarkers: Clinical Pharmacology's New 'PET'?" *Clinical Pharmacology and Therapeutics* 81, no. 6 (2007): 792–95.

O'Connor, Cliodhna, Geraint Rees, and Helene Joffe. "Neuroscience in the Public Sphere." *Neuron* 74, no. 2 (2012): 220–26.

O'Connor, John. "Joanne Woodward as an Alzheimer's Victim." *New York Times,* May 21, 1985, sec. Arts. http://www.nytimes.com/1985/05/21/arts/joanne-woodward-as-an-alzheimer-s-victim.html.

O'Dwyer, Siobhan T., Wendy Moyle, Tara Taylor, Jennifer Creese, and Melanie J. Zimmer-Gembeck. "Homicidal Ideation in Family Carers of People with Dementia." *Aging and Mental Health* 20, no. 11 (2016): 1174–81.

O'Dwyer, Siobhan T., Wendy Moyle, Melanie Zimmer-Gembeck, and Diego De Leo. "Suicidal Ideation in Family Carers of People with Dementia." *Aging and Mental Health* 20, no. 2 (2016): 222–30.

Office of Technology Assessment. *Losing a Million Minds.* Washington, D.C.: Office of Technology Assessment, 1987.

O'Hare, Kate. "Dr. Travis Stork Reflects on Hitting 1,000 Episodes." *Screener* (blog), April 29, 2014. http://screenertv.com/news-features/the-doctors-dr-travis-stork-reflects-on-hitting-1000-episodes/.

Oliver, Mike. "The Social Model of Disability: Thirty Years On." *Disability and Society* 28, no. 7 (2013): 1024–26.

Omalu, Bennet, Julian Bailes, Ronald L. Hamilton, M. Ilyas Kamboh, Jennifer Hammers, Mary Case, and Robert Fitzsimmons. "Emerging Histomorphologic Phenotypes of Chronic Traumatic Encephalopathy in American Athletes." *Neurosurgery* 69, no. 1 (2011): 173–83.

O'Neill, Desmond. "The Art of the Demographic Dividend." *The Lancet* 377, no. 9780 (2011): 1828–29.

Oprah Winfrey Network. "B. Smith on Living for the Moment with Alzheimer's." *SuperSoul.Tv* (blog), November 23, 2015. http://www.supersoul.tv/supersoul-short-films/b-smith-on-living-for-the-moment-with-alzheimers an-own-original.

Orr, Jackie. *Panic Diaries: A Genealogy of Panic Disorder.* Durham, N.C.: Duke University Press, 2006.

Osteen, Mark, ed. *Autism and Representation.* Reprint ed. New York: Routledge, 2008.

Pacella, Bernard L., and S. Eugene Barrera. "Electroencephalography: Its Applications in Neurology and Psychiatry." *Psychiatric Quarterly* 15, no. 3 (1941): 407–37.

Paddock, Nancy. *A Song of Twilight: Of Alzheimer's and Love.* Janesville, Minn.: Blueroad Press, 2011.

Parikka, Jussi. *What Is Media Archaeology?* Malden, Mass.: Polity, 2012.

Parker, Ashley, and William Wan. "Trump Keeps Boasting about Passing a Cognitive Test—but It Doesn't Mean What He Thinks It Does." *Washington Post*, July 22, 2020. https://www.washingtonpost.com/politics/trump-brag ging-cognitive-test-dementia/2020/07/22/6578e826-cb65-11ea-91f1-28aca 4d833a0_story.html.

Partridge, Bradley J., Stephanie K. Bell, Jayne C. Lucke, Sarah Yeates, and Wayne D. Hall. "Smart Drugs 'as Common as Coffee': Media Hype about Neuroenhancement." *PLoS ONE* 6, no. 11 (2011): e28416.

Pauwels, Luc, ed. *Visual Cultures of Science: Rethinking Representational Practices in Knowledge Building and Science Communication.* Hanover, N.H.: Dartmouth College Press, 2005.

Pear, Robert. "How a Single Disease Has Become a Political Cause." *New York Times*, June 3, 1983.

Peel, Elizabeth. "'The Living Death of Alzheimer's' versus 'Take a Walk to Keep Dementia at Bay': Representations of Dementia in Print Media and Carer Discourse." *Sociology of Health and Illness* 36, no. 6 (2014): 885–901.

Percoskie, Suzanne. "Art Therapy with the Alzheimer's Client." *Humanistic Psychologist* 25, no. 2 (1997): 208–11.

Perrin, Andrew, and Monica Anderson. "Share of U.S. Adults Using Social Media, Including Facebook, Is Mostly Unchanged since 2018." *Pew Research Center* (blog), April 10, 2019. https://www.pewresearch.org/fact-tank/2019/04/10/share-of-u-s-adults-using-social-media-including-facebook-is-most ly-unchanged-since-2018/.

Peters, John Durham. "Broadcasting and Schizophrenia." *Media, Culture, and Society* 32, no. 1 (2010): 123–40.

Peters, John Durham. *The Marvelous Clouds: Toward a Philosophy of Elemental Media.* Reprint ed. Chicago: University of Chicago Press, 2016.

Petersen, Ronald C., Rosebud O. Roberts, David S. Knopman, Bradley F. Boeve, Yonas E. Geda, Robert J. Ivnik, Glenn E. Smith, and Clifford R. Jack Jr. "Mild Cognitive Impairment: Ten Years Later." *Archives of Neurology* 66, no. 12 (2009): 1447–55.

Peterson, Nora, and Peter Martin. "Tracing the Origins of Success: Implications for Successful Aging." *The Gerontologist* 55, no. 1 (2015): 5–13.

Petsko, Gregory A. "The Coming Epidemic of Neurologic Disorders: What Science Is—and Should Be—Doing about It." *Daedalus* 141, no. 3 (2012): 98–107.

Phelps, R. M. "American Psychiatry (Perspectives in Medical Thought)." *Journal of Nervous and Mental Disease* 21, no. 12 (1896): 813–20.

Philley, Christopher. "'Away from Her': A Love Story in the Grip of Alzheimer Disease." *Neurology Today* 7, no. 12 (2007): 20–22.

Phillips, Lorraine J., Stephanie A. Reid-Arndt, and Youngju Pak. "Effects of a Creative Expression Intervention on Emotions, Communication, and Quality of Life in Persons with Dementia." *Nursing Research* 59, no. 6 (2010): 417–25.

Pias, Claus. "What's German about German Media Theory?" In *Media Transatlantic: Developments in Media and Communication Studies between North America and German-Speaking Europe,* edited by Norm Friesen, 15–27. Cham, Switzerland: Springer International, 2016.

Pickering, Neil. *The Metaphor of Mental Illness.* Oxford: Oxford University Press, 2006.

Pickett, William. "Senile Dementia: A Clinical Study of Two Hundred Cases with Particular Regard to Types of the Disease." *Journal of Nervous and Mental Disease* 31 (1904): 81–88.

Pickstone, John. *Ways of Knowing: A New History of Science, Technology, and Medicine.* Chicago: University of Chicago Press, 2001.

Pihlajamäki, Maija, and Reisa A. Sperling. "Functional MRI in Alzheimer's Disease and Other Dementias." In *The Handbook of Alzheimer's Disease and Other Dementias,* edited by Andrew E. Budson and Neil W. Kowall, 535–56. Malden, Mass.: Wiley-Blackwell, 2011.

Pinchevski, Amit, and John Durham Peters. "Autism and New Media: Disability between Technology and Society." *New Media and Society* 18, no. 11 (2016): 2507–23.

Pollen, Daniel A. *Hannah's Heirs: The Quest for the Genetic Origins of Alzheimer's Disease.* New York: Oxford University Press, 1996.

Polley, Sarah, dir. *Away from Her.* Lionsgate, 2007. DVD.

Portacolone, Elena, Clara Berridge, Julene K. Johnson, and Silke Schicktanz. "Time to Reinvent the Science of Dementia: The Need for Care and Social Integration." *Aging and Mental Health* 18, no. 3 (2014): 269–75.

Post, Stephen Garrard. *The Moral Challenge of Alzheimer Disease: Ethical Issues from Diagnosis to Dying*. 2nd ed. Baltimore: Johns Hopkins University Press, 2000.

Post, Stephen Garrard. "Stumbling on Joy: Not Always a 'Burden' of Care." *Alzheimer's Care Today* 8, no. 3 (2007): 247–50.

Postan, Emily. "Defining Ourselves: Personal Bioinformation as a Tool of Narrative Self-Conception." *Journal of Bioethical Inquiry* 13 (2016): 133–51.

Powell, Robert, and A. Pawloswki. "Dementia Day Care Looks Like 1950s Town to Stimulate Patients' Memories." *TODAY*, April 10, 2018. https://www.today.com/health/dementia-day-care-looks-1950s-stimulate-patients-brains-t126727.

Prevedel, Robert, Aart J. Verhoef, Alejandro J. Pernía-Andrade, Siegfried Weisenburger, Ben S. Huang, Tobias Nöbauer, Alma Fernández, et al. "Fast Volumetric Calcium Imaging across Multiple Cortical Layers Using Sculpted Light." *Nature Methods* 13 (2016): 1021–28.

Price, Margaret. *Mad at School: Rhetorics of Mental Disability and Academic Life*. Ann Arbor: University of Michigan Press, 2011.

Prince, Martin, and Jim Jackson. *World Alzheimer Report 2011*. London: Alzheimer Disease International, 2011.

Prince, Martin, Anders Wimo, Gemma-Claire Ali, Maëlenn Guerchet, Yu-Tzu Wu, and Matthew Prina. *World Alzheimer Report 2015: The Global Impact of Dementia*. London: Alzheimer Disease International, 2015. https://www.alz.co.uk/research/WorldAlzheimerReport2015.pdf.

Prounis, Charlene. "10 Steps to Product Positioning." *Medical Marketing and Media*, February 1, 2007.

Puar, Jasbir K. "The Cost of Getting Better: Suicide, Sensation, Switchpoints." *GLQ: A Journal of Lesbian and Gay Studies* 18, no. 1 (2012): 149–58.

Puar, Jasbir K. "Prognosis Time: Towards a Geopolitics of Affect, Debility and Capacity." *Women and Performance: A Journal of Feminist Theory* 19, no. 2 (2009): 161–72.

Quayson, Ato. *Aesthetic Nervousness: Disability and the Crisis of Representation*. New York: Columbia University Press, 2007.

Rabinovici, Gil D., Jason Karlawish, David Knopman, Heather M. Snyder, Reisa Sperling, and Maria C. Carrillo. "Testing and Disclosures Related to Amyloid Imaging and Alzheimer's Disease: Common Questions and Fact Sheet Summary." *Alzheimer's and Dementia* 12, no. 4 (2016): 510–15.

Rabinow, Paul. *Marking Time: On the Anthropology of the Contemporary*. Princeton, N.J.: Princeton University Press, 2008.

Rabinow, Paul, and Nikolas Rose. "Biopower Today." *Biosocieties* 1 (2006): 195–217.

Racine, Eric, Ofek Bar-Ilan, and Judy Illes. "fMRI in the Public Eye." *Nature Reviews Neuroscience* 6, no. 2 (2005): 159–64.

Racine, E., S. Waldman, J. Rosenberg, and J. Illes. "Contemporary Neuroscience in the Media." *Social Science and Medicine* 71, no. 4 (2010): 725–33.

Ramón y Cajal, Santiago. *Advice for a Young Investigator.* Cambridge, Mass.: MIT Press, 1999.

Rankin, Katherine P., Anli A. Liu, Sara Howard, Hilary Slama, Craig E. Hou, Karen Shuster, and Bruce L. Miller. "A Case-Controlled Study of Altered Visual Art Production in Alzheimer's and FTLD." *Cognitive and Behavioral Neurology* 20, no. 1 (2007): 48–61.

Rasmussen, Nicolas. *Picture Control: The Electron Microscope and the Transformation of Biology in America, 1940–1960.* Stanford, Calif.: Stanford University Press, 1997.

Ratcliff, Marc. *The Quest for the Invisible: Microscopy in the Enlightenment.* Farnham, U.K.: Ashgate, 2009.

Ratzan, Scott. "Editorial: Stamp Out Cancer." *Journal of Health Communication* 4, no. 3 (1999): 167–68.

Reagan, Nancy, and Ronald Reagan. *I Love You, Ronnie: The Letters of Ronald Reagan to Nancy Reagan.* New York: Random House, 2000.

Reagan, Ronald. "The Text of Reagan's Letter." *New York Times,* November 5, 1994. https://www.nytimes.com/1994/11/06/us/the-text-of-reagan-s-letter.html.

Reckwitz, Andreas. "The Status of the 'Material' in Theories of Culture: From 'Social Structure' to 'Artefacts.'" *Journal for the Theory of Social Behaviour* 32, no. 2 (2002): 195–217.

Reinhard, Susan C., Carol Levine, and Sarah Samis. *Home Alone: Family Caregivers Providing Complex Chronic Care.* Washington, D.C.: AARP Public Policy Institute, 2012. http://www.aarp.org/content/dam/aarp/research/pub lic_policy_institute/health/home-alone-family-caregivers-providing-com plex-chronic-care-rev-AARP-ppi-health.pdf.

Rich, Dayton A. "A Brief History of Positron Emission Tomography." *Journal of Nuclear Medicine Technology* 25, no. 1 (1997): 4–11.

Richter, Jochen. "The Brain Commission of the International Association of Academies: The First International Society of Neurosciences." *Brain Research Bulletin* 52, no. 6 (2000): 445–57.

Rijcke, Sarah de, and Anne Beaulieu. "Networked Neuroscience: Brain Scans and Visual Knowing at the Intersection of Atlases and Databases." In *Representation in Scientific Practice Revisited,* edited by Catelijne Coopmans, Janet Vertesi, and Michael E. Lynch, 131–52. Cambridge, Mass.: MIT Press, 2014.

Rippel, Amy. "Life Memoirs: 'Alzheimer's Albums' Protect History." *Daytona Beach News Journal,* November 19, 2007.

Riva, M. A., M. Manzoni, G. Isimbaldi, G. Cesana, and F. Pagni. "Histochemistry: Historical Development and Current Use in Pathology." *Biotechnic and Histochemistry* 89, no. 2 (2014): 81–90.

Roalf, David R., Paul J. Moberg, Sharon X. Xie, David A. Wolk, Stephen T. Moelter, and Steven E. Arnold. "Comparative Accuracies of Two Common Screening Instruments for Classification of Alzheimer's Disease, Mild Cognitive Impairment, and Healthy Aging." *Alzheimer's and Dementia* 9, no. 5 (2013): 529–37.

Roberts, K. B., and J. D. W. Tomlinson. *The Fabric of the Body: European Traditions of Anatomical Illustrations.* Oxford: Clarendon Press, 1992.

Robin, Harry. *The Scientific Image: From Cave to Computer.* New York: H. N. Abrams, 1992.

Rocca, Walter A., and Luigi A. Amaducci. "Letter to the Editors." *Alzheimer Disease and Associated Disorders* 2, no. 1 (1988): 56–57.

Roelcke, Volker. "Biologizing Social Facts: An Early 20th Century Debate on Kraepelin's Concepts of Culture, Neurasthenia, and Degeneration." *Culture, Medicine, and Psychiatry* 21, no. 4 (1997): 383–403.

Roelcke, Volker, Paul Weindling, and Louise Westwood. *International Relations in Psychiatry: Britain, Germany, and the United States to World War II.* Vol. 16. Rochester, N.Y.: University of Rochester Press, 2010.

Roizin, L. "Essay on the Origin and Evolution of Neuropathology." *Psychiatric Quarterly* 31 (1957): 531–55.

Romano, John, and Wallace C. Miller. "Clinical and Pneumo-encephalographic Studies in Pre-senile Dementia." *Radiology* 35, no. 2 (1940): 131–37.

Rose, F. Clifford. *The Neurobiology of Painting.* Vol. 74. San Diego, Calif.: Elsevier, 2006.

Rose, Nikolas S. *Inventing Our Selves: Psychology, Power, and Personhood.* Cambridge: Cambridge University Press, 1996.

Rose, Nikolas S. *The Politics of Life Itself: Biomedicine, Power, and Subjectivity in the Twenty-First Century.* Princeton, N.J.: Princeton University Press, 2007.

Rose, Nikolas, and Joelle Abi-Rached. *Neuro: The New Brain Sciences and the Management of the Mind.* Princeton, N.J.: Princeton University Press, 2013.

Rosen, George. *Madness in Society: Chapters in the Historical Sociology of Mental Illness.* Chicago: University of Chicago Press, 1968.

Rosenberg, Francesca, Amir Parsa, Laurel Humble, and Carrie McGee. *Meet Me: Making Art Accessible to People with Dementia.* New York: Museum of Modern Art, 2009.

Rosenberg, R. N., and R. C. Petersen. "The Human Alzheimer Disease Project: A New Call to Arms." *JAMA Neurology* 72, no. 6 (2015): 626–28.

Rossato-Bennett, Michael, dir. *Alive Inside.* Projector Media, 2014.

Roth, Martin, and J. D. Morrissey. "Problems in the Diagnosis and Classification of Mental Disorder in Old Age; with a Study of Case Material." *British Journal of Psychiatry* 98, no. 410 (1952): 66–80.

Roth, M., B. E. Tomlinson, and G. Blessed. "Correlation between Scores for Dementia and Counts of 'Senile Plaques' in Cerebral Grey Matter of Elderly Subjects." *Nature* 209, no. 5018 (1966): 109–10.

Rothman, Lily. "Read Ronald Reagan's Letter to the American People about His Alzheimer's Diagnosis." *Time*, September 1, 2016. https://time.com/4473625/ronald-reagan-alzheimers-letter/.

Rothschild, D. "Alzheimer's Disease: A Clinicopathologic Study of Five Cases." *American Journal of Psychiatry* 91, no. 3 (1934): 485–519.

Rothschild, D. "The Clinical Differentiation of Senile and Arteriosclerotic Psychoses." *American Journal of Psychiatry* 98, no. 3 (1941): 324–33.

Rothschild, D. "Pathologic Changes in Senile Psychoses and Their Psychobiologic Significance." *American Journal of Psychiatry* 93, no. 4 (1937): 757–88.

Rothschild, D., and J. Kasanin. "Clinicopathological Study of Alzheimer's Disease: Relationship to Senile Conditions." *Archives of Neurology and Psychiatry* 36, no. 2 (1936): 293.

Rothschild, David, and M. L. Sharp. "The Origin of Senile Psychoses: Neuropathological Factors and Factors of a More Personal Nature." *Diseases of the Nervous System* 2 (1941): Z19.

Rousseau, G. S., Miranda Gill, David Boyd Haycock, and Malte Christian Walter Herwig. *Framing and Imagining Disease in Cultural History*. New York: Palgrave Macmillan, 2003.

Rovner, Sandy. "Scientists Can Explain What Happens to the Brain, but Not Why." *Washington Post*, October 28, 1986, sec. Health.

Royal College of Psychiatrists. "On the Decline of the Moral Faculties in Old Age." *British Journal of Psychiatry* 19, no. 86 (1873): 259–64.

Rozelle, Ron. *Into That Good Night*. 1st ed. New York: Farrar, Straus, and Giroux, 1998.

Russell, Alec. "The Greatest Love Affair in the History of the Presidency." *Daily Telegraph*, June 7, 2004.

Russell, William. "Senility and Senile Dementia." *American Journal of Psychiatry* 58, no. 4 (1902): 625–33.

Rusted, Jennifer, Linda Sheppard, and Diane Waller. "A Multi-centre Randomized Control Group Trial on the Use of Art Therapy for Older People with Dementia." *Group Analysis* 39, no. 4 (2006): 517–36.

Sabat, Steven R. *The Experience of Alzheimer's Disease: Life through a Tangled Veil*. Oxford: Blackwell, 2001.

Sachdev, Ameet. "Alzheimer's Charities Fight over Money." *Chicago Tribune*, July 27, 2010.

Safar, Laura T., and Daniel Z. Press. "Art and the Brain: Effects of Dementia on Art Production in Art Therapy." *Art Therapy* 28, no. 3 (2011): 96–103.

Salisbury, Laura, and Andrew Shail, eds. *Neurology and Modernity: A Cultural History of Nervous Systems, 1800–1950.* Basingstoke, U.K.: Palgrave Macmillan, 2010.

Satizabal, Claudia L., Alexa S. Beiser, Vincent Chouraki, Geneviève Chêne, Carole Dufouil, and Sudha Seshadri. "Incidence of Dementia over Three Decades in the Framingham Heart Study." *New England Journal of Medicine* 374, no. 6 (2016): 523–32.

Savarese, Emily Thornton, and Ralph James Savarese. "'The Superior Half of Speaking': An Introduction." *Disability Studies Quarterly* 30, no. 1 (2010).

Savarese, Ralph James. "Cognition." In *Keywords for Disability Studies,* edited by Rachel Adams and David Serlin, 40–42. New York: New York University Press, 2015.

Schacter, Daniel L. *The Seven Sins of Memory: How the Mind Forgets and Remembers.* Boston: Houghton Mifflin, 2001.

Schickore, Jutta. *The Microscope and the Eye: A History of Reflections, 1740–1870.* Chicago: University of Chicago Press, 2007.

Schickore, Jutta. "'Through Thousands of Errors We Reach the Truth'—but How? On the Epistemic Roles of Error in Scientific Practice." *Studies in History and Philosophy of Science* 36, no. 3 (2005): 539–56.

Schmidgen, Henning. "Cinematography without Film Architectures and Technologies of Visual Instruction in Biology around 1900." In *Educated Eye: Visual Culture and Pedagogy in the Life Sciences,* edited by Nancy A. Anderson and Michael R. Dietrich, 94–120. Hanover, N.H.: Dartmouth College Press, 2012.

Schröter, Jens. "Disciplining Media Studies: An Expanding Field and Its (Self-)Definition." In *Media Transatlantic: Developments in Media and Communication Studies between North American and German-Speaking Europe,* edited by Norm Friesen, 29–48. Cham, Switzerland: Springer International, 2016.

Schwarz, Alan. "Dark Days Follow Hard-Hitting Career in NFL." *New York Times,* February 2, 2007. https://www.nytimes.com/2007/02/02/sports/football/02concussions.html.

Schwarz, Alan. "A Suicide, a Last Request, a Family's Questions." *New York Times,* February 22, 2011. http://www.nytimes.com/2011/02/23/sports/football/23duerson.html.

Sconce, Jeffrey. *Haunted Media: Electronic Presence from Telegraphy to Television.* 2nd ed. Durham, N.C.: Duke University Press, 2000.

Scott, Gregory, and James Toole. "1860—Neurology Was There." *Archives of Neurology* 55, no. 12 (1998): 1584–85.

Secomb, Linnell. *Philosophy and Love: From Plato to Popular Culture.* Edinburgh: Edinburgh University Press, 2007.

Sedgwick, Eve Kosofsky. "A Dialogue on Love." *Critical Inquiry* 24, no. 2 (1998): 611–31.

Sedgwick, Eve Kosofsky. *Touching Feeling: Affect, Pedagogy, Performativity.* Durham, N.C.: Duke University Press, 2003.

Segal, Lynne. *Out of Time: The Pleasures and Perils of Ageing.* London: Verso, 2013.

Segers, Kurt. "Degenerative Dementias and Their Medical Care in the Movies." *Alzheimer Disease and Associated Disorders* 21, no. 1 (2007): 55–59.

Selberg, Scott. "Dementia on the Canvas: Art and the Biopolitics of Creativity." In *Popularizing Dementia: Public Expressions and Representations of Forgetfulness,* edited by Aagje Swinnen and Mark Schweda, 137–62. Bielefeld, Germany: transcript, 2015.

Selberg, Scott. "Modern Art as Public Care: Alzheimer's and the Aesthetics of Universal Personhood." *Medical Anthropology Quarterly* 29, no. 4 (2015): 473–91.

Selberg, Scott. "Rhinestone Cowboy: Alzheimer's, Celebrity, and the Collusions of Self." *American Quarterly* 69, no. 4 (2017): 883–901.

Serlin, David, ed. *Imagining Illness: Public Health and Visual Culture.* Minneapolis: University of Minnesota Press, 2010.

Shankle, William Rodman, and Daniel Amen. *Preventing Alzheimer's: Ways to Help Prevent, Delay, Detect and Even Halt Alzheimer's Disease and Other Forms of Memory Loss.* New York: Penguin, 2004.

Shanley, Chris, Cherry Russell, Heather Middleton, and Virginia Simpson-Young. "Living through End-Stage Dementia: The Experiences and Expressed Needs of Family Carers." *Dementia* 10, no. 3 (2011): 325–40.

Sharma, Sarah. *In the Meantime: Temporality and Cultural Politics.* Durham, N.C.: Duke University Press, 2014.

Shen, Helen. "Neurotechnology: BRAIN Storm." *Nature* 503, no. 7474 (2013): 26–28.

Shenk, David. *The Forgetting: Alzheimer's, Portrait of an Epidemic.* New York: Doubleday, 2001.

Shepherd, Gordon M. *Creating Modern Neuroscience: The Revolutionary 1950s.* Oxford: Oxford University Press, 2010.

Sherry, Mark. "Crip Politics? Just . . . No." *The Feminist Wire* (blog), November 23, 2013. http://www.thefeministwire.com/2013/11/crip-politics-just-no/.

Shimamura, Arthur P., and Stephen E. Palmer, eds. *Aesthetic Science: Connecting Minds, Brains, and Experience.* 1st ed. Oxford: Oxford University Press, 2013.

Shirahama, Tsuranobu, and Alan S. Cohen. "High-Resolution Electron Microscopic Analysis of the Amyloid Fibril." *Journal of Cell Biology* 33, no. 3 (1967): 679–708.

Shirky, Clay. *Cognitive Surplus: How Technology Makes Consumers into Collabo-rators*. Reprint ed. New York: Penguin Books, 2011.

Shubin, Seymour. *The Man from Yesterday*. Chicago: Academy Chicago, 2005.

Siebers, Tobin. *Disability Aesthetics*. Ann Arbor: University of Michigan Press, 2010.

Siebers, Tobin. "Disability and the Theory of Complex Embodiment." In *The Disability Studies Reader*, 4th ed., edited by Lennard J. Davis, 316–35. New York: Routledge, 2013.

Siebers, Tobin. *Disability Theory*. Ann Arbor: University of Michigan Press, 2008.

Siebers, Tobin. "Introduction: Disability and Visual Culture." *Journal of Liter-ary and Cultural Disability Studies* 9, no. 3 (2015): 239–46.

Siegel, Lee. "Why Is America So Depressed?" *New York Times*, January 2, 2020, sec. Opinion. https://www.nytimes.com/2020/01/02/opinion/de pression-america-trump.html.

Sim, M., and W. Thomas Smith. "Alzheimer's Disease Confirmed by Cerebral Biopsy: A Therapeutic Trial with Cortisone and ACTH." *British Journal of Psychiatry* 101, no. 424 (1955): 604–9.

Simons, Daniel J., Walter R. Boot, Neil Charness, Susan E. Gathercole, Chris-topher F. Chabris, David Z. Hambrick, and Elizabeth A. L. Stine-Morrow. "Do 'Brain-Training' Programs Work?" *Psychological Science in the Public Interest* 17, no. 3 (2016): 103–86.

Simplican, Stacy Clifford. *The Capacity Contract: Intellectual Disability and the Question of Citizenship*. Minneapolis: University of Minnesota Press, 2015.

Singer, Ben. *Melodrama and Modernity: Early Sensational Cinema and Its Con-texts*. New York: Columbia University Press, 2001.

Skoller, Jeffrey. *Shadows, Specters, Shards: Making History in Avant-Garde Film*. 1st ed. Minneapolis: University of Minnesota Press, 2005.

Small, Gary, and Gigi Vorgan. *The Alzheimer's Prevention Program: Keep Your Brain Healthy for the Rest of Your Life*. New York: Workman, 2011.

Small, Gary, and Gigi Vorgan. *The Longevity Bible: Eight Essential Strategies for Keeping Your Mind Sharp and Your Body Young*. New York: Hyperion, 2007.

Small, Gary, and Gigi Vorgan. *The Memory Bible: An Innovative Strategy for Keeping Your Brain Young*. New York: Hyperion, 2002.

Small, Gary, and Gigi Vorgan. *The Memory Prescription: Dr. Gary Small's 14-Day Plan to Keep Your Brain and Body Young*. New York: Hyperion, 2004.

Smith, B., and Dan Gasby. *Before I Forget: Love, Hope, Help, and Acceptance in Our Fight against Alzheimer's*. New York: Harmony, 2016.

Smith, Patricia, Mary Michell Kenan, and Mark Edwin Kunik. *Alzheimer's for Dummies*. Hoboken, N.J.: John Wiley, 2004.

Smith, Stephen. "Be Well: The Toll Football Takes on the Brain." *Boston Globe,*
February 2, 2012. http://www.bostonglobe.com/lifestyle/style/2012/02/02/
GOZE2NEN8DLGBUmhlLddfJ/story.html.

Snyder, Heather, William R. Perlman, Robert Egge, and Maria C. Carrillo. "Alzheimer's Disease Public–Private Partnerships: Update 2017." *Alzheimer's
and Dementia* 14, no. 4 (2018): 522–31.

Snyder, Sharon L., Brenda Jo Brueggemann, and Rosemarie Garland Thomson. *Disability Studies: Enabling the Humanities.* New York: Modern Language
Association of America, 2002.

Snyder, Sharon L., and David T. Mitchell. *Cultural Locations of Disability.* 1st ed.
Chicago: University of Chicago Press, 2006.

Soldatic, Karen, and Shaun Grech. "Transnationalising Disability Studies:
Rights, Justice and Impairment." *Disability Studies Quarterly* 34, no. 2 (2014).

Solomon, Paul R., Aliina Hirschoff, Bridget Kelly, Mahri Relin, Michael Brush,
Richard D. DeVeaux, and William W. Pendlebury. "A 7 Minute Neurocogni-
tive Screening Battery Highly Sensitive to Alzheimer's Disease." *Archives of
Neurology* 55, no. 3 (1998): 349–55.

Soniat, Theodore L. L. "Histogenesis of Senile Plaques." *Archives of Neurology
and Psychiatry* 46, no. 1 (1941): 101.

Sontag, Susan. *AIDS and Its Metaphors.* New York: Farrar, Straus, and Giroux,
1988.

Sontag, Susan. *Illness as Metaphor.* New York: Farrar, Straus, and Giroux,
1978.

Sontag, Susan. *On Photography.* 1st Picador ed. New York: Picador, 1977.

Sourbati, Maria. "Disabling Communications? A Capabilities Perspective on
Media Access, Social Inclusion and Communication Policy." *Media, Culture,
and Society* 34, no. 5 (2012): 571–87.

Southard, E. E. "Anatomical Findings in Senile Dementia: A Diagnostic Study
Bearing Especially on the Group of Cerebral Atrophies." *American Journal
of Psychiatry* 66, no. 4 (1910): 673–708.

Southard, E. E. "On the Topographical Distribution of Cortex Lesions and
Anomalies in Dementia Pricox, with Some Account of Their Functional
Significance." *American Journal of Psychiatry* 71, no. 3 (1915): 603–71.

Southard, E. E., and H. W. Mitchell. "Clinical and Anatomical Analysis of 23
Cases of Insanity Arising in the Sixth and Seventh Decades with Especial
Relation to the Incidence of Arteriosclerosis and Senile Atrophy and to the
Distribution of Cortical Pigments." *American Journal of Psychiatry* 65 (Octo-
ber 1908): 293–336.

Sparks, Hannah. "Google's Super Bowl 2020 Commercial Will Make You Cry."
New York Post (blog), January 28, 2020. https://nypost.com/2020/01/28/
googles-super-bowl-2020-commercial-will-make-you-cry/.

Stafford, Barbara Maria. *Artful Science: Enlightenment, Entertainment, and the Eclipse of Visual Education.* Cambridge, Mass.: MIT Press, 1994.

Stafford, Barbara Maria. *Body Criticism: Imaging the Unseen in Enlightenment Art and Medicine.* Cambridge, Mass.: MIT Press, 1991.

Staiger, Janet, Janet Cvetkovich, and Ann Reynolds. "Introduction: Political Emotions and Public Feelings." In *Political Emotions: New Agendas in Communication,* edited by Janet Staiger, Janet Cvetkovich, and Ann Reynolds, 1–17. New York: Routledge, 2010.

Star, Susan. *Regions of the Mind: Brain Research and the Quest for Scientific Certainty.* Stanford, Calif.: Stanford University Press, 1989.

State Comprehensive Mental Health Services Plan Act, 99-660 § (1986).

Stengers, Isabelle. *The Invention of Modern Science.* Minneapolis: University of Minnesota Press, 2000.

Stern, Yaakov. "Cognitive Reserve in Ageing and Alzheimer's Disease." *The Lancet Neurology* 11, no. 11 (2012): 1006–12.

Stewart, Ellen Greene. "Art Therapy and Neuroscience Blend: Working with Patients Who Have Dementia." *Art Therapy* 21, no. 3 (2004): 148–55.

Stewart, Ellen Greene. "De Kooning's Dementia." *American Journal of Alzheimer's Disease and Other Dementias* 17, no. 5 (2002): 313–17.

Stewart, Ellen Greene. *Kaleidoscope—Color and Form Illuminate Darkness: An Exploration of Art Therapy and Exercises for Patients with Dementia.* Chicago: Magnolia Street, 2006.

Stewart, Kathleen. *Ordinary Affects.* Durham, N.C.: Duke University Press, 2007.

St. George-Hyslop, Peter H., Richard H. Myers, Jonathan L. Haines, Lindsay A. Farrer, Rudolph E. Tanzi, Koji Abe, Marianne F. James, P. Michael Conneally, Ronald J. Polinsky, and James F. Gusella. "Familial Alzheimer's Disease: Progress and Problems." *Neurobiology of Aging* 10, no. 5 (1989): 417–25.

Storr, Robert. "At Last Light." In *Willem de Kooning: The Late Paintings, the 1980s,* edited by Janet Jenkins and Siri Engberg, 39–80. San Francisco: San Francisco Museum of Art, 1995.

St. Pierre, Joshua. "Cripping Communication: Speech, Disability, and Exclusion in Liberal Humanist and Posthumanist Discourse." *Communication Theory* 25, no. 3 (2015): 330–48.

Sturken, Marita. *Tangled Memories: The Vietnam War, the AIDS Epidemic, and the Politics of Remembering.* Berkeley: University of California Press, 1997.

Sturken, Marita. *Tourists of History: Memory, Kitsch, and Consumerism from Oklahoma City to Ground Zero.* Durham, N.C.: Duke University Press, 2007.

Subramaniam, Ponnusamy, and Bob Woods. "The Impact of Individual Reminiscence Therapy for People with Dementia: Systematic Review." *Expert Review of Neurotherapeutics* 12, no. 5 (2012): 545–55.

Subramaniam, Ponnusamy, and Bob Woods. "Towards the Therapeutic Use of Information and Communication Technology in Reminiscence Work for People with Dementia: A Systematic Review." *International Journal of Computers in Healthcare* 1, no. 2 (2010): 106–25.

Suzuki, Kunihiko, Robert Katzman, and Saul R. Korey. "Chemical Studies on Alzheimer's Disease." *Journal of Neuropathology and Experimental Neurology* 24, no. 2 (1965): 211–24.

Sweeting, Helen, and Mary Gilhooly. "Dementia and the Phenomenon of Social Death." *Sociology of Health and Illness* 19, no. 1 (1997): 93–117.

Swinnen, Aagje. "Ageing in Film." In *Routledge Handbook of Cultural Gerontology*, edited by Julia Twigg and Wendy Martin, 69–76. Florence, Ky.: Routledge, 2015.

Swinnen, Aagje. "Dementia in Documentary Film: Mum by Adelheid Roosen." *The Gerontologist* 53, no. 1 (2013): 113–22.

Swinnen, Aagje, and Mark Schweda. *Popularizing Dementia: Public Expressions and Representations of Forgetfulness*. Bielefeld, Germany: transcript, 2015.

Takeda, Shinya, Kayo Tajime, and Toshiatsu Taniguchi. "The Takeda Three Colors Combination Test: A Screening Test for Detection of Very Mild Alzheimer's Disease." *Scientific World Journal* 2014 (2014): 1–5.

Talan, Jamie. "Neuroimaging Tracers for AD Detection Not Yet Ready for Prime Time, FDA Panel Advises." *Neurology Today* 8, no. 22 (2008): 1.

Taylor, Janelle S. "On Recognition, Caring, and Dementia." *Medical Anthropology Quarterly* 22, no. 4 (2008): 313–35.

Taylor, Janelle S. *The Public Life of the Fetal Sonogram: Technology, Consumption, and the Politics of Reproduction*. New Brunswick, N.J.: Rutgers University Press, 2008.

Taylor, Janelle S. "Surfacing the Body Interior." *Annual Review of Anthropology* 34, no. 1 (2005): 741–56.

Taylor, Richard. *Alzheimer's from the Inside Out*. Baltimore: Health Professions Press, 2007.

Taylor, Richard. "Alzheimer's from the Inside Out—Newsletter," January 11, 2012.

Taylor, Stuart, Jr. "CAT Scans Said to Show Shrunken Hinckley Brain." *New York Times*, June 2, 1982, sec. U.S. http://www.nytimes.com/1982/06/02/us/cat-scans-said-to-show-shrunken-hinckley-brain.html.

Tennstedt, Sharon L., and Frederick W. Unverzagt. "The ACTIVE Study: Study Overview and Major Findings." *Journal of Aging and Health* 25, no. 8 (2013): 3S–20S.

Terry, Robert. "Alzheimer's Disease at Mid-century (1927–1977) and a Little More." In *Alzheimer: 100 Years and Beyond*, edited by M. Jucker, K. Beyreuther, C. Haass, and R. M. Nitsch, 59–61. Berlin: Springer, 2006.

Terry, Robert D. "The Fine Structure of Neurofibrillary Tangles in Alzheimer's Disease." *Journal of Neuropathology and Experimental Neurology* 22, no. 4 (1963): 629–42.

Terry, Robert D., Nicholas K. Gonatas, and Martin Weiss. "Ultrastructural Studies in Alzheimer's Presenile Dementia." *American Journal of Pathology* 44, no. 2 (1964): 269–97.

Terry, R. D., N. K. Gonatas, and M. Weiss. "The Ultrastructure of the Cerebral Cortex in Alzheimer's Disease." *Transactions of the American Neurological Association* 89 (1964): 12.

Terry, Robert D., and Carlos Peña. "Experimental Production of Neurofibrillary Degeneration." *Journal of Neuropathology and Experimental Neurology* 24, no. 2 (1965): 200–210.

Thewlis, Malford. *The Care of the Aged (Geriatrics)*. St. Louis, Mo.: Mosby, 1941.

Thiher, Allen. *Revels in Madness*. Ann Arbor: University of Michigan Press, 1999.

Thomas, Kelly Devine. "Shaping de Kooning's Legacy." *ARTnews*, September 8, 2011. http://www.artnews.com/2011/09/08/shaping-de-koonings-legacy/.

Thomsen, Dorthe Kirkegaard, and Dorthe Berntsen. "The Cultural Life Script and Life Story Chapters Contribute to the Reminiscence Bump." *Memory* 16, no. 4 (2008): 420–35.

Thomsen, Michael. "Ether One: The Video Game That Tries to Simulate Dementia." *New Yorker*, November 19, 2014. http://www.newyorker.com/business/currency/ether-one-video-game-tries-simulate-dementia.

Thomson, Rosemarie Garland. *Extraordinary Bodies: Figuring Physical Disability in American Culture and Literature*. 1st ed. New York: Columbia University Press, 1996.

Thorndike, John. *The Last of His Mind: A Year in the Shadow of Alzheimer's*. Athens, Ohio: Swallow Press, 2009.

Thorne, Will, and Will Thorne. "TV Ratings: Super Bowl LIV Draws 102 Million Viewers, Up a Fraction on 2019." *Variety* (blog), February 3, 2020. https://variety.com/2020/tv/news/super-bowl-liv-ratings-1203490564/.

Tiffany, William J. "The Occurrence of Miliary Plaques in Senile Brains." *American Journal of Insanity* 70, no. 3 (1914): 695–740.

Time. "How to Live Longer Better." February 26, 2018.

Titford, Michael. "A Short History of Histopathology Technique." *Journal of Histotechnology* 29, no. 2 (2006): 99–110.

Tomes, Nancy. "Merchants of Health: Medicine and Consumer Culture in the United States, 1900–1940." *Journal of American History* 88, no. 2 (2001): 519–47.

Tomlinson, B. E., G. Blessed, and M. Roth. "Observations on the Brains of Demented Old People." *Journal of the Neurological Sciences* 11, no. 3 (1970): 205–42.

Tomlinson, B. E., G. Blessed, and M. Roth. "Observations on the Brains of Non-demented Old People." *Journal of the Neurological Sciences* 7, no. 2 (1968): 331–56.

Torack, Richard M. "Adult Dementia: History, Biopsy, Pathology." *Neurosurgery* 4, no. 5 (1979): 434–42.

Torack, Richard M. "The Early History of Senile Dementia." In *Alzheimer's Disease*, edited by Barry Reisberg, 23–28. New York: Free Press, 1983.

Torrance, Kelly Jane. "Director Shows Deft Touch." *Washington Times*, May 10, 2007.

Treichler, Paula A. *How to Have Theory in an Epidemic: Cultural Chronicles of AIDS*. Durham, N.C.: Duke University Press, 1999.

Treichler, Paula A., Lisa Cartwright, and Constance Penley. *The Visible Woman: Imaging Technologies, Gender, and Science*. New York: New York University Press, 1998.

Tremain, Shelley. "This Is What a Historicist and Relativist Feminist Philosophy of Disability Looks Like." *Foucault Studies*, no. 19 (2015): 7–42.

Tumbelaka, R. "Alzheimer's Disease." *Journal of Nervous and Mental Disease* 56, no. 5 (1922): 482–503.

Turda, Marius. *Modernism and Eugenics*. New York: Palgrave Macmillan, 2010.

Tuschling, Anna. "Historical, Technological and Medial a Priori: On the Belatedness of Media." *Cultural Studies* 30, no. 4 (2016): 680–703.

Twigg, Julia. *Routledge Handbook of Cultural Gerontology*. London: Routledge, Taylor and Francis Group, 2015.

Uchihara, Toshiki. "Silver Diagnosis in Neuropathology: Principles, Practice and Revised Interpretation." *Acta Neuropathologica* 113, no. 5 (2007): 483–99.

Ulrich, Jürg. *Histochemistry and Immunohistochemistry of Alzheimer's Disease*. Progress in Histochemistry and Cytochemistry 27. Stuttgart, Germany: Gustav Fischer, 1993.

Ulrich, Jürg. *Histology and Histopathology of the Aging Brain*. Interdisciplinary Topics in Gerontology 25. New York: Karger, 1988.

U.S. Weekly. "30 Most Romantic Movies of All Time." February 14, 2012. http://www.usmagazine.com/entertainment/pictures/30-most-romantic -movies-of-all-time-2012102/20669.

Väliaho, Pasi. *Biopolitical Screens: Image, Power, and the Neoliberal Brain*. Cambridge, Mass.: MIT Press, 2014.

Van Buren, Abigail. "Advice to You." *Atlanta Constitution*, October 23, 1980.

Van Dijck, José. *The Transparent Body: A Cultural Analysis of Medical Imaging*. Seattle: University of Washington Press, 2005.

Van Gorp, Baldwin, and Tom Vercruysse. "Frames and Counter-frames Giving Meaning to Dementia: A Framing Analysis of Media Content." *Social Science and Medicine* 74, no. 8 (2012): 1274–81.

Vidal, F. "Brainhood, Anthropological Figure of Modernity." *History of the Human Sciences* 22, no. 1 (2009): 5–36.

Vradenburg, George. "Alzheimer's: Google Glass as Brain Prosthetic." *Huffington Post,* January 21, 2014. http://www.huffingtonpost.com/george-vradenburg/alzheimers-google-glass-as-brain-prosthetic_b_4637488.html.

Wagner, Henry N. "A Brief History of Positron Emission Tomography (PET)." *Seminars in Nuclear Medicine* 28, no. 3 (1998): 213–20.

Waldby, Cathy. *The Visible Human Project: Informatic Bodies and Posthuman Medicine.* London: Routledge, 2000.

Waller, Diane. *Arts Therapies and Progressive Illness: Nameless Dread.* New York: Brunner-Routledge, 2002.

Walz, Steffen P., and Sebastian Deterding, eds. *The Gameful World: Approaches, Issues, Applications.* Cambridge, Mass.: MIT Press, 2015.

Warner, John Harley. "The Fall and Rise of a Professional Mystery: Epistemology, Authority, and the Emergence of Laboratory Medicine in Nineteenth Century Medicine." In *The Laboratory Revolution in Medicine,* edited by Andrew Cunningham and Perry Williams, 110–41. Cambridge: Cambridge University Press, 1992.

Wasserman, Todd. "A Facebook Campaign Simulated Alzheimer's, and It Will Stop You in Your Tracks." *Mashable,* January 28, 2014. http://mashable.com/2014/01/28/holland-alzheimers-facebook/.

Wasson, Haidee. *Museum Movies: The Museum of Modern Art and the Birth of Art Cinema.* Berkeley: University of California Press, 2005.

Wayne, Randy. *Light and Video Microscopy.* San Diego, Calif.: Academic Press, 2014.

Wayne, Randy. "Photomicrography." In *Light and Video Microscopy,* 2nd ed., 97–110. San Diego, Calif.: Academic Press, 2014.

Wearing, Sadie. "Dementia and the Biopolitics of the Biopic: From Iris to the Iron Lady." *Dementia* 12, no. 3 (2013): 315–25.

Webb, Steve. *From the Watching of Shadows: The Origins of Radiological Tomography.* Bristol, U.K.: A. Hilger, 1990.

Weber, Leonard J. *Profits before People? Ethical Standards and the Marketing of Prescription Drugs.* Bloomington: Indiana University Press, 2006.

Weiner, Michael W., Paul S. Aisen, Clifford R. Jack, William J. Jagust, John Q. Trojanowski, Leslie Shaw, Andrew J. Saykin, et al. "The Alzheimer's Disease Neuroimaging Initiative: Progress Report and Future Plans." *Alzheimer's and Dementia* 6, no. 3 (1010): 202–11.

Weiner, Michael W., and Dallas P. Veitch. "Introduction to Special Issue: Overview of Alzheimer's Disease Neuroimaging Initiative." *Alzheimer's and Dementia* 11, no. 7 (2015): 730–33.

Weiner, Michael W., Dallas P. Veitch, Paul S. Aisen, Laurel A. Beckett, Nigel J. Cairns, Jesse Cedarbaum, Michael C. Donohue, et al. "Impact of the Alzheimer's Disease Neuroimaging Initiative, 2004 to 2014." *Alzheimer's and Dementia* 11, no. 7 (2015): 865–84.

Weiner, Michael W., Dallas P. Veitch, Paul S. Aisen, Laurel A. Beckett, Nigel J. Cairns, Jesse Cedarbaum, Robert C. Green, et al. "2014 Update of the Alzheimer's Disease Neuroimaging Initiative: A Review of Papers Published since Its Inception." *Alzheimer's and Dementia* 11, no. 6 (2015): e1–e120.

Weingarten, M. D., A. H. Lockwood, S. Y. Hwo, and M. W. Kirschner. "A Protein Factor Essential for Microtubule Assembly." *Proceedings of the National Academy of Sciences of the United States of America* 72, no. 5 (1975): 1858–62.

Weisberg, Deena Skolnick, Frank C. Keil, Joshua Goodstein, Elizabeth Rawson, and Jeremy R. Gray. "The Seductive Allure of Neuroscience Explanations." *Journal of Cognitive Neuroscience* 20, no. 3 (2007): 470–77.

Weuve, Jennifer, Liesi E. Hebert, Paul A. Scherr, and Denis A. Evans. "Prevalence of Alzheimer Disease in US States." *Epidemiology* 26, no. 1 (2015): e4–e6.

Wexler, Alice. *Art and Disability: The Social and Political Struggles Facing Education.* New York: Palgrave Macmillan, 2009.

Weyl, M. "Love Song at the End of the Day: A Wife's Journey." *Dementia* 8, no. 1 (2009): 9–15.

Whelehan, Imelda, and Joel Gwynne. *Ageing, Popular Culture and Contemporary Feminism Harleys and Hormones.* Basingstoke, U.K.: Palgrave Macmillan, 2014.

White, William Alanson. *The Principles of Mental Hygiene.* New York: Macmillan, 1917.

White Paper Games. *Ether One.* 2016. PlayStation 4.

Whitehouse, Peter J. "Why I No Longer Consult for Drug Companies." *Culture, Medicine, and Psychiatry* 32, no. 1 (2008): 4–10.

Whitehouse, P. J., and W. E. Deal. "Situated beyond Modernity: Lessons for Alzheimer's Disease Research." *Journal of the American Geriatrics Society* 43, no. 11 (1995): 1314–15.

Whitehouse, Peter J., Atwood D. Gaines, Heather Lindstrom, and Janice E. Graham. "Anthropological Contributions to the Understanding of Age-Related Cognitive Impairment." *The Lancet Neurology* 4, no. 5 (2005): 320–26.

Whitehouse, Peter, and Daniel George. *The Myth of Alzheimer's: What You Aren't Being Told about Today's Most Dreaded Diagnosis.* New York: St. Martin's Press, 2008.

Whitehouse, Peter J., Konrad Maurer, and Jesse F. Ballenger, eds. *Concepts of Alzheimer Disease: Biological, Clinical, and Cultural Perspectives.* Baltimore: Johns Hopkins University Press, 2000.

Whitson, Jennifer. "Foucault's Fitbit." In *The Gameful World: Approaches, Issues, Applications,* edited by Steffen P. Walz and Sebastian Deterding, 339–58. Cambridge, Mass.: MIT Press, 2015.

Williams, Jeannie. "For Winslet: A Story of Absolute Love." *USA Today,* December 14, 2001.

Williams, Simon J., Paul Higgs, and Stephen Katz. "Neuroculture, Active Ageing and the 'Older Brain': Problems, Promises and Prospects." *Sociology of Health and Illness* 34, no. 1 (2012): 64–78.

Wilson, Catherine. *The Invisible World: Early Modern Philosophy and the Invention of the Microscope.* Princeton, N.J.: Princeton University Press, 1995.

Wilson, Duncan. "Quantifying the Quiet Epidemic: Diagnosing Dementia in Late 20th-Century Britain." *History of the Human Sciences* 27, no. 5 (2014): 126–46.

Wilson, Robert S., Kristin R. Krueger, Steven E. Arnold, Julie A. Schneider, Jeremiah F. Kelly, Lisa L. Barnes, Yuxiao Tang, and David A. Bennett. "Loneliness and Risk of Alzheimer Disease." *Archives of General Psychiatry* 64, no. 2 (2007): 234–40.

Wise, M. Norton. "Making Visible." *Isis* 97, no. 1 (2006): 75–82.

Wisniewski, Henryk M., and Robert D. Terry. "Reexamination of the Pathogenesis of the Senile Plaque." *Progress in Neuropathology* 2 (1973): 1–26.

Wisniewski, Henryk, Robert D. Terry, and Asao Hirano. "Neurofibrillary Pathology." *Journal of Neuropathology and Experimental Neurology* 29, no. 2 (1970): 163–76.

Witte, Michael M., Norman L. Foster, Adam S. Fleisher, Monique M. Williams, Kimberly Quaid, Michael Wasserman, Gail Hunt, et al. "Clinical Use of Amyloid-Positron Emission Tomography Neuroimaging: Practical and Bioethical Considerations." *Alzheimer's and Dementia: Diagnosis, Assessment, and Disease Monitoring* 1, no. 3 (2015): 358–67.

Wolbarst, Anthony B. *Looking Within: How X-Ray, CT, MRI, Ultrasound, and Other Medical Images Are Created, and How They Help Physicians Save Lives.* Berkeley: University of California Press, 1999.

Wolff, Jennifer L., Sydney M. Dy, Kevin D. Frick, and Judith D. Kasper. "End of Life Care: Findings from a National Survey of Informal Caregivers." *Archives of Internal Medicine* 167 (2007): 40–46.

Wolff, Jennifer L., John Mulcahy, Jin Huang, David L. Roth, Kenneth Covinsky, and Judith D. Kasper. "Family Caregivers of Older Adults, 1999–2015: Trends in Characteristics, Circumstances, and Role-Related Appraisal." *The Gerontologist* 58, no. 6 (2018): 1021–32.

Wollin, Lonnie. "Dear Abby: A Voice for People Facing Alzheimer's Long before Own Diagnosis." *Alzheimer's Association* (blog), January 18, 2013. http://blog.alz.org/dear-abby-voice-for-alzheimers/.

Woloshin, S. "The U.S. Postal Service and Cancer Screening—Stamps of Approval?" *New England Journal of Medicine* 340, no. 11 (1999): 884–87.

Woodard, J. S. "Alzheimer's Disease in Late Adult Life." *American Journal of Pathology* 49, no. 6 (1966): 1157–69.

Woodward, James. *Between Remembering and Forgetting: The Spiritual Dimensions of Dementia.* 1st ed. New York: Mowbray, 2010.

Wren, Adam. "The Unblinding: Has Lilly Solved the Alzheimer's Puzzle?" *Indianapolis Monthly,* November 2, 2016. http://www.indianapolismonthly.com/longform/alzheimers-eli-lilly-unblinding/.

Wright, Helen. *Introduction to Scientific Visualization.* New York: Springer, 2006.

Wu, Shinyi, William A. Vega, Jason Resendez, and Haomiao Jin. *Latinos and Alzheimer's Disease: New Numbers behind the Crisis.* US Against Alzheimer's. http://www.usagainstalzheimers.org/sites/default/files/Latinos-and-AD_USC_UsA2-Impact-Report.pdf.

Wurtman, Richard J. "Alzheimer's Disease." *Scientific American* 252, no. 1 (1985): 62–74.

Wurtman, Richard J. "Some Philosophical Aspects of Alzheimer's Discovery: An American Perspective." In *Alzheimer's Disease: Epidemiology, Neuropathology, Neurochemistry, and Clinics,* edited by H. Beckmann, K. Maurer, and P. Riederer, 3–5. Vienna: Springer, 1990.

Wyatt, Rupert. *Rise of the Planet of the Apes.* 20th Century Fox, 2011. DVD.

Xu, Wei, Jin-Tai Yu, Meng-Shan Tan, and Lan Tan. "Cognitive Reserve and Alzheimer's Disease." *Molecular Neurobiology* 51, no. 1 (2015): 187–208.

Yarkony, Lisa. "Whisper Your Way into Their World: A Loving and Gentle Approach to Those with Alzheimer's Disease." *Caring* 29, no. 6 (2010): 14–19.

Yasuda, Kiyoshi, Kazuhiro Kuwabara, Noriaki Kuwahara, Shinji Abe, and Nobuji Tetsutani. "Effectiveness of Personalised Reminiscence Photo Videos for Individuals with Dementia." *Neuropsychological Rehabilitation* 19, no. 4 (2009): 603–19.

Yeo, Jing Ming, Briony Waddell, Zubair Khan, and Suvankar Pal. "A Systematic Review and Meta-analysis of 18F-Labeled Amyloid Imaging in Alzheimer's Disease." *Alzheimer's and Dementia: Diagnosis, Assessment, and Disease Monitoring* 1, no. 1 (2015): 5–13.

Young, Carol Ann. "First My Mother, Then My Aunt: A Caregiver's Diary of Alzheimer's Disease." In *Always on Call: When Illness Turns Families into*

Caregivers, edited by Carol Levine, 23–33. Nashville, Tenn.: Vanderbilt University Press, 2004.

Zeisel, John. *I'm Still Here: A Breakthrough Approach to Understanding Someone Living with Alzheimer's.* New York: Avery, 2009.

Zhao, Qing-Fei, Lan Tan, Hui-Fu Wang, Teng Jiang, Meng-Shan Tan, Lin Tan, Wei Xu, et al. "The Prevalence of Neuropsychiatric Symptoms in Alzheimer's Disease: Systematic Review and Meta-analysis." *Journal of Affective Disorders* 190 (January 15, 2016): 264–71.

Index

neurofibrils, 62
neuroimage aesthetic, 32–33,
    140–48, 156–57
neuroimaging: authority of, 19, 116;
    barriers to, 1; biomarkers and,
    100; clinical evaluation and, 118;
    diagnostic, 96, 107; popular
    culture and, 142, 144; public
    and, 18–20, 31, 75–76, 84, 87,
    88–89; representation and, 24,
    145–46, 148; technologies, 3, 6,
    83, 86, 94; truth and, 43; in vivo,
    8, 90, 92–94, 102
neurology, 44, 257n31
neuronal staining, 52–53
neuronal theory, 38, 257n31
neuropathologists, 30, 50, 54, 76–77,
    250n13
neuropathology, 10, 26, 41, 43–44,
    57–58, 61, 72, 90–91
neuropharmacology, 45
neuroplasticity, 128
neuroscience: brain tissue and
    early, 50; early German, 46–47;
    faith and, 147; investments
    in, 107; neuroculture and, 3;
    proleptic structure of, 43, 90,
    241; public's trust in, 145–46,
    274n17; reductive allure of,
    274n17; technologization of
    early, 44
neuroscientific aesthetic, 141–48,
    156–57
Nevelson, Louise, 165–66
Newcastle research, 80–81, 100,
    263n39
New England Society of Psychiatry, 61
"New Face of Alzheimer's, The"
    (article), 119–20
news coverage of Alzheimer's, 1, 32,
    118, 120, 142, 228, 240

New York Museum of Modern Art
    (MoMA): de Kooning shows at,
    204–8; Meet Me program at, 34,
    165–69, 171–74, 190–92, 277n7,
    277n12; Robert Terry at, 79
New York Times, 118, 200, 221, 228
New York University, 167
Nissl, Franz, 51
Nobel Prize recipients, 53, 64
non-senile dementia, 57
nosology, 42, 55, 56, 57, 59, 84
nostalgia, 33, 141, 150, 155
Notebook, The (film), 230, 283n38,
    283n44
"Not Gonna Miss You" (Campbell),
    217

Obama, Barack, 98–99, 103–4, 107,
    229
objectivity, mechanical, 54
O'Connor, Sandra Day, 283n42
older bodies. *See* aging
Once Invisible (exhibition), 79
O'Neill, Desmond, 202
Oprah.com, 124
Oprah Winfrey Network (OWN),
    227–28
optimism, 35, 125, 271n45
Ordon, Dr., 134
origin myth, 40, 68, 261n104
othering, medical, 67
othering stigma, 108, 268n11
Oz, Mehmet (Dr. Oz), 114–15, 125,
    142–44, 269n23

pathologized self, 3, 14, 19
pathology of Alzheimer's, 8, 11–12,
    13, 58, 66, 75, 79–80, 207–8, 235
Peanuts comic strip, 169–70
people of color, 13, 108, 159
Perlmutter, David, 142–44

SCOTT SELBERG is a member of the faculty of the Department of Communication at Portland State University.